T0259394

Tinnitus

Editors

CAROL A. BAUER
RONNA HERTZANO
DIDIER DEPIREUX

OTOLARYNGOLOGIC CLINICS OF NORTH AMERICA

www.oto.theclinics.com

Consulting Editor
SUJANA S. CHANDRASEKHAR

August 2020 • Volume 53 • Number 4

ELSEVIER

1600 John F. Kennedy Boulevard • Suite 1800 • Philadelphia, Pennsylvania, 19103-2899

http://www.oto.theclinics.com

OTOLARYNGOLOGIC CLINICS OF NORTH AMERICA Volume 53, Number 4
August 2020 ISSN 0030-6665, ISBN-13: 978-0-323-73288-8

Editor: Stacy Eastman
Developmental Editor: Laura Fisher

© 2020 Elsevier Inc. All rights reserved.

This periodical and the individual contributions contained in it are protected under copyright by Elsevier, and the following terms and conditions apply to their use:

Photocopying
Single photocopies of single articles may be made for personal use as allowed by national copyright laws. Permission of the Publisher and payment of a fee is required for all other photocopying, including multiple or systematic copying, copying for advertising or promotional purposes, resale, and all forms of document delivery. Special rates are available for educational institutions that wish to make photocopies for non-profit educational classroom use. For information on how to seek permission visit www.elsevier.com/permissions or call: (+44) 1865 843830 (UK)/(+1) 215 239 3804 (USA).

Derivative Works
Subscribers may reproduce tables of contents or prepare lists of articles including abstracts for internal circulation within their institutions. Permission of the Publisher is required for resale or distribution outside the institution. Permission of the Publisher is required for all other derivative works, including compilations and translations (please consult www.elsevier.com/permissions).

Electronic Storage or Usage
Permission of the Publisher is required to store or use electronically any material contained in this periodical, including any article or part of an article (please consult www.elsevier.com/permissions). Except as outlined above, no part of this publication may be reproduced, stored in a retrieval system or transmitted in any form or by any means, electronic, mechanical, photocopying, recording or otherwise, without prior written permission of the Publisher.

Notice
No responsibility is assumed by the Publisher for any injury and/or damage to persons or property as a matter of products liability, negligence or otherwise, or from any use or operation of any methods, products, instructions or ideas contained in the material herein. Because of rapid advances in the medical sciences, in particular, independent verification of diagnoses and drug dosages should be made.

Although all advertising material is expected to conform to ethical (medical) standards, inclusion in this publication does not constitute a guarantee or endorsement of the quality or value of such product or of the claims made of it by its manufacturer.

Otolaryngologic Clinics of North America (ISSN 0030-6665) is published bimonthly by Elsevier, Inc., 360 Park Avenue South, New York, NY 10010-1710. Months of issue are February, April, June, August, October, and December. Business and Editorial Offices: 1600 John F. Kennedy Blvd., Suite 1800, Philadelphia, PA 19103-2899. Customer Service Office: 6277 Sea Harbor Drive, Orlando, FL 32887-4800. Periodicals postage paid at New York, NY and additional mailing offices. Subscription prices are $424.00 per year (US individuals), $947.00 per year (US institutions), $100.00 per year (US & Canadian student/resident), $548.00 per year (Canadian individuals), $1200.00 per year (Canadian institutions), $592.00 per year (international individuals), $1200.00 per year (international institutions), $270.00 per year (international student/resident). Foreign air speed delivery is included in all *Clinics'* subscription prices. All prices are subject to change without notice. **POSTMASTER:** Send address changes to *Otolaryngologic Clinics of North America*, Elsevier Health Sciences Division, Subscription Customer Service, 3251 Riverport Lane, Maryland Heights, MO 63043. **Telephone: 1-800-654-2452 (U.S. and Canada); 314-447-8871 (outside U.S. and Canada). Fax: 314-447-8029. E-mail: journalscustomerservice-usa@elsevier.com (for print support); journalsonlinesupport-usa@elsevier.com (for online support).**

Reprints. For copies of 100 or more of articles in this publication, please contact the Commercial Reprints Department, Elsevier Inc., 360 Park Avenue South, New York, NY 10010-1710. Tel.: 212-633-3874; Fax: 212-633-3820; E-mail: reprints@elsevier.com.

Otolaryngologic Clinics of North America is also published in Spanish by McGraw-Hill Interamericana Editores S.A., P.O. Box 5-237, 06500 Mexico D.F., Mexico.

Otolaryngologic Clinics of North America is covered in *MEDLINE/PubMed (Index Medicus), Current Contents/Clinical Medicine, Excerpta Medica, BIOSIS, Science Citation Index,* and *ISI/BIOMED.*

Contributors

CONSULTING EDITOR

SUJANA S. CHANDRASEKHAR, MD, FACS, FAAOHNS
Past President, American Academy of Otolaryngology–Head and Neck Surgery, Secretary-Treasurer, American Otological Society, Partner, ENT & Allergy Associates, LLP, Clinical Professor, Department of Otolaryngology–Head and Neck Surgery, Zucker School of Medicine at Hofstra-Northwell, Hempstead, New York, USA; Clinical Associate Professor, Department of Otolaryngology–Head and Neck Surgery, Icahn School of Medicine at Mount Sinai, New York, New York, USA

EDITORS

CAROL A. BAUER, MD
Professor Emerita, Department of Otolaryngology–Head and Neck Surgery, Southern Illinois University School of Medicine, Springfield, Illinois, USA

DIDIER DEPIREUX, PhD
Chief Scientific Officer, R&D OtolithLabs, Adjunct Faculty, Department of Otorhinolaryngology–Head and Neck Surgery, University of Maryland School of Medicine, Baltimore, Maryland, USA; Otolithlabs, Washington, DC, USA

RONNA HERTZANO, MD, PhD
Associate Professor, Department of Otolaryngology–Head and Neck Surgery, Associate Professor, Department of Anatomy and Neurobiology, Affiliate Member, Institute for Genome Sciences, University of Maryland School of Medicine, Baltimore, Maryland, USA

JENNIFER A. VILLWOCK, MD
Department of Otolaryngology– Head and Neck Surgery, Kansas University, University of Kansas Medical Center, Kansas City, Kansas, USA

AUTHORS

MEREDITH E. ADAMS, MD, MS
Associate Professor, Department of Otolaryngology–Head and Neck Surgery, University of Minnesota, Minneapolis, Minnesota, USA

SANA AMANAT, MSc. PhD
Student, Otology and Neurotology Group CTS495, Department of Genomic Medicine, GENYO - Centre for Genomics and Oncological Research – Pfizer, University of Granada, Junta de Andalucía, Andalusian Regional Government, PTS Granada, Granada, Spain

SEILESH BABU, MD
Department of Otology, Neurotology, and Skull Base Surgery, Michigan Ear Institute, Farmington Hills, Michigan, USA; Program Director, Ascension Macomb Otolaryngology Residency, Warren, Michigan, USA; Associate Professor, Department of Otolaryngology, Wayne State University, Detroit, Michigan, USA

MARIE-SARAH BAILLARGEON
École d'orthophonie et d'audiologie, Faculty of Medicine, Université de Montréal, Montreal, Canada

CAROL A. BAUER, MD
Professor Emerita, Department of Otolaryngology–Head and Neck Surgery, Southern Illinois University School of Medicine, Springfield, Illinois, USA

THOMAS J. BROZOSKI, PhD
Research Professor, Emeritus, Department of Otolaryngology–Head and Neck Surgery, Southern Illinois University School of Medicine, Springfield, Illinois, USA

KADJA FERRAZ CAMPARA, MBBS
College of Medicine, Universidade do Vale do Taquari-UNIVATES, Lajeado, Brazil

KATHLEEN F. CARLSON, PhD
United States Department of Veterans Affairs Rehabilitation Research & Development, National Center for Rehabilitative Auditory Research, Veterans Affairs Portland Health Care System, School of Public Health, Oregon Health & Science University, Center to Improve Veteran Involvement in Care, Portland, Oregon, USA

CHRISTOPHER R. CEDERROTH, PhD
Associate Professor, Department of Physiology and Pharmacology, KarolinskaInstitutet, Stockholm, Sweden

SUJANA S. CHANDRASEKHAR, MD, FACS, FAAOHNS
Past President, American Academy of Otolaryngology -Head and Neck Surgery, Secretary-Treasurer, American Otological Society, Partner, ENT & Allergy Associates, LLP, Clinical Professor, Department of Otolaryngology -Head and Neck Surgery, Zucker School of Medicine at Hofstra-Northwell, Hempstead, New York, USA; Clinical Associate Professor, Department of Otolaryngology -Head and Neck Surgery, Icahn School of Medicine at Mount Sinai, New York, New York, USA

STEVEN W. CHEUNG, MD
Professor, Department of Otolaryngology–Head and Neck Surgery, University of California, San Francisco, San Francisco, California, USA

CLAUDIA BARROS COELHO, MD, PhD
Postgraduate Program in Medical Sciences, College of Medicine, Universidade do Vale do Taquari-UNIVATES, Lajeado, Brazil; Department of Otolaryngology–Head and Neck Surgery, University of Iowa, Iowa City, Iowa, USA

DIDIER DEPIREUX, PhD
Chief Scientific Officer, R&D OtolithLabs, Adjunct Faculty, Department of Otorhinolaryngology–Head and Neck Surgery, University of Maryland School of Medicine, Baltimore, Maryland, USA; Otolithlabs, Washington, DC, USA

VICTORIA DUDA, MScS, PhD
Post-doctoral Fellow, École d'orthophonie et d'audiologie, Faculty of Medicine, Université de Montréal, Montreal, Canada

JONAS DYHRFJELD-JOHNSEN, PhD
Vice President, Research and Translational Development, Sensorion SA, Montpellier, France

DAVID J. EISENMAN, MD
Associate Professor, Department of Otorhinolaryngology–Head and Neck Surgery, University of Maryland School of Medicine, Baltimore, Maryland, USA

ALEXANDER GALAZYUK, PhD
Associate Professor, Department of Anatomy and Neurobiology, Northeast Ohio Medical University, Rootstown, Ohio, USA

SUSAN E. GRIEST, MPH
United States Department of Veterans Affairs Rehabilitation Research & Development, National Center for Rehabilitative Auditory Research, Veterans Affairs Portland Health Care System, Department of Otolaryngology–Head and Neck Surgery, Oregon Health & Science University, Portland, Oregon, USA

LESLIE D. GRUSH, AuD
United States Department of Veterans Affairs Rehabilitation Research & Development, National Center for Rehabilitative Auditory Research, Veterans Affairs Portland Health Care System, Portland, Oregon, USA

SYLVIE HÉBERT, PhD
Professor, École d'orthophonie et d'audiologie, Faculty of Medicine, Université de Montréal,]Montreal, Canada; International Laboratory for Brain, Music and Sound Research (BRAMS), Outremont, Quebec, Canada

JAMES A. HENRY, PhD
United States Department of Veterans Affairs Rehabilitation Research & Development, National Center for Rehabilitative Auditory Research, Veterans Affairs Portland Health Care System, Department of Otolaryngology–Head and Neck Surgery, Oregon Health & Science University, Portland, Oregon, USA

RONNA HERTZANO, MD, PhD
Associate Professor, Department of Otolaryngology–Head and Neck Surgery, Associate Professor, Department of Anatomy and Neurobiology, Affiliate Member, Institute for Genome Sciences, University of Maryland School of Medicine, Baltimore, Maryland, USA

TINA C. HUANG, MD
Assistant Professor, Department of Otolaryngology–Head and Neck Surgery, University of Minnesota, Minneapolis, Minnesota, USA

FATIMA T. HUSAIN, PhD
Department of Speech and Hearing Science, The Neuroscience Program, The Beckman Institute for Advanced Science and Technology, University of Illinois at Urbana-Champaign, Champaign, Illinois, USA

TOBIAS KLEINJUNG, MD
Department of Otorhinolaryngology and Head and Neck Surgery, University Hospital Zurich, University of Zurich, Zurich, Switzerland

DAWN KONRAD-MARTIN, PhD
Associate Director, United States Department of Veterans Affairs Rehabilitation Research & Development, National Center for Rehabilitative Auditory Research, Veterans Affairs Portland Health Care System, Associate Professor, Department of Otolaryngology–Head and Neck Surgery, Oregon Health & Science University, Portland, Oregon, USA

BERTHOLD LANGGUTH, MD
Department of Psychiatry and Psychotherapy, Interdisciplinary Tinnitus Center, University of Regensburg, Regensburg, Germany

K.J. LEE, MD, FACS
Associate Clinical Professor, Donald and Barbara Zucker School of Medicine at Hofstra/ Northwell; Quinnipiac University Frank H. Netter MD School of Medicine; Yale School of Medicine

MARK E. LEE, MBA
CEO, Halo Media Group

ERIKA L. LIPFORD, BSc
Department of Otorhinolaryngology–Head and Neck Surgery, University of Maryland School of Medicine, Baltimore, Maryland, USA

JOSE A. LOPEZ-ESCAMEZ, MD, PhD
Otology & Neurotology Group CTS495, Department of Genomic Medicine, GENYO - Centre for Genomics and Oncological Research – Pfizer, University of Granada, Junta de Andalucía, Andalusian Regional Government, PTS Granada, Department of Otolaryngology, Instituto de Investigación Biosanitaria ibs, GRANADA, Hospital Universitario Virgen de las Nieves, Department of Surgery, Division of Otolaryngology, Universidad de Granada, Granada, Spain

FRIEDERIKE S. LUETZENBERG, BS
MD/MBA Candidate Class of 2022, University of Central Florida College of Medicine, Orlando, Florida, USA

ELIZABETH MARKS, ClinPsyD
ClinPsyD, Lecturer, Clinical Psychologist, University of Bath, Claverton Down, Bath, United Kingdom

LAURENCE McKENNA, PhD, MClinPsychol
MClinPsychol, Consultant Clinical Psychologist, Department Clinical Psychology, Royal National Ear Nose Throat and Eastman Dental Hospital, University College London Hospital, Honorary Clinical Lecturer, University College London Ear Institute, London, United Kingdom

SRIKANTAN NAGARAJAN, PhD
Professor, Departments of Radiology and Biomedical Imaging, and Otolaryngology–Head and Neck Surgery, University of California, San Francisco, San Francisco, California, USA

KELLY M. REAVIS, MPH
United States Department of Veterans Affairs Rehabilitation Research & Development, National Center for Rehabilitative Auditory Research, Veterans Affairs Portland Health Care System, School of Public Health, Oregon Health & Science University, Portland, Oregon, USA

ROBERTO SANTOS, MBBS
College of Medicine, Universidade do Vale do Taquari-UNIVATES, Lajeado, Brazil

OLIVIA SCULLY, BSc
École d'orthophonie et d'audiologie, Faculty of Medicine, Université de Montréal, Montreal, Canada

MICHAEL D. SEIDMAN, MD, FACS
Director, Otologic/Neurotologic/Skull Base Surgery, Medical Director, Wellness and Integrative Medicine, Advent Health (Celebration and South Campuses), Professor, Otolaryngology–Head and Neck Surgery, University of Central Florida College of Medicine, Collaborative Professor, Otolaryngology Head and Neck Surgery, University of South Florida, AdventHealth Medical Group Otolaryngology–Head and Neck Surgery, Celebration, Florida, USA

LAGUINN P. SHERLOCK, AuD
Research Audiologist, Army Hearing Program, US Army Public Health Center, Aberdeen, Research Audiologist, Audiology and Speech Pathology Center, Walter Reed National Military Medical Center, Bethesda, Maryland, USA

SARAH M. THEODOROFF, PhD
Research Investigator, United States Department of Veterans Affairs Rehabilitation Research & Development, National Center for Rehabilitative Auditory Research, Veterans Affairs Portland Health Care System, Assistant Professor, Department of Otolaryngology–Head and Neck Surgery, Oregon Health & Science University, Portland, Oregon, USA

EMILY J. THIELMAN, MS
United States Department of Veterans Affairs Rehabilitation Research & Development, National Center for Rehabilitative Auditory Research, Veterans Affairs Portland Health Care System, Portland, Oregon, USA

RICHARD TYLER, PhD, MSc
Departments of Otolaryngology–Head and Neck Surgery, and Speech Pathology and Audiology, University of Iowa, Iowa City, Iowa, USA

FLORIAN VOGT, PhD, ClinPsyD
ClinPsyD, Clinical Psychologist, Royal National Ear Nose Throat and Eastman Dental Hospital, University College London Hospital, London, United Kingdom

Contents

Animal models have significantly contributed to understanding the pathophysiology of chronic subjective tinnitus. They are useful because they control etiology, which in humans is heterogeneous; employ random group assignment; and often use methods not permissible in human studies. Animal models can be broadly categorized as either operant or reflexive, based on methodology. Operant methods use variants of established psychophysical procedures to reveal what an animal hears. Reflexive methods do the same using elicited behavior, for example, the acoustic startle reflex. All methods contrast the absence of sound and presence of sound, because tinnitus cannot by definition be perceived as silence.

Tinnitus is commonly referred to as "ringing in the ears." Epidemiologic studies highlight challenges associated with clinical determination of tinnitus and ascertainment of its etiology, functional effects, temporal characteristics, psychoacoustic parameters, and risk factors. Because no standards exist for capturing these factors as measures, direct comparison of data between studies is not possible. This report suggests terminology and definitions to promote standardization, with a brief overview of findings from selected population-based epidemiologic studies. Tinnitus-specific data are presented from the Noise Outcomes in Servicemembers Epidemiology study. Further epidemiologic studies are needed to develop tinnitus treatment and a cure for this chronic condition.

Tinnitus is the perception of sound in the absence of an external source. Genetic studies on families, twins, and adoptees cohorts have been conducted supporting tinnitus heritability, with higher heritability in men with bilateral tinnitus at any age, and young women with bilateral tinnitus, but not in unilateral tinnitus. The condition is associated with several comorbidities such as hearing loss, Meniere disease, sleep disorders, depression, and migraine and may lead toward suicidal attempts in extreme cases. Several studies have reported few regulatory allelic variants in candidate genes and pathways associated with tinnitus development, but replication studies are needed to validate them.

Tinnitus is spoken of as if it were a single thing, but there are many different causes, likely many different mechanisms, and many different subtypes. This article reviews a broad range of approaches to understand and demarcate different tinnitus subtypes, which will be critical for exploring and finding cures for different subtypes.

Cochlear damage is often thought to result in hearing thresholds shift, whether permanent or temporary. The report of tinnitus in the absence of any clear deficit in cochlear function was believed to indicate that hearing loss and tinnitus, while comorbid, could arise independently from each other. In all likelihood, tinnitus that is not of central nervous system origin is associated with hearing loss. As a correlate, although a treatment of most forms of tinnitus will likely emerge in the years to come, curing tinnitus will first require curing hearing loss.

Tinnitus is commonly experienced by military Service Members and Veterans, especially by the newest generation who served in Iraq and Afghanistan. When patients seek health care for tinnitus, it is important to determine its type, check for comorbid conditions that might be triggering or exacerbating the condition, and to address its functional and psychosocial effects. Otolaryngologists are usually the first health care professional to evaluate a patient with tinnitus, and it is essential to provide appropriate referrals for this high-burden condition. Noise-induced tinnitus is multifaceted; by performing a thorough assessment, appropriate action can be taken to best meet the needs of patients.

Tinnitus is the perception of a self-generated sound and an individual's psychological reaction to it. This article discusses one element of the reaction: depression. Epidemiologic studies have noted high comorbidity of tinnitus and depression. Findings from recent brain imaging studies have noted shared neural networks in depression and severe tinnitus. As further evidence of this overlaps, antidepressants, counseling, and psychology-based approaches have been used to treat tinnitus. Multifaceted treatment strategies, using both sound-based therapies (not discussed in this paper) and psychology-based approaches, are a necessary part of the treatment options, with the aim of enhancing self-efficacy in patients with tinnitus.

The results showed a trend of increased post-gap amplitudes and reduced gap salience; however, the small number of articles yield and limited consensus prohibit any conclusions for clinical use. Nevertheless, gap-induced EPs may be further explored as a potential tool for tinnitus detection.

This article reviews the use of human neuroimaging for chronic subjective tinnitus. Evidence-based guidance on the clinical use of imaging to identify relevant auditory lesions when evaluating tinnitus patients is given. After introducing the anatomy and imaging modalities most pertinent to the neuroscience of tinnitus, the article reviews tinnitus-associated alterations in key auditory and nonauditory networks in the central nervous system. Emphasis is placed on how these findings support proposed models of tinnitus and how this line of investigation is relevant to practicing clinicians.

Tinnitus distress results from a weave of physical and psychological processes. Reducing the power of the psychological processes will therefore reduce the degree of suffering. The main psychological therapy in this context is cognitive behavioral therapy (CBT). This seeks to understand and change the influence of thinking processes, including information processing biases, and the behaviors that these motivate, on the experience of tinnitus. The results of systematic reviews and meta-analyses indicate that CBT is the tinnitus management approach for which there is the most robust evidence. In spite of this, it remains difficult to access for people with tinnitus.

The search for an effective medication that will eliminate tinnitus has a long history. Currently, no drugs exist that universally cure tinnitus. Pharmacologic interventions that have been investigated can be divided into those that attempt to eliminate the perception of tinnitus, and those that are designed to treat the negative comorbidities associated with tinnitus, thereby mitigating tinnitus' negative impact on quality of life. A third category of drugs can also be considered that addresses an identified pathologic condition that has tinnitus as an associated symptom (for example, Meniere's disease, otosclerosis, migraine-associated vertigo). This third category is not addressed.

Device-based clinical treatments for tinnitus are predominantly sound based and include ear-level sound generators, hearing aids, cochlear implants, and tinnitus treatment devices. They are intended for patients with bothersome tinnitus. Bothersome tinnitus is characterized by problems with sleep, concentration, and mood. Most people with bothersome tinnitus have hearing loss and would benefit from amplification; however, not all patients are willing to use hearing aids. Tinnitus treatment devices are available to assist those who are not good candidates for amplification, and include devices used while sleeping and devices used for specified periods during the day.

Because Western medicine has remained largely unsuccessful at treating tinnitus symptoms, many physicians as well as patients have turned to alternative treatment options to decrease patients' suffering and improve their quality of life. Although research in complementary/integrative medicine continues to be scarce and inconclusive, studies are pointing toward the positive effects of acupuncture, herbal remedies, dietary supplements, antioxidants, melatonin, and hypnosis on tinnitus. Although the efficacies of these treatments are inconsistent and may depend on a patient's unique circumstances, studies acknowledge that each treatment is worth trying in light of the potential benefits while being both noninvasive and well tolerated.

Despite recent, major steps forward in our understanding of tinnitus pathophysiology and improved research methodology, tinnitus remains a clear unmet clinical need. Here, the authors identify current active clinical and preclinical development programs of tinnitus drug candidates using publications, databases, and company communications. The current drug development programs hold promise for new therapeutic options for tinnitus patients, but further fundamental research is needed to validate additional targets for treating tinnitus.

Tinnitus is a common symptom. Standard therapies aim at improving the quality of life and reducing the psychological stress associated with tinnitus. Most interventions have little or no effect on the main symptom. Those affected subjects, however, want such a change and prefer a specific solution, such as pharmacologic therapy to other modalities. Scientific efforts have not yet led to significant improvement in the range of therapies. This article outlines existing efforts and develops ideas on how research for improved tinnitus therapy might look in the future.

Otolaryngologists are in a good position to advocate for our patients and our specialty. We can do it as a volunteer or as a full-time job running for political office at the state or federal level. To be taken seriously, we need to offer solutions besides citing the problems. We encourage otolaryngologists to work with our Academy and its ENT-PAC (Ear, Nose, Throat Political Action Committee). Medicine is a great profession and Otolaryngology–Head and Neck Surgery is an even better specialty.

In 2018, the Joint Councils of the American Otological Society and the American Neurotology Society adopted a statement on diversity and inclusion for programs henceforth. That statement stands as a landmark touch point in our societies that heralds the engagement of all our members as we all work to advance knowledge and skills in otology and neurotology. I was asked to write this piece for Otology & Neurotology, and republication in this Clinics series establishes a baseline understanding of the historical limitations in organized otolaryngology and the willingness of societies to adapt and lead in shaping our profession's future.

OTOLARYNGOLOGIC CLINICS
OF NORTH AMERICA

SERIES OF RELATED INTEREST

Facial Plastic Surgery Clinics
Available at: https://www.facialplastic.theclinics.com/

THE CLINICS ARE AVAILABLE ONLINE!
Access your subscription at:
www.theclinics.com

Foreword

Tinnitus: Current Understanding of an Age-Old Problem

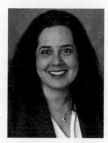

Sujana S. Chandrasekhar, MD, FACS, FAAOHNS
Consulting Editor

Tinnitus, the perception of sound where there is no external sound stimulus, has long been part of the human experience. Because of our current noisy society, this condition affects 1 in 10 adults.[1] However, it did not begin with the Industrial Age. There are references to it in Hindu ayurvedic medicine, where it is considered an imbalance of vata dosha, or the wind element, and in classical China, where it was thought to be caused by an imbalance of yin and yang. Mesopotamian remedies included exorcism and chants dedicated to the god of water. The ancient Egyptians tried treating it by infusing a mixture of oil, frankincense, tree sap, herbs, and soil through a reed stalk into the external ear. Greek and Roman treatments included exercise, rubbing, gargling, dieting, and the application of balms. Aristotle and Hippocrates advised masking the inner sound with an outer sound, which is still commonly advised today. A medieval Welsh remedy was to apply a hot loaf of bread to each ear. One Renaissance writer hypothesized that tinnitus was the wind trapped in the ear and recommended surgery.[2] The myriad of treatments matches that offered to patients today.

Tinnitus is one of those medical conditions that can vex both sufferer and health care professional. It is common and persistent, with 27% of people experiencing it for over 15 years and 36% of tinnitus sufferers having near constant symptoms. However, only 7.2% of individuals with tinnitus in the 2007 National Health Interview Survey (raw N = 75,764) reported their tinnitus as a "big" or "very big" problem versus 41.6% reporting it as a "small" problem.[1] In the half who actually had discussed their tinnitus with a physician, medications were recommended in 46%, and the other interventions discussed included hearing aids (9.2%), masking devices (4.9%), and cognitive-behavioral therapy (0.2%). This, to me, indicates some dearth of knowledge of the latest information regarding tinnitus, described in the American Academy of Otolaryngology–Head and Neck Surgery Clinical Practice Guidelines on Tinnitus[3]

Otolaryngol Clin N Am 53 (2020) xv–xvi
https://doi.org/10.1016/j.otc.2020.04.004
0030-6665/20/© 2020 Published by Elsevier Inc.

and in terrific detail here in this issue of *Otolaryngologic Clinics of North America*, guest edited by Drs Carol Bauer, Ronna Hertzano, and Didier Depireux.

The articles in this issue approach tinnitus in a systematic manner. There are animal models for this condition, which show promise for pharmacotherapy. Understanding epidemiology and genetics allows the professional to then move on to classifying tinnitus for the particular patient in front of them. We are all aware of the association of noise exposure with tinnitus and hearing loss. The articles devoted to this dive deeply into the matter. Tinnitus is a subjective experience, without a one-to-one correlation with hearing loss or noise exposure. However, we now have some objective measures, electrophysiologically and with imaging, that can help us both understand its impact on the individual and assess efficacy of interventions.

Validated interventions for tinnitus include cognitive behavioral therapy, certain pharmacotherapies, and auditory devices, such as ear-level maskers, hearing aids, and cochlear implants. Nonallopathic or complementary and alternative medicine treatments, as alluded to in the first paragraph, have a long history in both the United States and overseas. The wealth of basic science and research on tinnitus has resulted in development of novel modalities that are in trials. The final series of articles describe these in detail.

I commend Drs Bauer, Hertzano, and Depireux on tackling this difficult and important problem, both in their professional lives and in guest editing this issue of *Otolaryngologic Clinics of North America* . Once you read the articles they have compiled, you will feel much more comfortable when that next patient walks in complaining of tinnitus. And you will be able to embark on a mutual plan of understanding the symptom and shared decision making in coming up with a treatment plan. The pat answer to tinnitus, "You'll just have to learn to live with it," can be stricken from our vocabulary.

Sujana S. Chandrasekhar, MD, FACS, FAAOHNS
Consulting Editor, Otolaryngologic Clinics of North America

Past President, American Academy of Otolaryngology-Head and Neck Surgery

Secretary-Treasurer, American Otological Society

Partner, ENT & Allergy Associates LLP
18 East 48th Street, 2nd Floor, New York, NY 10017, USA

Clinical Professor, Department of Otolaryngology-Head and Neck Surgery
Zucker School of Medicine at Hofstra-Northwell, Hempstead, NY, USA

Clinical Associate Professor, Department of Otolaryngology-Head and Neck Surgery
Icahn School of Medicine at Mount Sinai, New York, NY, USA

E-mail address:
ssc@nyotology.com

REFERENCES

1. Bhatt JM, Lin HW, Bhattacharyya N. Prevalence, severity, exposures, and treatment patterns of tinnitus in the United States. JAMA Otolaryngol Head Neck Surg 2016;142(10):959–65.
2. Landragin A. The organ of the universe: on living with tinnitus. Los Angeles (CA): Los Angeles Review of Books; 2017.
3. Tunkel DE, Bauer CA, Sun GH, et al. Clinical practice guideline: tinnitus executive summary. Otolaryngol Head Neck Surg 2014;151(4):533–41.

Preface

Tinnitus: Clinical, Basic Science, Audiologic and Industry Updates

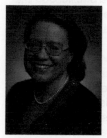
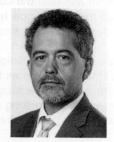
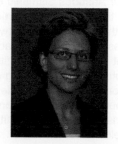

Carol A. Bauer, MD   Didier Depireux, PhD   Ronna Hertzano, MD, PhD

Editors

Tinnitus, the perception of sound without an external source, is a phenomenon that interests people from many backgrounds and disciplines. In the United States, it is estimated that 30 million adults experience tinnitus on a daily basis, and for upward of 5% of them, the experience is severely disruptive and negatively impacts quality of life. Therefore, there are many individuals with tinnitus who may benefit from this issue by learning what is currently known about tinnitus cause and treatments. Although *Otolaryngologic Clinics of North America* issues are geared primarily for physicians and other auditory/neural health care providers, the material herein can be accessed effectively by patients, either directly or as communicated by their hearing health professional.

Tinnitus treatment begins with the very first interaction a patient has with their provider, whether they are a primary care physician, an advanced practice nurse or physician's assistant, an audiologist, or an otolaryngologist head and neck surgeon. Many providers are frequently frustrated when evaluating patients with tinnitus and are uncertain when determining how to evaluate and select the best treatment approach for the individual. While tinnitus is one of the most frequent symptoms experienced by patients who present to the office of an otolaryngologist, the pathophysiology of tinnitus and its treatments are not routinely taught or tested as part of the official training in Otolaryngology Head and Neck Surgery. Not surprisingly, patients are frustrated and disturbed when they are told as a blanket statement that there is no cure or treatment for them, and they must learn to live with their tinnitus.

This issue is not a "how I do it" manual, but a collection of what is currently known about tinnitus from a variety of perspectives. As such, we hope it will serve as a resource and guide for patients and practitioners alike. Each article provides a clear summary on a specific aspect of tinnitus, including basic science theories and research techniques, genetics and heritability, and a review of the impact of damaging

Otolaryngol Clin N Am 53 (2020) xvii–xviii
https://doi.org/10.1016/j.otc.2020.04.003
0030-6665/20/© 2020 Published by Elsevier Inc.

noise and how it relates to tinnitus. Also included are practical reviews of the role of alternative or complementary medicine and current evidence for the 3 broad areas of traditional tinnitus treatment approaches: sound therapy, behavioral therapy, and pharmacologic therapy. Finally, a summary of the factors that are barriers in the field frames promising areas for research to unravel the mechanisms of tinnitus and leverage that information into development of new therapeutics.

The *Otolaryngologic Clinics of North America* last published an issue dedicated to tinnitus in 2003. Dr Aristides Sismanis organized and edited a superb collection that is a classic in the tinnitus field. The articles on the patient's perspective (Dr Stephen M. Nagler) and the relationship between depression and tinnitus (Dr Robert A. Dobie) are timeless and well worth reading.

It is self-evident that patients benefit from well-informed clinicians and the expert knowledge they utilize when providing care. This issue provides the clinician with an up-to-date and comprehensive overview of the subject. It is our hope that this work will form a solid foundation for practitioners interested in knowing more about tinnitus. We also hope this issue will be of benefit to patients and will inspire continued research to advance the field.

Carol A. Bauer, MD
Department of Otolaryngology Head
and Neck Surgery
Southern Illinois University School of Medicine
720 N. Bond Street, Springfield, IL 62702, USA

Didier Depireux, PhD
Chief Scientific Officer, OtolithLabs
1875 Connecticut Avenue
Washington, DC 20009, USA

Department of Otorhinolaryngology
Head and Neck Surgery
University of Maryland
School of Medicine
Baltimore, MD 21201, USA

Ronna Hertzano, MD, PhD
Department of Otolaryngology
Head and Neck Surgery
Department of Anatomy and Neurobiology
Institute for Genome Sciences
University of Maryland School of Medicine
16 South Eutaw Street, Suite 500
Baltimore, MD 21201, USA

E-mail addresses:
cbauer@siumed.edu (C.A. Bauer)
depireux@gmail.com (D. Depireux)
rhertzano@som.umaryland.edu (R. Hertzano)

Animal Models of Tinnitus
A Review

Alexander Galazyuk, PhD[a],*, Thomas J. Brozoski, PhD[b]

KEYWORDS

- Animal models • Tinnitus • Acoustic startle reflex • Operant behavioral methods
- Psychophysics

KEY POINTS

- At present there is no standard animal model of tinnitus. Two contemporary types of models are reflexive and operant; each has positive and negative features.
- Reflexive models trace their origin to an experiment of Turner and colleagues; operant models trace theirs to an experiment of Jastreboff and colleagues.
- Caution is advised to distinguish between animal tinnitus studies that independently confirm the presence of tinnitus and those that do not.

INTRODUCTION

Tinnitus in this review refers to chronic subjective tinnitus, which has no identifiable acoustic correlate. Despite the common name, "ringing in the ears," its source(s) appear to be primarily in the central nervous system rather than the auditory periphery. Acute tinnitus commonly follows a single exposure to high-level sound or a high dose of aspirin and typically resolves within minutes to hours. As such, it is not of medical concern. In contrast, chronic tinnitus, estimated to affect 35 million to 50 million adults in the United States,[1] most commonly follows auditory trauma or chronic hearing loss and often persists for a lifetime.[2] It has been estimated that approximately 5% of those experiencing chronic tinnitus seek medical treatment. Although common, and recognized since the time of Galen,[3] the pathophysiology of tinnitus is incompletely understood. This contributes to the absence of generally effective treatments, although a standard of care has been established.[4,5] Tinnitus typically is perceived as a simple sound or a ringing or buzzing sensation, but its pathophysiology is far from simple.

[a] Department of Anatomy and Neurobiology, Northeast Ohio Medical University, 4209 State Route 44, Rootstown, OH 44272-9698, USA; [b] Emeritus, Department of Otolaryngology Head and Neck Surgery, Southern Illinois University School of Medicine, 801 North Rutledge Street, PO Box 19629, Springfield, IL 62794, USA
* Corresponding author.
E-mail address: agalaz@neomed.edu

Otolaryngol Clin N Am 53 (2020) 469–480
https://doi.org/10.1016/j.otc.2020.03.001
0030-6665/20/Published by Elsevier Inc.

ANIMAL TINNITUS MODELS

Tinnitus appears to be a primitive hearing disorder. This is not to say that its pathology is simple but rather that it derives from basic neurophysiologic mechanisms likely to be present in animals as well as humans.[6] Animal models have been available since 1988[7] and have contributed significantly to understanding the neuroscience of tinnitus.[8,9] Although animal models only approximate the human condition, their advantages over clinical studies are several. Notably, (1) they directly control etiology; (2) they permit application of many experimental tools, from behavioral to molecular; and (3) random assignment to experimental groups enables the use of more powerful inferential statistics as well as attribution of cause.

The key problem in developing an animal tinnitus model is objective and reliable assessment rather than induction. In humans, tinnitus can be induced by many conditions. These conditions have in common the reduction of peripheral signal to the brain.[10–12] In animals, tinnitus has been induced using systemic treatment with salicylates,[7,13–16] ototoxic exposure,[17–19] surgical disruption of the cochlea,[20] and acoustic over exposure.[18,21–23] These methods draw on factors known to affect tinnitus in humans.

The key to solving the assessment problem was provided by Jastreboff and colleagues.[24] Although tinnitus might sound like anything to an animal (or human), it can never sound like silence. All animal models of tinnitus use behavioral methods that differentiate how animals respond to sound versus silence. Typically, animal studies also include 1 or more normal-hearing control groups. Although considerable effort has been invested in finding valid and reliable direct measures of tinnitus that do not involve behavior, at present behavioral methods are used exclusively for at least 2 reasons: there is no procedure for either reliably producing or determining tinnitus alone, without potential confounds; and a presumptive tinnitus state might be derived from associated phenomena, such as hearing loss, hyperacusis, or drug side effects. Behavioral methods enable such confounds to be more clearly sorted out.

Many presumptive tinnitus animal experiments have examined the effects of conditions likely to cause tinnitus, such as high-level sound exposure or ototoxic damage, without directly confirming the presence of tinnitus. These experiments can be informative about the consequences of auditory insults but should be interpreted cautiously with respect to tinnitus. Not all humans exposed to acoustic trauma or other insults develop tinnitus.[25] Similarly it has been shown that not all animals exposed to tinnitus-inducing procedures display evidence of tinnitus.[26–28] Therefore, experiments that examine only the consequence of manipulations that typically produce tinnitus, without objective confirmation, are likely to include animals without tinnitus and, therefore, could be reporting the effects of something other than tinnitus.

Unfortunately, there is no generally accepted, or standard, animal model of tinnitus against which others can be validated. Existent models have their respective strengths and weaknesses. For overview purposes, animal models can be divided into 2 broad categories: models that interrogate animals about their auditory experience and models that examine alteration of an auditory reflex. Interrogative models, hereafter called operant models, loosely following the terminology of Skinner,[29] examine the effect of tinnitus on voluntary, or emitted behavior that is modified by training in an acoustic environment. These models have the general advantage of relying on auditory perception. As such, animals evaluate what they are hearing and differentially respond on the basis of their evaluation. Because operant methods require animals to report what they are hearing, they have conceptual features in common with the interrogation of humans with tinnitus, that is, analogous to asking, "What do you hear?" Operant models tap into functions in many brain areas, including areas outside those commonly defined as auditory. Although this aspect of operant models might be considered a shortcoming, it also is a strength, in that contemporary research has shown tinnitus to be mediated by widely distributed alterations in brain function.[10,30–33] A shortcoming of operant models is that they require training and motivating subjects, interventions that can be both time consuming and require careful experimental control. In contrast, reflexive animal models rely on unconditioned reflexes, such as the acoustic startle response, and do not require either training or motivation management. Reflexive methods, such as sound gap-prepulse inhibition of the acoustic startle (GPIAS), also are rapid, and, therefore, are well suited to determining the time course of tinnitus development. These features probably account for the current widespread use of GPIAS in animal tinnitus experiments. Although widely used, GPIAS models are not without their own issues and complexities. A further consideration is that the acoustic startle reflex, on which GPIAS is based, depends primarily on brainstem circuits.[34] Therefore, the neurophysiologic substrate driving the reflexive behavior assessed by GPIAS, might not have the same substrate indicated by operant models.

GAP-PREPULSE INHIBITION OF THE ACOUSTIC STARTLE MODELS
Animal Research

More than 10 years ago, a new method for tinnitus screening in laboratory animals was introduced by Turner and colleagues.[35] This paradigm utilizes the acoustic startle reflex, which is ubiquitously expressed in mammals and consists of contraction of the major muscles of the body following a loud and unexpected sound[36] (**Fig. 1**A). This reflex is reduced when preceded by a silent gap embedded in a soft background noise or tone (**Fig. 1**B). Gap detection typically is assessed by the ratio between the magnitude of the startle stimulus presented alone (no-gap trial) and trials in which a gap preceded startle stimulus (gap trials), also GPIAS.[35] Reduced inhibition, after acoustic trauma or sodium salicylate treatments, is assumed to reflect tinnitus perception: when tinnitus is qualitatively similar to the background noise, it fills in the gap and, hence, reduces inhibition (**Fig. 1**C).

This method was adopted enthusiastically and is now used widely by many scientists in the field due to its relative simplicity over other methods of tinnitus assessment. Because it is based on a reflex, the method is much cheaper and faster than other methods requiring training animals for weeks or months.[21,37] It also allows for tinnitus screening of a large number of animals testing simultaneously in multiple testing boxes. Comparing animals' gap detection performances before and after tinnitus induction allows to separate tinnitus positive from tinnitus negative animals. The possibility of using this method for scientists with little experience in animal behavior and an opportunity to apply this methodology for tinnitus assessment in humans,made GPIAS the dominant assessment method in the field of tinnitus research.

The GPIAS methodology has been improved on over the past decade.[38,39] It has been shown that careful considerations of GPIAS parameters, such as the startle stimulus and background intensities, acoustical parameters of the gap of silence preceding the startle, and overall duration of a testing session, greatly improve results of GPIAS testing in laboratory animals.[40] Recent research also demonstrated large variability in GPIAS measurements between different days of testing, especially in mice.[41] Therefore, averaging these results across multiple testing sessions greatly increases statistical power of the obtained data and improves the reliability of tinnitus assessments. Recent improvements to startle response magnitude assessments[42,43] and

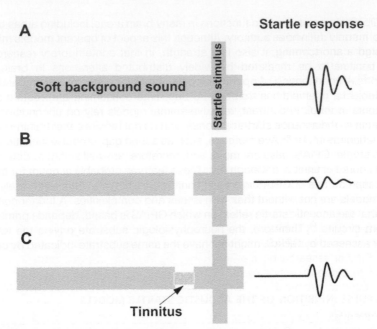

Fig. 1. Schematic description of the GPIAS assay for tinnitus. A startle wideband noise stimulus, 20-ms duration (*vertical bars*), is inserted into a narrowband noise or pure tone background (*horizontal bars*) without a gap of silence (A) or with the gap (B and C). The gap has a 20-ms to 50-ms duration, and is presented 50 ms before the startle. Animal startle response waveforms to the startle stimulus are shown on the right. The startle amplitude is represented by the height of the waveform. If a startle stimulus is presented during continuous background the animal's startle response is strong (A). If a gap of silence occurs before the startle stimulus, the startle response is greatly suppressed (B). In animals with tinnitus (C), the gap is filled by the tinnitus (*shaded rectangle within the gap*) and therefore the startle response in these animals is less suppressed by the preceding gap compared to the tinnitus-free animals (compare the startle amplitudes in B and C).

various methods of startle response separation from animals' ambient movements[42,44] greatly improve GPIAS data analysis. In small rodents, the whole-body startle reflex is relatively easy to measure, but in larger, less active mammals, such as the guinea pig, it habituates rapidly. Therefore, the pinna reflex measurement technique has been suggested to be used instead of whole-body startle reflex during GPIAS sessions.[45,46]

Despite years of using GPIAS for tinnitus assessment in various laboratory animals, the field continues to debate the original filling-in interpretation of the paradigm. In a study conducted on mice, the placement of the gap of silence either closer or further away from the proceeding startle stimulus could dramatically alter gap detection performance in mice.[47] Therefore, the investigators raised a doubt as to whether tinnitus is filling-in the gap; otherwise, the gap placement before the startle should not have a large effect on an animal's gap detection performance. Importantly, however, the most significant debates concerning GPIAS methodology on animals largely depend on successful demonstration that the method is capable of assessing tinnitus in humans.

Human Research

One of the main advantages of GPIAS over other methods is that it can be used in both laboratory animals and humans.[38] Several research laboratories have attempted to apply GPIAS method to humans for tinnitus assessment. Eye blink was proposed to be used instead of whole-body startle reflex in these studies. These experiments had a significant advantage over the animals' studies because in humans, exact tinnitus parameters, such as intensity and spectrum, can be identified by tinnitus self-reports. If so, during GPIAS testing, it is possible to match the background sound parameters to a person's tinnitus characteristics, which theoretically would optimize the success of the GPIAS. Unfortunately, in one of these studies it was found that gap detection performance in tinnitus patients did not depend on whether the individuals have tinnitus or not.[48] Another study showed a difference in gap detection performance between tinnitus patients and controls.[49] This deficit was not linked, however, to the tinnitus frequency. Although these studies raised concerns and emphasized caution, they did not rule out a possibility that GPIAS deficits can be interpreted as an indication of tinnitus. If animals or humans constantly experience a phantom sound, it still must be present during the silent gap during GPIAS testing. Therefore, a gap, even partially filled by tinnitus, still would be making gap detection more challenging, especially when the background spectrum would closely match the spectrum of tinnitus. Further research on the improvements of GPIAS testing paradigm might help to detect gap detection challenges in tinnitus patients. The most recent work has attempted to directly measure human neurophysiologic correlates of gap detection with cortical auditory evoked potentials recorded in the electroencephalogram.[50] The N1 potentials in response to gaps of silence were recorded from scalp in normal tinnitus-free individuals. Such an approach does not require overt responses from the participant nor measures responses modulated by gaps. Gap-evoked cortical responses were identified in all conditions for the vast majority of participants. The N1 responses were independent of background noise frequencies or background levels. The authors[50] concluded that this experimental design potentially could be used in both animals and humans to identify tinnitus objectively.

EARLY OPERANT MODELS

A variety of operant methods for tinnitus determination in animals have been developed. Two early operant models, those developed by Jastreboff and colleagues[7] and by Bauer and Brozoski,[21] illustrate many features common to these models. Operant models examine the effect of tinnitus on emitted behavior that has been modified by auditory training. Both methods are interrogative, in that they require subjects to respond differentially to auditory events. In the Jastreboff model, tinnitus was induced by high systemic doses of sodium salicylate. Rats were conditioned to stop licking a water spout by imposing a mild electric shock, at the end of random periods when the continuous background sound (broadband noise [BBN], 60dB sound pressure level [SPL]) was turned off, that is, during periods of external silence. The animals then were tested with randomly inserted silent periods, without shocks, after acute salicylate exposure (300 mg/kg). The salicylate-treated animals showed more persistent licking during the sound-off periods than controls without salicylate.[7] The interpretation was that salicylate induced tinnitus, as it is well known to do in humans, and masked the sound-off silence; therefore, the rats continued to lick as they would have if sound were present. In an informative variant procedure, Jastreboff and colleagues[7] demonstrated the obverse effect with animals that were lick-suppression trained while on salicylate. In this variant, the rats suppressed licking more during sound-off test periods than nonsalicylate controls. The interpretation was that suppression training, with tinnitus present, conditioned the animals to not lick when their tinnitus, a salient internal sound, was heard. A limitation of the Jastreboff salicylate lick-suppression model is that it was suitable only for determining acute tinnitus. Reasons for this limitation are two-fold: tinnitus induced by salicylate treatment is temporary, subsiding within a day or so after discontinuing the drug, and, more importantly, the tinnitus influence on licking was measured during extinction of conditioned suppression (there were no shocks when tinnitus testing). Extinction is a transient behavioral state.

A derivative operant method, well suited to assessing chronic tinnitus and still in use, was developed by Bauer and colleagues.[13,21,22] In the Bauer model, chronic tinnitus was induced using a single unilateral exposure to moderate-level tones (4 kHz at 80dB SPL) in chinchillas or high-level band-limited noise centered at 16 kHz (116–120dB SPL) in rats, for 1 hour, 3 or more months prior to tinnitus assessment. Unilateral exposure was used to preserve normal hearing in 1 ear. It also reflects a condition commonly associated with tinnitus in humans. Asymmetric acoustic trauma or hearing loss in humans is commonly associated with chronic tinnitus, including bilateral tinnitus.[51] All animals were trained to lever press for food pellets in the presence of BBN (60dB SPL) and were tested for tinnitus using randomly introduced 1-minute periods of either sound off, or tones at various levels. Lever pressing during sound-off periods was suppressed by delivering a lever press–contingent foot shock at the end of sound-off periods. In other words, the animals could avoid the foot shock by not lever pressing during sound off. Tinnitus was indicated by decreased lever pressing when tested with tones in the vicinity of 20 kHz (**Fig. 2**A), although tones of various frequency at various levels were tested. Control animals were not exposed to tinnitus induction but otherwise were treated and tested in parallel. The interpretation was that animals with chronic tinnitus could not hear true silence but instead heard their tinnitus. Because they were trained to suppress lever pressing when their tinnitus was audible (during sound-off periods), they suppressed lever pressing to stimulus-driven sensations that resembled their tinnitus.[6,21] In the Bauer model, testing and training are integrated into every session. This meant that chronic tinnitus could be measured with undiminished sensitivity over long periods. The model has been used to assess tinnitus in rats for as long as 17 months.[21] It also was found that a proportion of the exposed animals, typically 30% to 40%, did not develop tinnitus, although the audiometric profile of all exposed animals was equivalent (**Fig. 2**B). The Bauer model also has been used to determine acute tinnitus induced by systemic salicylate[13] as well as chronic tinnitus induced by ototoxic exposure.[18]

OPERANT MODEL VARIATIONS

Experimenters have examined several variations in an attempt to improve operant models. Several excellent reviews of tinnitus models may be consulted for variant features.[52–54] The extended training required by the Bauer model has a negative impacts on throughput and can be shortened by using an unconditioned indicator, such as licking a spout for water. Several researchers have adopted this modification. Zheng and colleagues[55] developed a model that incorporated many features of the Bauer model, using water-deprived rats required to lick a spout for water instead of pressing a lever for food. This considerably decreased training time, although it did not decrease the time required for tinnitus to appear after acoustic induction. A wrinkle that must be addressed when substituting licking for lever pressing is the episodic nature of licking. Spontaneous pauses in licking must be taken into account, so as not to count them as false-positive suppressions. Zheng and colleagues[55] used shortened test sessions to reduce this error. In another operant variation, using licking behavior, Jones and May[56] trained rats to lick to sound resembling their tinnitus, rather than

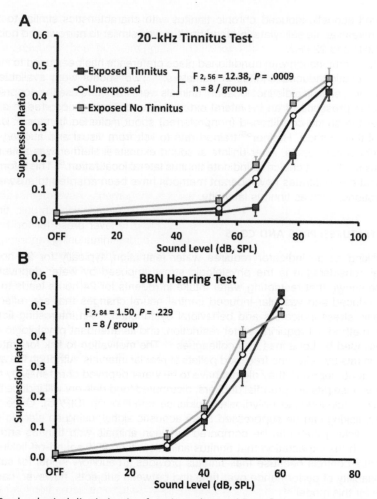

Fig. 2. Psychophysical discrimination functions obtained from 3 groups of rats; relative lever pressing, recorded as a suppression ratio (Y axis) is plotted against test-stimulus sound level (X axis). A suppression ratio of 0 reflects no lever presses, whereas a suppression ratio of 0.5 reflects lever pressing at baseline rate preceding the test stimulus. Both experimental groups (n = 8 each [*filled square data points*]) were unilaterally exposed to band-limited noise (120dB SPL, octave band centered at 16 kHz) 6 months prior to testing. The unexposed controls (n = 8 [*unfilled circular data points*]) were trained and tested in parallel. (*A*) Shows the average of 5 sessions using 20kHz test tones. A subset of exposed subjects suppressed significantly more to the 20kHz stimuli. The statistical difference between the exposed-with-tinnitus and unexposed groups is shown. (*B*) Suppression behavior (average of 5 sessions) of the same animals tested with BBN, diagnostic for free-field hearing but not tinnitus is shown. Data points are group means averaged over 5 test sessions; error bars indicate the standard error of the mean. Significance levels were determined using a mixed analysis of variance (n = 8 per group).

suppressing to tinnitus-like sound. Chronic tinnitus was induced using high-level sound exposure whereas acute tinnitus was induced using high-dose salicylate treatment. Episodic features of licking were controlled by using test periods of only a few minutes and by using a tinnitus score normalized to each animal's nontest lick rate.

They found acoustic-induced chronic tinnitus with characteristics similar to 16kHz tones, whereas acute salicylate induced tinnitus was similar to narrowband noise between 8 kHz and 22 kHz.

Licking in combination with conditioned place preference has been used to indicate chronic acoustic-induced tinnitus in hamsters.[57] Two spouts were available from which to drink, each in a distinct location; animals were trained to use the nonpreferred spout in the presence of an ipsilateral external sound. Testing occurred in silence. Licking at the sound-conditioned (nonpreferred) spout indicated tinnitus.[28] Using a variant of this method, Heffner[58] trained rats to lick from visual and auditory–cued left or right water spouts. After unilateral sound exposure, Heffner was able to use left versus right spout choice to indicate tinnitus lateral localization.[58] This informative experiment demonstrates how operant methods have been adapted to answer specific questions, such as tinnitus laterality.

MODEL FEATURES: PROS AND CONS

Using licking as an indicator requires water restriction, typically for 24 hours. A nontrivial consideration is the physiologic stress imposed by water deprivation. It has been shown that restricting water intake in rodents for 24 hours leads to vasopressin-induced and vascular-induced central neural changes that are reflected in physiologic stress indicators and behavioral dysfunction.[59] An interesting lick suppression method not requiring water restriction, and its attendant physiologic stress, was developed by Lobarinas and colleagues.[37] The motivation to lick for water was induced in rats by delivering free food pellets at regular intervals. Although the animals had to be food deprived, they did not have to be water deprived or extensively trained to lick. Because rats are prandial drinkers, distributed food delivery will induce licking, hence, schedule-induced polydipsia avoidance conditioning (SIPAC). Once SIPAC stabilizes, licking can be suppressed to an acoustic signal, using an electric shock. Sound-off licking then can be compared between animals with tinnitus and those without, with the expectation that tinnitus animals will do less sound-off licking than non-tinnitus controls because their tinnitus provides an auditory signal for suppression. Variability of performance over time and between subjects, however, has been an issue for this model.[52]

Unlike reflex-based animal models, operant models are obliged to motivate subjects to respond appropriately to sensory events. As some pet owners and all animal trainers know, animals do not comply with human requests unless they are motivated. Typically, motivation is established experimentally by restricting access to food or water or by imposing an aversive stimulus. These 3 strategies may be used singularly or in combination to comprise a given method.

Operant models described so far have in common the combined use of positive reinforcement, such as food or water, and punishment procedures, such as foot shock. It is well known that aversive stimulus control lends itself to more rapid conditioning than positive control.[60] With that in mind, some animal models have exclusively used aversive stimulus control to improve efficiency. Guitton and colleagues[61] trained rats to jump from an electrified floor to an insulated pole when an auditory signal was present. Because the task was moderately strenuous, the animals had a low spontaneous rate of jumping without foot shock. After salicylate treatment, the animals were tested without sound and spontaneous pole jumps were recorded; an elevated number of jumps indicated tinnitus. Using this model, both group and individual comparisons could be made, with animals serving as their own control. A limitation was that the method does not lend itself cleanly to testing chronic tinnitus, and, as a discrete trial procedure, the animals typically had to be handled between trials in order for a new trial to be initiated. Handling introduces a potential source of error that may not be entirely controlled by treatment blinding, because an increased number of spontaneous jumps would unblind the experimenter. Relying exclusively on aversive control also interjects a stress factor. Stress could be considered a positive feature, however, because humans frequently comment that stress exacerbates their tinnitus.

SUMMARY: FEATURES OF AN IDEAL ANIMAL TINNITUS MODEL

Criteria of validity, sensitivity, and reliability have to be balanced against efficiency, cost, and throughput, in any animal model. An ideal model would be sensitive enough to detect low levels of tinnitus yet clearly separate tinnitus from confounds, such as hearing loss and hyperacusis. The sensitivity of an ideal model would not diminish with repeated testing, allowing measurement of chronic tinnitus and the use of extended test series necessary to test therapeutics. Sensitive and reliable models also should require a low number of animals. Determining validity is never as clear cut as determining reliability; however, animal models should be validated against one another and against quantitative human data whenever possible. Tinnitus features, such as pitch, loudness, and duration, should be reflected in all models. Finally, a more direct, and ideally noninvasive, measure of tinnitus, not requiring extended psychophysical testing, would be advantageous.

ACKNOWLEDGMENTS

Preparation of this article was supported by research grant R01 DC016918 from the National Institute on Deafness and Other Communication Disorders of the US Public Health Service (A. Galazyuk.)

REFERENCES

1. Shargorodsky J, Curhan GC, Farwell WR. Prevalence and characteristics of tinnitus among US adults. Am J Med 2010;123:711–8.
2. Bauer CA. Tinnitus. N Engl J Med 2018;378:1224–31.
3. Dan B. Titus's tinnitus. J Hist Neurosci 2005;14:210–3.
4. Tunkel DE, Bauer CA, Sun GH, et al. Clinical practice guideline: tinnitus executive summary. Otolaryngol Head Neck Surg 2014;151:533–41.
5. Tunkel DE, Jones SL, Rosenfeld RM. Guidelines for tinnitus. JAMA 2016;316: 1214–5.
6. Brozoski TJ, Bauer CA. Learning about tinnitus from an animal model. Semin Hear 2008;29:242–58.
7. Jastreboff PJ, Brennan JF, Coleman JK, et al. Phantom auditory sensation in rats: an animal model for tinnitus. Behav Neurosci 1988;102:811–22.
8. Kaltenbach JA. Tinnitus: models and mechanisms. Hear Res 2011;276:52–60.
9. Brozoski TJ, Bauer CA. Animal models of tinnitus. Hear Res 2016;338:88–97.
10. Norena AJ, Farley BJ. Tinnitus-related neural activity: theories of generation, propagation, and centralization. Hear Res 2013;295:161–71.
11. Schaette R. Tinnitus in men, mice (as well as other rodents), and machines. Hear Res 2014;311:63–71.
12. Yang S, Bao S. Homeostatic mechanisms and treatment of tinnitus. Restor Neurol Neurosci 2013;31:99–108.
13. Bauer CA, Brozoski TJ, Rojas R, et al. Behavioral model of chronic tinnitus in rats. Otolaryngol Head Neck Surg 1999;121:457–62.

14. Mahlke C, Wallhausser-Franke E. Evidence for tinnitus-related plasticity in the auditory and limbic system, demonstrated by arg3.1 and c-fos immunocytochemistry. Hear Res 2004;195:17–34.
15. Ruttiger L, Ciuffani J, Zenner HP, et al. A behavioral paradigm to judge acute sodium salicylate-induced sound experience in rats: a new approach for an animal model on tinnitus. Hear Res 2003;180:39–50.
16. Yang G, Lobarinas E, Zhang L, et al. Salicylate induced tinnitus: behavioral measures and neural activity in auditory cortex of awake rats. Hear Res 2007;226:244–53.
17. Alkhatib A, Biebel UW, Smolders JW. Reduction of inhibition in the inferior colliculus after inner hair cell loss. Neuroreport 2006;17:1493–7.
18. Bauer CA, Turner JG, Caspary DM, et al. Tinnitus and inferior colliculus activity in chinchillas related to three distinct patterns of cochlear trauma. J Neurosci Res 2008;86:2564–78.
19. Kaltenbach JA, Rachel JD, Mathog TA, et al. Cisplatin-induced hyperactivity in the dorsal cochlear nucleus and its relation to outer hair cell loss: relevance to tinnitus. J Neurophysiol 2002;88:699–714.
20. Zacharek MA, Kaltenbach JA, Mathog TA, et al. Effects of cochlear ablation on noise induced hyperactivity in the hamster dorsal cochlear nucleus: implications for the origin of noise induced tinnitus. Hear Res 2002;172:137–43.
21. Bauer CA, Brozoski TJ. Assessing tinnitus and prospective tinnitus therapeutics using a psychophysical animal model. J Assoc Res Otolaryngol 2001;2:54–64.
22. Brozoski TJ, Bauer CA, Caspary DM. Elevated fusiform cell activity in the dorsal cochlear nucleus of chinchillas with psychophysical evidence of tinnitus. J Neurosci 2002;22:2383–90.
23. Dehmel S, Pradhan S, Koehler S, et al. Noise overexposure alters long-term somatosensory-auditory processing in the dorsal cochlear nucleus–possible basis for tinnitus-related hyperactivity? J Neurosci 2012;32:1660–71.
24. Jastreboff PJ, Brennan JF, Sasaki CT. An animal model for tinnitus. Laryngoscope 1988;98:280–6.
25. Tyler RS, Erlandsson S. Management of the tinnitus patient. In: Luxon Linda M, editor. Textbook of audiological medicine. Oxford (England): Isis; 2000. p. 571–8.
26. Ahlf S, Tziridis K, Korn S, et al. Predisposition for and prevention of subjective tinnitus development. PLoS One 2012;7:e44519.
27. Bauer CA, Wisner K, Sybert LT, et al. The cerebellum as a novel tinnitus generator. Hear Res 2013;295:130–9.
28. Heffner HE, Harrington IA. Tinnitus in hamsters following exposure to intense sound. Hear Res 2002;170:83–95.
29. Skinner BF. The behavior of organisms; an experimental analysis. New York: D. Appleton-Century Company; 1938.
30. Eggermont JJ, Roberts LE. The neuroscience of tinnitus. Trends Neurosci 2004;27:676–82.
31. Roberts LE, Eggermont JJ, Caspary DM, et al. Ringing ears: the neuroscience of tinnitus. J Neurosci 2010;30:14972–9.
32. Brozoski TJ, Ciobanu L, Bauer CA. Central neural activity in rats with tinnitus evaluated with manganese-enhanced magnetic resonance imaging (MEMRI). Hear Res 2007;228:168–79.
33. Brozoski TJ, Wisner KW, Odintsov B, et al. Local NMDA receptor blockade attenuates chronic tinnitus and associated brain activity in an animal model. PLoS One 2013;8:e77674.

34. Gomez-Nieto R, Horta-Junior Jde A, Castellano O, et al. Origin and function of short-latency inputs to the neural substrates underlying the acoustic startle reflex. Front Neurosci 2014;8:216.
35. Turner JG, Brozoski TJ, Bauer CA, et al. Gap detection deficits in rats with tinnitus: a potential novel screening tool. Behav Neurosci 2006;120:188–95.
36. Koch M. The neurobiology of startle. Prog Neurobiol 1999;59:107–28.
37. Lobarinas E, Sun W, Cushing R, et al. A novel behavioral paradigm for assessing tinnitus using schedule-induced polydipsia avoidance conditioning (SIP-AC). Hear Res 2004;190:109–14.
38. Galazyuk A, Hébert S. Gap-prepulse inhibition of the acoustic startle reflex (GPIAS) for tinnitus assessment: current status and future directions. Front Neurol 2015;6:88.
39. Shore SE, Roberts LE, Langguth B. Maladaptive plasticity in tinnitus–triggers, mechanisms and treatment. Nat Rev Neurol 2016;12:150–60.
40. Longenecker R, Galazyuk AV. Methodological optimization of tinnitus assessment using prepulse inhibition of the acoustic startle reflex. Brain Res 2012;1485:54–62.
41. Longenecker RJ, Galazyuk AV. Variable effects of acoustic trauma on behavioral and neural correlates of tinnitus in individual animals. Front Behav Neurosci 2016;10:207.
42. Grimsley CA, Longenecker RJ, Rosen MJ, et al. An improved approach to separating startle data from noise. J Neurosci Methods 2015;253:206–17.
43. Gerum R, Rahlfs H, Streb M, et al. Open(G)PIAS: r tinnitus screening and threshold estimation in rodents. Front Behav Neurosci 2019;13:140.
44. Choe Y, Park I. Proposal of conditional random interstimulus interval method for unconstrained enclosure based GPIAS measurement systems. Biomed Eng Lett 2019;9:367–74.
45. Berger JI, Coomber B, Shackleton TM, et al. A novel behavioural approach to detecting tinnitus in the guinea pig. J Neurosci Methods 2013;213:188–95.
46. Wu C, Martel DT, Shore SE. Increased synchrony and bursting of dorsal cochlear nucleus fusiform cells correlate with tinnitus. J Neurosci 2016;36:2068–73.
47. Hickox AE, Liberman MC. Is noise-induced cochlear neuropathy key to the generation of hyperacusis or tinnitus? J Neurophysiol 2014;111:552–64.
48. Fournier P, Hébert S. Gap detection deficits in humans with tinnitus as assessed with the acoustic startle paradigm: does tinnitus fill in the gap? Hear Res 2013;295:16–23.
49. Gilani VM, Ruzbahani M, Mahdi P, et al. Temporal processing evaluation in tinnitus patients: results on analysis of gap in noise and duration pattern test. Iran J Otorhinolaryngol 2013;25:221–6.
50. Paul BT, Schoenwiesner M, Hébert S. Towards an objective test of chronic tinnitus: Properties of auditory cortical potentials evoked by silent gaps in tinnitus-like sounds. Hear Res 2018;366:90–8.
51. Davis A, El Refaie A. Epidemiology of tinnitus. In: Tyler RS, editor. Tinnitus handbook. Clifton Park (NY): Delmar Cengage Learning; 2000. p. 1–24.
52. Hayes SH, Radziwon KE, Stolzberg DJ, et al. Behavioral models of tinnitus and hyperacusis in animals. Front Neurol 2014;5:179.
53. von der Behrens W. Animal models of subjective tinnitus. Neural Plast 2014;2014:741452.
54. Stolzberg D, Salvi RJ, Allman BL. Salicylate toxicity model of tinnitus. Front Syst Neurosci 2012;6:28.

55. Zheng Y, Vagal S, McNamara E, et al. A dose-response analysis of the effects of L-baclofen on chronic tinnitus caused by acoustic trauma in rats. Neuropharmacology 2012;62:940–6.
56. Jones A, May BJ. Improving the reliability of tinnitus screening in laboratory animals. J Assoc Res Otolaryngol 2017;18:183–95.
57. Heffner HE, Koay G. Tinnitus and hearing loss in hamsters (Mesocricetus auratus) exposed to loud sound. Behav Neurosci 2005;119:734–42.
58. Heffner HE. A two-choice sound localization procedure for detecting lateralized tinnitus in animals. Behav Res Methods 2011;43:577–89.
59. Faraco G, Wijasa TS, Park L, et al. Water deprivation induces neurovascular and cognitive dysfunction through vasopressin-induced oxidative stress. J Cereb Blood flow Metab 2014;34:852–60.
60. LeDoux JE. Emotion circuits in the brain. Annu Rev Neurosci 2000;23:155–84.
61. Guitton MJ, Caston J, Ruel J, et al. Salicylate induces tinnitus through activation of cochlear NMDA receptors. J Neurosci 2003;23:3944–52.

Tinnitus
An Epidemiologic Perspective

James A. Henry, PhD[a,b],*, Kelly M. Reavis, MPH[a,c],
Susan E. Griest, MPH[a,b], Emily J. Thielman, MS[a],
Sarah M. Theodoroff, PhD[a,b], Leslie D. Grush, AuD[a],
Kathleen F. Carlson, PhD[a,c,d]

KEYWORDS

- Tinnitus • Epidemiology • Risk factors • Prevalence • Ototoxicity • Noise
- Hearing loss

KEY POINTS

- Tinnitus, often referred to as "ringing in the ears," is a health condition that is estimated to affect 10% to 15% of adults worldwide.
- Epidemiologic studies have attempted to describe tinnitus and its many facets, such as its psychoacoustic characteristics and functional effects.
- Data and findings cannot be compared between studies due to lack of standardization in tinnitus assessment.
- One of the goals of this article is to provide definitions and assessment tools that can promote standardization and data that are comparable between studies.
- The Noise Outcomes in Servicemembers Epidemiology study has a specific focus on tinnitus; this study can serve as a model for the capture of uniform and comparable measures.

[a] United States Department of Veterans Affairs Rehabilitation Research & Development, National Center for Rehabilitative Auditory Research, Veterans Affairs Portland Health Care System, 3710 Southwest US Veterans Hospital Road, Portland, OR 97239, USA; [b] Department of Otolaryngology–Head & Neck Surgery, Oregon Health & Science University, 3181 Southwest Sam Jackson Park Road, PV01, Portland, Oregon 97239, USA; [c] School of Public Health, Oregon Health & Science University, MC: GH230, 3181 Southwest Sam Jackson Park Road, PV01, Portland, Oregon 97239, USA; [d] Center to Improve Veteran Involvement in Care, Veterans Affairs Portland Health Care System, 3710 Southwest US Veterans Hospital Road, Portland, OR 97239, USA
* Corresponding author. VA RR&D National Center for Rehabilitative Auditory Research, Veterans Affairs Portland Health Care System, 3710 Southwest US Veterans Hospital Road, Portland, OR 97239.
E-mail address: james.henry@va.gov

INTRODUCTION

Tinnitus is the perception of sound—in the head and/or ears—that does not have a source outside of the body. The 2 basic types of tinnitus are primary and secondary.[1] The sensation of primary tinnitus is entirely subjective, originating somewhere in the auditory system and confined to the auditory pathways. The American Academy of Otolaryngology–Head and Neck Surgery Foundation (AAO-HNSF) defines primary tinnitus as "idiopathic and may or may not be associated with sensorineural hearing loss."[1] Secondary tinnitus involves an underlying mechanical source within the head or neck that transmits an actual acoustic signal by bone conduction to the auditory end organ, where it is detected and processed as would be any external sound. This article focuses on the epidemiology of primary tinnitus, which is by far the most prevalent type.[1] Throughout the rest of this article, references to tinnitus indicate primary tinnitus unless otherwise specified. This article includes an overview of characteristics and epidemiologic findings from studies that have focused on tinnitus and describes pertinent results from the authors' own, ongoing epidemiology study.

Purpose

The overarching purpose of epidemiologic research is to develop knowledge of the distribution and determinants of health conditions across populations.[2] More specifically, the objective is to obtain data associated with a particular health condition or disease to improve the effectiveness of its prevention, management, or cure. Tinnitus is a health condition, not a disease. It is the symptom of pathologic neural activity that manifests as an unwanted phantom auditory sensation. To advance the development of methodologies that can restore normal neural function, research attempts to explain which mechanisms trigger tinnitus and sustain its underlying pathologic neural activity. This is difficult because tinnitus is associated most often with a permanently damaged auditory system. Thus, it may be necessary first to determine how damaged components of the auditory system can be restored. Epidemiologic research is 1 component of the larger effort to understand tinnitus etiology and to work toward a cure, or cures. Tinnitus-focused epidemiologic research examines risk factors to further inform determination of etiology and to advance prevention efforts. The integration of epidemiologic investigative methodologies and findings with those of other scientific endeavors can strengthen understanding of the causal mechanisms and drivers of tinnitus and allows elucidating populations at risk.

Because epidemiologic research requires precise definitions, the different parameters of tinnitus that must be defined are described first. These parameters include temporal characteristics, functional and emotional effects, and perceptual (including psychoacoustic) attributes.

Temporal Characteristics of Tinnitus

Temporal characteristics of tinnitus include how long the sensation lasts, how often it occurs, and for what length of time (duration) it has been experienced. Defining these characteristics is essential due to the many possible variations within these parameters. First, tinnitus must be distinguished from transient ear noise, which is the sudden unilateral sensation of a phantom tonal sound that decays within a minute or so. Transient ear noise, also referred to as spontaneous tinnitus,[3] often is described as a whistling sound and typically is accompanied by a sense of ear fullness and hearing loss. These symptoms decay simultaneously and the ear returns to normal function. Transient ear noise is experienced on an occasional basis by practically everyone and is not considered pathologic tinnitus.

If a phantom auditory sensation lasts at least 5 minutes; this normally distinguishes it from transient ear noise.[4] If tinnitus lasting at least 5 minutes is experienced infrequently, however, it is considered as a different category of tinnitus than tinnitus experienced on a regular basis. This distinction is somewhat arbitrary, but, for the epidemiology study the authors have undertaken, *regular* is defined tinnitus as tinnitus that occurs at least weekly.[5] Regular tinnitus can further be classified as *intermittent* (occurring on a daily or weekly basis) or *constant* (always present), either of which indicates a pathologic condition necessitating assessment. Ideally, assessment is performed by both an otolaryngologist and an audiologist due to the high likelihood of comorbid hearing loss.[6]

The duration of a person's tinnitus (how long it has been experienced) can vary from 1 day to many decades. The dividing point between acute tinnitus and chronic tinnitus (referred to, respectively, by the AAO-HNSF as recent-onset and persistent) usually is considered 6 months.[1] To reasonably ensure that tinnitus is chronic, a great majority of tinnitus clinical trials require their research participants to have experienced tinnitus for at least 6 months. Tinnitus of less than 6 months duration is considered more labile. The typical natural history of tinnitus is to habituate to both awareness of, and reactions to, the auditory sensation within 1 year to 2 years.[3] The AAO-HNSF guideline makes the point that a person whose tinnitus is bothersome after 6 months is more likely in need of management than if the tinnitus has been bothersome for less than 6 months.

Functional and Emotional Effects of Tinnitus

Although primary tinnitus mainly involves the auditory pathways, its sensation can cause disturbing effects of activation in the limbic and autonomic nervous systems.[7] Such tinnitus may be considered "bothersome" because it is reported to be for approximatively 20% of people who experience chronic tinnitus.[1,8] Tinnitus can be mildly, moderately, or severely bothersome.[3] For some individuals, tinnitus is considered debilitating. When tinnitus becomes bothersome, it most broadly affects sleep, concentration, and emotional stability. Sleep disturbance is the most common effect of bothersome tinnitus.[9,10] Tinnitus also can affect tasks adversely that involve concentration, such as reading and writing. Finally, there is ample evidence that tinnitus may be associated with mental distress, namely depression and anxiety.[11] Tinnitus does not reduce hearing sensitivity but it can distract from listening, which may exacerbate the perception of a hearing problem.

Perceptual Attributes of Tinnitus

The perception of tinnitus can be described with respect to its loudness, pitch, spectral quality, number of sounds perceived, and lateralization. None of these parameters can be evaluated or quantified objectively, so their study relies on patient self-report.

It seems that the loudness of tinnitus might be its most significant source of distress. Loudness of tinnitus can be reported on a numeric 0 to 10 scale, with 10 representing the "loudest sound imaginable." High ratings of tinnitus loudness tend to be associated with high index scores on tinnitus outcome questionnaires; hence, self-rated loudness and tinnitus functional and emotional effects are strongly correlated.[12] Tinnitus loudness can also be assessed by asking tinnitus patients to match the level of an external tone or noise to the loudness of their tinnitus. Because tinnitus cannot be objectively observed, however, this approach cannot be proved accurate or reliable. Likewise, it is not possible to validate that post-treatment changes in tinnitus loudness matches represent meaningful and reliable changes or even that post-treatment changes are related specifically to treatment.[13] To evaluate whether a treatment can effectively suppress the tinnitus percept, it is helpful to be able to objectively quantify tinnitus loudness before and after treatment.

Pitch matching is a common clinical procedure but cannot be objectively validated and has not been proved to have clinical relevance. Pitch matching is done using various methods with the common objective to match the frequency of a tone to the perceived pitch of the tinnitus. It is known that repeated pitch matches tend to be variable, often spanning a range of 2 to 3 octaves.[13] This high variability calls into question the validity of sound therapies that rely on pitch matching to establish acoustic parameters with respect to the perceived pitch of tinnitus. It seems likely that tinnitus often is not perceived as a pure tone but rather as a sound spectrum, which could explain why repeated pitch matches can vary so much within a given frequency range. Any tone within the range of an individual's tinnitus spectrum might be judged to match the tinnitus percept.[14] The perceived tinnitus pitch usually is within the frequency range of hearing loss,[15–17] and patients typically match their tinnitus to a tone greater than 3 kHz.[9]

People with tinnitus often report that they hear multiple sounds.[9] They can distinguish and describe each sound and how the different sounds relate to each other with respect to their loudness and pitch. For example, a tinnitus sufferer might hear a high-pitched sound along with a low-pitched hum. The high-pitched sound might be noticeable in most situations if it is above the frequency range of typical ambient sound. By contrast, the hum might be easily masked by ambient sound and, therefore, be noticeable only in very quiet environments.

Finally, tinnitus can be perceived as occurring in various locations with respect to the head and ears. The tinnitus may be heard as unilateral, bilateral, as symmetric, as asymmetric, in the head, in the ears, and/or outside of the head.[9] The localization or lateralization of tinnitus might yield clues as to its underlying mechanism. For example, it can be postulated that tinnitus that is heard in both ears might originate in 2 different locations distal (peripheral) to the medial superior olive where sounds have not binaurally converged below this level of the brainstem.[18,19] In contrast, tinnitus that is perceived as a fused binaural percept might originate somewhere proximal (central) to the medial superior olive. This example illustrates how precise definitions for tinnitus parameters of interest can inform understanding of its distribution and determinants in various populations.

EPIDEMIOLOGIC STUDIES: PREVALENCE OF AND RISK FACTORS FOR TINNITUS

This overview of findings from tinnitus epidemiologic studies is limited to a few population-based studies that the authors selected as representative of the field. Hoffman and Reed[8] conducted a survey of epidemiologic studies relating to tinnitus prior to the year 2000. Their review was thorough, and interested readers are advised to refer to their publication for more detailed analysis. Their main findings were as follows: (1) factors highly associated with the presence and severity of tinnitus include degree of hearing loss, exposure to high levels of both occupational and nonoccupational noise, and overall general health; (2) additional factors associated with tinnitus include cardiovascular and cerebrovascular disease, pharmaceutical medications, ear infections and inflammation, head or neck trauma including traumatic brain injury, hyperthyroidism and hypothyroidism, Meniere's disease, otosclerosis, sudden deafness, and vestibular schwannoma; (3) genetic factors may be associated with tinnitus; (4) once hearing loss is taken into account, age may have no association with tinnitus; (5) chronic tinnitus has a 10% to 15% prevalence in the adult population; and (6) military veterans (vs nonveterans) are at significantly greater risk for developing chronic tinnitus.

Baguley and colleagues[20] searched for relevant tinnitus studies published between 1987 and 2012, with a focus on studies published within the previous 5 years. Consistent with Hoffman and Reed,[8] they found that a majority of studies reported 10% to 15% prevalence of tinnitus in adults. They found the main risk factor for tinnitus to be hearing loss but pointed out that people with hearing loss may not report tinnitus and that people with bothersome tinnitus may have hearing sensitivity within audiometrically normal limits. Another identified major risk factor was noise due to occupational or recreational exposure. Additional risk factors included various prescription and nonprescription drugs, otosclerosis, Meniere's disease, vestibular schwannoma, head injuries, smoking, alcohol consumption, arthritis, obesity, and hypertension. Baguley and colleagues[20] listed comorbidities, including depression, anxiety, temporomandibular joint disorder, and hyperacusis. Among studies that reported the localization of tinnitus, most found that for approximately half of tinnitus patients, tinnitus was perceived in the middle of the head or in both ears. For all others, tinnitus was perceived as predominantly left-sided. Some patients perceived their tinnitus to come from outside of the head. The authors found only 1 longitudinal study that reported incidence data.[21] In that study, which included a cohort between 48 years and 92 years of age, baseline prevalence was approximately 8%. Incidence of new tinnitus was approximately 6% and 13% for 5 years and 10 years in duration, respectively. Baguley and colleagues[20] highlighted the fact that epidemiologic studies use inconsistent definitions of tinnitus and different questions, resulting in heterogeneous data.

McCormack and colleagues[4] conducted a systematic review of all studies between 1980 and 2015 that reported the prevalence of tinnitus in adults; 39 studies, representing 16 countries, met their criteria for data extraction. Approximately 3 of every 5 studies were conducted in Europe, and approximately half of the studies had been conducted since 2010. Across all the studies, reported prevalence of tinnitus was 5% to 43%. Only 12 of these studies used a consistent definition of tinnitus, and their prevalence levels ranged between 12% and 30%. Otherwise, there were 8 different definitions used for tinnitus; approximately one-third (34%) of the studies defined tinnitus as "lasting for more than 5 minutes at a time." The investigators pointed out the widespread inconsistency in how tinnitus is defined and reported, which may account for the extreme variability among prevalence estimates. Furthermore, heterogeneity of the data prevented pooling data across studies to perform meta-analyses. The studies used different tinnitus diagnostic criteria, considered different age groups, and analyzed and reported their data differently. It, therefore, was not possible to estimate a global prevalence of tinnitus. The authors concluded that epidemiologic studies of tinnitus should utilize standardized questions for measuring, reporting, and defining tinnitus.

DATA FROM THE NATIONAL HEALTH AND NUTRITION EXAMINATION SURVEY

Table 1 shows 2009 to 2012 data from the population-based National Health and Nutrition Examination Survey (NHANES) study, which reviews commonly examined demographic associations as an up-to-date presentation of the state of US community dwelling adults (20 years and older) with tinnitus.[11] In this study, participants were asked, "In the past 12 months, have you been bothered by ringing, roaring, or buzzing in your ears or head that lasts for 5 minutes or more?" Those who responded affirmatively then were asked, "How long have you been bothered by this ringing,

Table 1
Characteristics of US adults ages 20 and older by tinnitus status, National Health and Nutrition Examination Survey, 2009-2012. Prevalence is shown as percentages and 95% confidence intervals. All results are weighted using NHANES 2009-2012 examination weights. Row percentages are shown.

Characteristic	Sample Size (n = 5550)	Tinnitus (%)	No Tinnitus (%)
Sex			
Male	2732	19 (16–22)	81 (78–84)
Female	2818	16 (14–18)	84 (82–86)
Missing	0	—	—
Age			
20–39 y	1876	9 (7–11)	91 (89–93)
40–59 y	1754	21 (17–24)	79 (76–83)
60–79 y	1525	25 (21–28)	75 (72–79)
80+ y	395	24 (19–30)	76 (70–82)
Missing	0	—	—
Race/ethnicity			
Non-Hispanic white	2184	20 (17–22)	80 (78–83)
Non-Hispanic black	1387	13 (11–15)	87 (85–89)
Mexican American	588	13 (10–16)	87 (84–90)
Other Hispanic	524	12 (9–15)	88 (85–91)
Other	867	13 (8–18)	87 (82–92)
Missing	0	—	—
Education			
<High school	1338	21 (16–26)	79 (74–84)
High school graduate	1164	20 (15–24)	80 (76–85)
>High school	3045	16 (14–17)	84 (83–86)
Missing	3	—	—
Income (federal poverty level)			
≤100%	1696	16 (14–18)	84 (82–86)
101%–200%	1324	23 (18–27)	77 (73–82)
>200%	2530	16 (15–18)	84 (82–85)
Missing	0	—	—
Marital status			
Married	2712	17 (15–19)	83 (81–85)
Widowed/divorced/separated	1273	26 (21–31)	74 (69–79)
Never married	1143	13 (10–15)	87 (85–90)
Living with partner	420	13 (8–18)	87 (82–92)
Missing	2	—	—
Veteran status			
Veteran	625	27 (20–33)	73 (8–10)
Nonveteran	4925	16 (15–18)	84 (82–85)
Missing	0	—	—

(continued on next page)

Table 1
(continued)

Characteristic	Sample Size (n = 5550)	Tinnitus (%)	No Tinnitus (%)
Occupational noise exposure			
Yes	1870	24 (20–28)	76 (72–80)
No	3678	14 (12–16)	86 (84–88)
Missing	2	—	—
Self-reported hearing ability			
Excellent/good	4216	11 (9–13)	89 (87–91)
Little trouble	825	35 (29–41)	65 (59–71)
Moderate trouble	315	45 (36–55)	55 (45–64)
Severe trouble/deaf	192	49 (43–59)	51 (43–59)
Missing	2	—	—
General health status			
Excellent/very good	1836	14 (12–16)	86 (84–88)
Good	1951	19 (16–22)	81 (78–84)
Fair	903	27 (21–32)	73 (68–79)
Poor	179	29 (22–36)	71 (64–78)
Missing	681	—	—
Smoking			
Never	3137	15 (13–17)	85 (83–87)
Former	1331	19 (16–23)	81 (77–84)
Current	1076	23 (18–28)	77 (72–82)
Missing	6	—	—
Hypertension			
Yes	2079	25 (21–28)	75 (72–79)
No	3464	14 (12–16)	86 (84–88)
Missing	7	—	—
Hyperlipidemia			
Yes	1861	23 (18–29)	77 (71–82)
No	3550	14 (12–17)	86 (83–88)
Missing	139	—	—
Diabetes			
Yes	700	26 (19–32)	74 (68–81)
No	4723	16 (15–18)	84 (82–85)
Borderline	123	23 (7–38)	77 (62–93)
Missing	4	—	—
Cardiovascular disease			
Yes	608	27 (21–34)	73 (66–79)
No	4942	17 (15–19)	83 (81–85)
Missing	0	—	—
Cancer history			
Yes	545	21 (15–27)	79 (73–85)

(continued on next page)

	Sample Size (n = 5550)	Tinnitus (%)	No Tinnitus (%)
Table 1 *(continued)*			
Characteristic			
No	5000	17 (15–19)	83 (81–85)
Missing	5	—	—

Data are shown as percentages (95% CI). All results are weighted using NHANES 2009 to 2012 examination weights. Row percentages are shown. From Prevalence of Self-Reported Depression Symptoms and Perceived Anxiety among Community-Dwelling US Adults Reporting Tinnitus," by Reavis K., 2020, Perspectives of the ASHA Special Interest Groups.11 https://perspectives.pubs.asha.org/.

roaring, or buzzing in your ears or head?" Response options for tinnitus duration were less than 3 months, 3 months to 1 year, 1 year to 4 years, 5 years to 9 years, greater than or equal to 10 years, and unknown. For the NHANES data presented in this article, tinnitus was defined as lasting greater than or equal to 3 months, a notably shorter time frame than the greater than or equal to 6 months suggested by the AAO-HNSF guidelines.[1]

NHANES 2009 to 2012 data (see **Table 1**) suggest that 15% (95% CI, 13%–17%) of US adults were "bothered by" tinnitus lasting 3 months or longer. A majority of adults with tinnitus were white, widowed or divorced, less academically accomplished, and at or slightly above the federal poverty line. Compared with adults without tinnitus, those with tinnitus tended to be older. Of the health behaviors and comorbidities examined, adults with tinnitus were more likely to be former or current smokers, to self-report poorer hearing, and to report having cardiovascular disease, hypertension, hyperlipidemia, diabetes, and cancer. Additionally, those who were military veterans were more likely to report tinnitus (26%; 95% CI, 19%–32%) than those without a history of military service (14%; 95% CI, 12%–16%).[11]

TINNITUS DATA FROM THE NOISE OUTCOMES IN SERVICE MEMBERS EPIDEMIOLOGY STUDY

Since 2007, tinnitus has been the most prevalent service-connected disability for US military veterans (Veterans Benefits Administration annual reports, 2007–2018, https://www.benefits.va.gov/REPORTS/abr/). Similar to the NHANES 2009 to 2012 data discussed previously, an analysis of NHANES data from 1999 to 2006 showed that veterans have twice the prevalence of tinnitus as nonveterans.[22] These results are not surprising, given that military service often involves exposure to hazardous noise, chemicals, and head injury. As of fiscal year 2018, more than 1.9 million veterans had a service-connected disability claim approved (awarded) for tinnitus (**Fig. 1**). From 2017 to 2018, this number increased by 184,221 in just 1 year.

Department of Veterans Affairs (VA) audiologists routinely conduct compensation and pension examinations for veterans claiming to have tinnitus linked to military service. These claims often are made many years after separating from the military, raising the question whether the onset of tinnitus might be delayed by years after noise and chemical exposures. In response to veterans' concerns about tinnitus and hearing loss, Congress mandated that the Institute of Medicine (now known as the Heath and Medicine Division of the National Academy of Sciences) produce a report including recommendations for research "to fill the void for prospective, longitudinal,

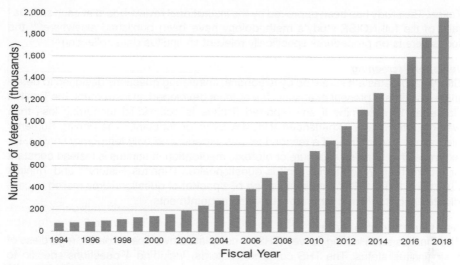

Fig. 1. Numbers of Veterans with a service-connected tinnitus disability in each of fiscal years, 1994 to 2018.

epidemiologic data on noise-induced hearing loss and tinnitus in military personnel."[23(p208)] Among the report's findings was the recommendation to

> *Establish cohorts of military veterans with various documented noise exposures, immediately upon discharge, and survey them periodically for ototoxic exposures, subsequent nonmilitary noise exposures, and hearing function, as well as presence and severity of tinnitus, in order to determine whether there is a delay in the effects of military noise exposure. These cohorts will need to be followed through the remainder of members' lifetimes, but this longitudinal study will reveal elements of the natural history of noise-induced hearing loss and tinnitus that otherwise will not be determined.*[23(p208)]

Heeding the Institute of Medicine recommendations, the authors' research group initiated a longitudinal epidemiologic study to address the etiology, prevalence, and effects of tinnitus and hearing loss among active-duty service members and veterans recently separated from military service (within approximately 2.5 years). The NOISE study, which began in early 2014, is building a longitudinal cohort that will enable long-term assessments of changes in tinnitus and hearing relative to military experiences and occupational and recreational exposures experienced since military separation. To date, more than 900 participants have enrolled as members of this study cohort. Data from the NOISE study that are specific to tinnitus are discussed later. The authors are careful in this study to use precise tinnitus, measurement, and reporting definitions that apply measurement best practices even when this sometimes has required the development of new instruments.

Method

Study sites
The NOISE study is being performed at 2 sites. The main study site is the National Center for Rehabilitative Auditory Research (NCRAR), which is part of the VA Portland Health Care System in Portland, Oregon. NOISE data also are collected at the Department of Defense Hearing Center of Excellence at Joint Base San Antonio–Lackland,

Texas. The study has been approved by the institutional review board at each site. Details of the full NOISE study's methodology have been published elsewhere[24]; the focus here is on procedures specifically relevant to tinnitus data collection.

Telephone screening

Study candidates are screened by telephone, answering questions designed to determine if tinnitus is present or absent. The authors developed an instrument, the Tinnitus Screener, to determine if any reported tinnitus is occasional (occurring less than weekly), intermittent (experienced at least weekly), or constant.[5] The Tinnitus Screener also allows ascertaining if a respondent has experienced only temporary tinnitus, for example, due to noise exposure or ototoxic medication. If tinnitus is instead constant or intermittent, 2 additional tinnitus questionnaires (Tinnitus History[25] and Tinnitus Functional Index [TFI][26]) are sent as part of a packet of questionnaires mailed to candidates prior to their in-laboratory baseline appointments.

Assessment questionnaires

The Tinnitus and Hearing Survey (THS) is completed by all participants, regardless of their tinnitus status. The THS contains 10 items, including 4 questions specific to tinnitus, 4 specific to hearing, and 2 specific to sound tolerance.[27] For nontinnitus participants, the 4 tinnitus items are ignored for reporting purposes. The tinnitus data, discussed later, were derived from the Tinnitus Screener, TFI, THS, and Tinnitus History. These data were obtained from NOISE study participants who were deemed to have intermittent or constant tinnitus according to the results of the initial Tinnitus Screener.

The accuracy of the initial phone screening is verified when participants present for audiologic testing. The research audiologist asks if they hear tinnitus. If they answer yes, then the audiologist works to determine the location of their tinnitus and whether it is "typical today." If a participant who screened negative for tinnitus over the phone is found to test positive for tinnitus during the in-person examination, that participant then completes the additional tinnitus questionnaires as part of the baseline appointment.

The 25-item TFI[26,28] has been tested extensively to support the classification of TFI scores (on a scale of 0–100) below a value of 25 as indicating relatively mild tinnitus, typically requiring little or no intervention. TFI scores from 25 to 50 suggest more significant problems with tinnitus, indicating possible or borderline need for professional attention. Scores above 50 indicate tinnitus that is severe enough to qualify for more aggressive clinical intervention, possibly involving referral to specialty tinnitus care.

The THS was designed primarily to distinguish tinnitus-specific from hearing-specific complaints.[27] The THS contains 3 sections: section A contains 4 items that assess self-reported functional effects of tinnitus that are not confounded by hearing difficulties; section B contains 4 items that query hearing difficulties that are not confounded by tinnitus problems; and section C contains 2 items that screen for a sound tolerance problem (hyperacusis, misophonia, or noise sensitivity).[29]

The Tinnitus History[25] establishes factors associated with tinnitus history (duration, onset rapidity, onset associations, changes since onset in intermittency, localization, and loudness), tinnitus attributes (present intermittency, localization, number and type of sounds heard, and loudness rating), and tinnitus impact/severity (relating to sleep disturbance, concentration difficulties, emotional reactions, and intrusiveness).

Data analysis

To ensure completeness of tinnitus-related data, all questionnaires were reviewed by a member of the study team during the participants' visits. If missing items were

Table 2
Demographics of Noise Outcomes in Servicemembers Epidemiology study participants (n = 690)

	Service Members With No Tinnitus (n = 176)	Service Members With Tinnitus (n = 111)	Veterans No Tinnitus (n = 151)	Veterans Tinnitus (n = 252)
Age (y), mean (SD), range	33.6 (8.6), 19–59	36.5 (8.8), 22–60	33.2 (8.2), 21–55	34.8 (9.6), 21–61
Gender: male (%)	56	85	82	89
Race/ethnicity: non-Hispanic, white (%)	62	65	79	80
Military branch, n (%)				
Army	48 (47)	54 (53)	53 (28)	138 (72)
Marines	3 (60)	2 (40)	27 (42)	38 (58)
Navy	8 (53)	7 (47)	40 (50)	40 (50)
Air Force	117 (71)	48 (29)	31 (46)	67 (54)
Tinnitus screener status, n (%)				
No tinnitus	152 (86)	0	126 (83)	0
Occasional/temporary tinnitus	24 (14)	0	25 (17)	0
Intermittent tinnitus	0	25 (22)	0	71 (28)
Constant tinnitus	0	86 (78)	0	181 (72)
Hearing loss (average >20 dB), n (%)				
Low frequency (0.25–2 kHz)	9 (5)	22 (20)	13 (9)	50 (20)
High frequency (3–8 kHz)	24 (14)	39 (35)	29 (19)	86 (34)
Extended high frequency (9–16 kHz)	45 (26)	62 (56)	49 (33)	115 (46)
Screened positive for depression, n (%)[a]	11 (6)	20 (18)	23 (15)	78 (31)
Screened positive for anxiety, n (%)[a]	35 (20)	51 (46)	59 (39)	143 (57)
Screened positive for sleepiness, n (%)[b]	67 (38)	58 (53)	58 (39)	153 (44)

[a] Hospital Anxiety and Depression Scale.
[b] Epworth Sleepiness Scale.

detected prior to data entry and verification, attempts were made to contact the participant by phone to complete and verify the data. To minimize data entry errors, all questionnaires were scanned twice into a study database using TeleForm (Hewlett Packard, Palo Alto, California). Any discrepancies noted between the 2 scans were resolved by the NOISE study data manager using an established protocol. The audiometric data were entered manually, with 1 audiologist reading the data from the source document and another entering the data and orally reporting the entry being made.

Tinnitus data were obtained from the first 690 NOISE study participants (287 service members and 403 veterans). Data analyses were conducted using SPSS, version 22, with the goal of describing characteristics of service members and veterans with and without tinnitus on factors related to demographics, tinnitus and hearing status, mental health screening, and tinnitus characteristics. Observations of similarities and differences between groups are discussed later.

Results

Table 2 shows baseline demographic data for 690 NOISE study participants, broken down for service members and veterans with and without tinnitus. The average age for these 4 cohorts was between 33.2 years and 36.5 years. In each category, most participants were men. Among service members, most were in the Air Force. Among veterans, most had served in the Army. More than one-third (39%) of service members and approximately two-thirds (63%) of veterans reported intermittent or constant tinnitus. The prevalence of tinnitus was highest for participants who serve/served in the Army. Among all participants, the percent of hearing loss (mean hearing thresholds >20-dB HL [hearing level]) across all 3 frequency ranges (low-frequency, 0.25–2 kHz; high-frequency, 3–8 kHz; and extended high-frequency, 9–16 kHz) was higher for those who reported tinnitus. Hearing loss was most prevalent in the extended high-frequency range (56% of service members and 46% of veterans with tinnitus). The prevalence of depression, anxiety, and sleepiness also was higher for those who reported tinnitus (depression: an additional 12% of service members and 16% of veterans; anxiety: an additional 26% of service members and 18% of veterans; and sleepiness: an additional 15% of service members and 5% of veterans).

Table 3 shows data from the Tinnitus History that describe characteristics of tinnitus for 360 NOISE study participants with constant or intermittent tinnitus. Most service members and veterans reported having experienced tinnitus for 3 years to 5 years. Tinnitus was reported most often as linked with noise exposure; however, most participants were uncertain what caused their tinnitus. Most service members and veterans reported their tinnitus location in "both ears." When asked, "How much of a problem is your tinnitus?" 43% of service members and 56% of veterans rated their tinnitus as at least "a moderate problem." Slightly more than half of service members (54%) and almost half of veterans described their tinnitus as "one sound." Service members and veterans both reported that their tinnitus caused difficulties performing work or other activities (22% of service members and 29% of veterans).

Table 3 also shows results of the Tinnitus Functional Index (TFI) and Tinnitus and Hearing Survey (THS). The mean score for the TFI (range of possible scores: 0–100) was 30.5 for service members and 36.6 for veterans, whereas the mean score for the THS section A (tinnitus section; range of possible scores: 0–16) was 2.9 for service members and 3.6 for veterans.

Discussion of Noise Outcomes in Service Members Epidemiology Study Results

The authors have been reporting tinnitus data from the NOISE study since they evaluated the first 100 veteran participants, 67% of whom met the definition for chronic tinnitus.[5] Since then, the authors have refined methods of identifying the presence of tinnitus by administering the Tinnitus Screener over the telephone as well as verifying results during in-laboratory testing by an audiologist. The "occasional" category was also added, to differentiate tinnitus that occurs irregularly (occasional = less than weekly) versus regularly (intermittent = at least weekly). Current results reveal a tinnitus prevalence estimate of 63% in the veteran cohort. Although this is reduced from the previous estimate of 67%, current data are consistent in showing that approximately two-thirds of the 403 veteran participants experienced chronic tinnitus. This high prevalence is remarkable considering that these veterans are young (average 34.8 years of age) and have been separated from the military for less than 3 years.

Among adults who experience tinnitus, only approximately 20% are bothered enough by it to seek clinical intervention.[1,8] Those who seek help report effects ranging from mild to severe.[3] The NOISE study participants (service members and veterans) with tinnitus responded to the question, "How much of a problem is tinnitus?" Service members' and veterans' responses to this question were similar with respect to tinnitus being "not a problem" (13% of service members and 12% of veterans) or a "big" or "very big problem" (combined: 9% of service members and 11% of veterans) (see **Table 3**). Where the service member and veteran cohorts were less comparable was in their descriptions of tinnitus as a "small problem" (44% of service members and 32% of veterans) or "moderate problem" (34% of service members and 45% of veterans). It is reasonable to assume that individuals with at least a "big problem" would be most likely to seek clinical services and that those with a "moderate problem" would be less likely to seek intervention (though some might). The findings to date comport generally with overall estimates that approximately 20% of adults with tinnitus are likely to seek clinical services.[1,8] It is further noted that the mean index score for the TFI was 30.5 (SD 20.7; range 0–90.8) for service members and 36.6 (SD 21.9; range 0–96.8) for veterans, indicating that for both cohorts, tinnitus is a relatively mild problem overall, with large variability appearing as a range of scores spanning almost the entire range of possible scores on the TFI (0–100).

DISCUSSION

This article includes a relatively cursory review of epidemiologic studies that have included data on tinnitus. Most of these studies addressed general health, including tinnitus as 1 of many specific health conditions. Definitions of tinnitus have varied widely between studies, although most studies attempt to distinguish acute versus chronic and nonbothersome versus bothersome tinnitus. Although it may seem straightforward to ask individuals whether or not they experience tinnitus, this was not always the case in the NOISE study. Participants occasionally were confused as to what actually constitutes tinnitus, and some were unreliable with their responses. It was evident that precise definitions were needed, and this is what motivated development of the Tinnitus Screener.[5] As described previously, the Tinnitus Screener categorizes tinnitus as temporary, occasional, intermittent, or constant. It also can categorize the absence of tinnitus (which indicates the person has experienced only transient ear noise, also known as spontaneous tinnitus).

Any epidemiologic study reporting tinnitus prevalence data must at least differentiate between subjects who do and do not have tinnitus. A common definition is needed to develop findings that can be compared between studies. Adhering to the suggestion that tinnitus must exceed 5 minutes in duration[30–32] rules out spontaneous tinnitus (transient ear noise). Tinnitus of 5 minutes duration that occurs irregularly (eg, every few weeks) does not constitute pathologic tinnitus.

Table 3
Tinnitus characteristics of Noise Outcomes in Servicemembers Epidemiology study participants with constant or intermittent tinnitus (n = 360)

Tinnitus Characteristic	Service Members (n = 110)	Veterans (n = 250)
Tinnitus duration (%)		
<1 y	11	4
1–2 y	23	18
3–5 y	26	41
6–10 y	22	21
11+ y	18	16
Tinnitus onset associations (%)[a]		
Accident	2	7
Illness	0	2
Loud noise	30	44
Other	10	7
Not sure	63	54
Tinnitus localization (%)[a]		
Left ear only	15	7
Right ear only	8	6
Both ears	66	78
In head, right	6	5
In head, left	4	3
Fills head	21	23
Other location	0	1
Number of tinnitus sounds (%)		
1 sound	54	49
2 sounds	17	17
3+ sounds	28	34
How much of a problem is tinnitus? (%)		
Not a problem	13	12
Small problem	44	32
Moderate problem	34	45
Big problem	8	7
Very big problem	1	4
Because of tinnitus, over the past 6 mo have you found that you (%)		
Had to take frequent rests when doing work or other activities?	3	11
Cut down the amount of time you spend on work or other activities?	7	15
Accomplished less than you would like?	12	20
Did not do work or other activities as carefully as usual?	11	17
Were limited in the kind of work you do or other activities?	8	15
Had difficulty performing work or other activities?	22	29
Needed special assistance?	6	11
TFI, mean (SD), range	30.5 (20.7), 0–90.8	36.6 (21.9), 0–96.8
THS section A—tinnitus, mean (SD), range	2.9 (2.9) 0–14	3.6 (3.3) 0–16

[a] Participants may report more than 1 response.

Dauman and Tyler[33] proposed that tinnitus of at least 5 minutes duration, however, must occur at least twice per week to be considered pathologic. For the NOISE study, the authors required that in order to place participants in the tinnitus group, their tinnitus of at least 5 minutes duration must be experienced at least weekly. For future epidemiologic studies, the authors recommend that "tinnitus lasting at least 5 minutes and occurring at least weekly" be used to define the presence of tinnitus. It also should be determined if the tinnitus has been experienced for 6 months or more, to distinguish between tinnitus that is persistent/chronic versus recent-onset/acute.[1]

Once it is established that a person experiences pathologic tinnitus, chronic or otherwise, the next task is to determine if the tinnitus is bothersome and, if so, to what degree. A global question that has been used for this purpose is, "How much of a problem is tinnitus?"[25,26] Response options are "not a problem," "small problem," "moderate problem," "big problem," and "very big problem." The authors' concern with this question is that individuals who experience both tinnitus and hearing loss might be bothered primarily by the hearing loss, attributing their problem instead to the presence of tinnitus. Blaming tinnitus for a hearing problem is a common mistake.[34] For this reason, epidemiologic studies examining the association between problematic tinnitus and any outcome of interest may be confounded by hearing loss. To address this concern, the authors recommend using the THS,[27] which is ideal for epidemiologic research because of its brevity, validation, and demonstrated value in separating self-perceived hearing problems from tinnitus problems.[5,35–37]

Despite the many epidemiologic studies that have reported data on tinnitus, much remains to be learned. The science of epidemiology can help elucidate causes of tinnitus and point to promising methods of prevention, treatment, and/or cures. Because many epidemiologic studies are observational in nature (ie, they do not involve controlled conditions), however, care in their design and conduct is of the utmost importance. Heterogeneity in the findings of epidemiologic studies reported to date underscores the importance and the need for consistent definitions and precise measures.

Despite the inconsistent use of definitions and questions in epidemiologic studies, some findings have been consistent. The prevalence of tinnitus in adult populations tends consistently to be in the 10% to 15% range. It appears that military experience increases the prevalence of tinnitus, as seen by the NHANES analyses and the NOISE study. It appears, therefore, that veteran status represents a collection of military risk factors, along with predictable risk factors, such as poorer health status, hearing loss, gender, posttraumatic stress disorder, and traumatic brain injury.[38] As discussed previously, Hoffman and Reed[8] concluded that, once hearing loss is accounted for, age is not a risk factor for tinnitus. Other studies consistently have identified age as a risk factor.[4,20,38,39]

Although a majority of people with chronic tinnitus are not significantly bothered by the phantom sound, many experience tinnitus-related functional limitations and seek help from health care providers. A study of veterans using VA health care found that, among all veterans who had used VA health care in the prior 5 years, 11% had been diagnosed with and received clinical services for tinnitus at least once and 3% at least twice.[40] Comorbid hearing loss, traumatic brain injury, and mental health and substance use outcomes were highly prevalent among these patients. A random sample of these veterans (those diagnosed at least once with tinnitus) found that the majority had TFI scores in the severe or very severe range of tinnitus severity. Therefore, health care providers (otolaryngologists) should be prepared with tools to help these patients, including collaborative relationships with other key clinicians, including audiologists and mental health providers.

Although there currently is no cure for tinnitus,[41] that is, no method demonstrated by evidence to consistently reduce or eliminate the perception of the phantom sound, it is a common misconception that nothing can be done for those who suffer from this condition. Evidence-based practices for reducing tinnitus-related distress do exist, so patients should never be told that "nothing can be done" or they should "learn to live with it." Cognitive behavioral therapy has the strongest research evidentiary support for management of tinnitus-related distress.[1,42] Because of the common comorbidity of mental health conditions, cognitive behavioral therapy is a logical choice for intervention especially for those with the most problematic tinnitus. Other methods may be equally effective despite not being vetted by systematic reviews. These methods include Tinnitus Retraining Therapy,[43] Progressive Tinnitus Management,[37] and Tinnitus Activities Treatment.[44] There also is considerable evidence that hearing aids and combination instruments (hearing aids with a built-in sound generator) are effective tools for tinnitus management.[45–47]

SUMMARY

The study of tinnitus is, in many ways, still in its infancy, with much to be gained through ongoing and future research. Prevalence data are needed to understand the distribution of tinnitus in various populations. Longitudinal studies are needed to address gaps in the understanding of how tinnitus prevalence changes over time and how tinnitus characteristics change within individuals and to establish the determinants of new-onset tinnitus. Cross-sectional studies can estimate prevalence to speculate about tinnitus determinants, but incidence studies are needed to confirm theories of etiology. Prevalence over time can be estimated by examining a series of cross-sectional studies. For instance, NHANES data over the years can be used to determine how prevalence is changing. Epidemiology research is essential to answer these key questions and inform best practices.

DISCLOSURE

This work was supported by a Department of Defense Congressionally Directed Medical Research Program Investigator-Initiated Research Award (PR121146), a Joint Warfighter Medical Research Program Award (JW160036), and a US VA Rehabilitation Research and Development (RR&D) Research Career Scientist Award (1 IK6 RX002990-01). This material is the result of work supported with resources and the use of facilities at the VA RR&D National Center for Rehabilitative Auditory Research (VA RR&D NCRAR Center Award; C9230C) at the VA Portland Health Care System in Portland, Oregon, as well as the United States Department of Defense Hearing Center of Excellence in San Antonio, Texas. The views expressed in this article are those of the authors and do not necessarily represent the official policy or position of the Defense Health Agency, Department of Defense, or any other US government agency. This work was prepared as part of official duties as US Government employees and, therefore, is defined as US Government work under Title 17 U.S.C.§101. Per Title 17 U.S.C.§105, copyright protection is not available for any work of the US Government.

REFERENCES

1. Tunkel DE, Bauer CA, Sun GH, et al. Clinical practice guideline: tinnitus. Otolaryngol Head Neck Surg 2014;151(2 Suppl):S1–40.
2. Frerot M, Lefebvre A, Aho S, et al. What is epidemiology? Changing definitions of epidemiology 1978-2017. PLoS One 2018;13(12):e0208442.

3. Dobie RA. Overview: suffering from tinnitus. In: Snow JB, editor. Tinnitus: theory and management. Lewiston (NY): BC Decker Inc.; 2004. p. 1–7.
4. McCormack A, Edmondson-Jones M, Somerset S, et al. A systematic review of the reporting of tinnitus prevalence and severity. Hear Res 2016;337:70–9.
5. Henry JA, Griest S, Austin D, et al. Tinnitus screener: results from the first 100 participants in an epidemiology study. Am J Audiol 2016;25(2):153–60.
6. Nondahl DM, Cruickshanks KJ, Huang GH, et al. Tinnitus and its risk factors in the Beaver Dam offspring study. Int J Audiol 2011;50(5):313–20.
7. Jastreboff PJ. Phantom auditory perception (tinnitus): mechanisms of generation and perception. Neurosci Res 1990;8:221–54.
8. Hoffman HJ, Reed GW. Epidemiology of tinnitus. In: Snow JB, editor. Tinnitus: theory and management. Lewiston (NY): BC Decker Inc.; 2004. p. 16–41.
9. Meikle M, Taylor-Walsh E. Characteristics of tinnitus and related observations in over 1800 tinnitus patients. J Laryngol Otol 1984;(Suppl. 9):17–21. Proceedings of the Second International Tinnitus Seminar, New York 1983. Ashford, Kent: Invicta Press.
10. Erlandsson S. Psychological profiles of tinnitus patients. In: Tyler RS, editor. Tinnitus handbook. San Diego (A): Singular Publishing Group; 2000. p. 25–57.
11. Reavis KM, Henry JA, Carlson KF. Prevalence of self-reported Depression Symptoms and Perceived Anxiety among Community-Dwelling US Adults Reporting Tinnitus. Perspectives of the ASHA Special Interest Groups. (In press).
12. Manning C, Grush L, Thielman E, et al. Comparison of tinnitus loudness measures: matching, rating, and scaling. Am J Audiol 2019;28(1):137–43.
13. Henry JA. "Measurement" of tinnitus. Otol Neurotol 2016;37(8):e276–85.
14. Henry JA, Flick CL, Gilbert A, et al. Comparison of manual and computer-automated procedures for tinnitus pitch-matching. J Rehabil Res Dev 2004; 41(2):121–38.
15. Schaette R, Konig O, Hornig D, et al. Acoustic stimulation treatments against tinnitus could be most effective when tinnitus pitch is within the stimulated frequency range. Hear Res 2010;269(1–2):95–101.
16. Norena A, Micheyl C, Chery-Croze S, et al. Psychoacoustic characterization of the tinnitus spectrum: implications for the underlying mechanisms of tinnitus. Audiol Neurootol 2002;7(6):358–69.
17. Roberts LE, Moffat G, Baumann M, et al. Residual inhibition functions overlap tinnitus spectra and the region of auditory threshold shift. J Assoc Res Otolaryngol 2008;9(4):417–35.
18. Feldmann H. Mechanisms of tinnitus. In: Vernon JA, Møller AR, editors. Mechanisms of tinnitus. Needham Heights (MA): Allyn & Bacon; 1995. p. 35–56.
19. Gelfand SA. Hearing—an introduction to psychological and physiological acoustics. New York: Marcel Dekker, Inc.; 1998.
20. Baguley D, McFerran D, Hall D. Tinnitus. Lancet 2013;382(9904):1600–7.
21. Nondahl DM, Cruickshanks KJ, Wiley TL, et al. The ten-year incidence of tinnitus among older adults. Int J Audiol 2010;49(8):580–5.
22. Folmer RL, McMillan GP, Austin DF, et al. Audiometric thresholds and prevalence of tinnitus among male veterans in the United States: Data from the National Health and Nutrition Examination Survey, 1999-2006. J Rehabil Res Dev 2011; 48(5):503–16.
23. Humes LE, Joellenbeck LM, Durch JS, editors. Noise and military service: implications for hearing loss and tinnitus. Washington, DC: The National Academies Press; 2006.

24. Gordon JS, Griest SE, Thielman EJ, et al. Audiologic characteristics in a sample of recently-separated military Veterans: The Noise Outcomes in Servicemembers Epidemiology Study (NOISE Study). Hear Res 2017;349:21–30.
25. Johnson RM. The masking of tinnitus. In: Vernon JA, editor. Tinnitus treatment and relief. Needham Heights (MA): Allyn & Bacon; 1998. p. 164–86.
26. Meikle MB, Henry JA, Griest SE, et al. The tinnitus functional index: development of a new clinical measure for chronic, intrusive tinnitus. Ear Hear 2012;33(2): 153–76.
27. Henry JA, Griest S, Zaugg TL, et al. Tinnitus and hearing survey: a screening tool to differentiate bothersome tinnitus from hearing difficulties. Am J Audiol 2015; 24(1):66–77.
28. Carlson KF, Griest S, Lewis MS, et al. Associations between Traumatic Brain Injury, Tinnitus, and Hearing Loss: An Epidemiologic Study of Recently Discharged Service Members. Military Health System Research Symposium. Fort Lauderdale, FL, August 19, 2015.
29. Theodoroff SM, Reavis KM, Griest SE, et al. Decreased sound tolerance associated with blast exposure. Sci Rep 2019;9(1):10204.
30. Coles RRA. Epidemiology of tinnitus: (2) demographic and clinical features. J Laryngol Otol 1984;(Suppl. 9):195–202.
31. Hazell JWP. Models of tinnitus: generation, perception, clinical implications. In: Vernon JA, Møller AR, editors. Mechanisms of tinnitus. Needham Heights (MA): Allyn & Bacon; 1995. p. 57–72.
32. Davis AC. Hearing in adults. London: Whurr Publishers, Ltd.; 1995.
33. Dauman R, Tyler RS. Some considerations on the classification of tinnitus. In: Aran J-M, Dauman R, editors. Proceedings of the fourth international tinnitus seminar. Bordeaux, France: Kugler Publications; 1992. p. 225–9.
34. Ratnayake SA, Jayarajan V, Bartlett J. Could an underlying hearing loss be a significant factor in the handicap caused by tinnitus? Noise Health 2009;11(44): 156–60.
35. Raj-Koziak D, Gos E, Rajchel J, et al. Tinnitus and hearing survey: a Polish study of validity and reliability in a clinical population. Audiol Neurootol 2017;22(4–5): 197–204.
36. Scheffer AR, Mondelli M. Tinnitus and hearing survey: cultural adaptation to Brazilian Portuguese. Braz J Otorhinolaryngol 2019. https://doi.org/10.1016/j.bjorl. 2019.06.009.
37. Henry JA, Thielman EJ, Zaugg TL, et al. Randomized controlled trial in clinical settings to evaluate effectiveness of coping skills education used with progressive tinnitus management. J Speech Lang Hear Res 2017;60(5):1378–97.
38. Theodoroff SM, Lewis MS, Folmer RL, et al. Hearing impairment and tinnitus: prevalence, risk factors, and outcomes in US service members and veterans deployed to the Iraq and Afghanistan wars. Epidemiol Rev 2015;37:71–85.
39. Lew HL, Garvert DW, Pogoda TK, et al. Auditory and visual impairments in patients with blast-related traumatic brain injury: Effect of dual sensory impairment on Functional Independence Measure. J Rehabil Res Dev 2009;46(6):819–26.
40. Carlson KF, Gilbert TA, O'Neil ME, et al. Health care utilization and mental health diagnoses among veterans with tinnitus. Am J Audiol 2019;28(1S):181–90.
41. McFerran DJ, Stockdale D, Holme R, et al. Why is there no cure for tinnitus? Front Neurosci 2019;13:802.
42. Fuller TE, Haider HF, Kikidis D, et al. Different teams, same conclusions? a systematic review of existing clinical guidelines for the assessment and treatment of tinnitus in adults. Front Psychol 2017;8:206.

43. Jastreboff PJ. Tinnitus retraining therapy. Prog Brain Res 2007;166:415–23.
44. Tyler RS, editor. Tinnitus treatment: clinical protocols. New York: Thieme Medical Publishers, Inc.; 2005.
45. Shekhawat GS, Searchfield GD, Stinear CM. Role of hearing AIDS in tinnitus intervention: a scoping review. J Am Acad Audiol 2013;24(8):747–62.
46. Henry JA, Frederick M, Sell S, et al. Validation of a novel combination hearing aid and tinnitus therapy device. Ear Hear 2015;36(1):42–52.
47. Henry JA, McMillan G, Dann S, et al. Tinnitus management: randomized controlled trial comparing extended-wear hearing aids, conventional hearing aids, and combination instruments. J Am Acad Audiol 2017;28(6):546–61.

Heritability and Genetics Contribution to Tinnitus

Jose A. Lopez-Escamez, MD, PhD[a,b,c],*, Sana Amanat, MSc[a]

KEYWORDS

• Genetics • Tinnitus • Prevalence • Genotyping • Genetic heritability

KEY POINTS

- Tinnitus is a condition affecting more than 15% of the adult population, being more prevalent in adults older than 65 years.
- Epidemiologic studies with twins and adoptees support tinnitus heritability.
- Tinnitus is associated with hearing loss, sleep disorders, migraine, anxiety, depression, and suicide risk.
- The evidence to support a genetic contribution to tinnitus, including an association of common or rare variants in certain genes, such as *BDNF or GDNF*, is weak.

INTRODUCTION

Tinnitus is the perception of an auditory noise that can take various forms from ringing in the ear to beeping, hissing, roaring, or buzzing; the condition involves more than 15% of an adult population.[1,2] Evidence supporting a genetic contribution to common disorders is usually inferred from prevalence studies comparing different populations with diverse ethnic backgrounds, the observation of familial clustering, and twin studies showing higher concordance between monozygotic than dizygotic twins in bilateral cases. Tinnitus is a complex condition associated with several disorders and its heritability is conditioned by the genetic contribution to the associated disorder. Variations in the human genome may contribute to different disorders, that is, common allelic variations contributing to tinnitus may also contribute to hearing

[a] Otology & Neurotology Group CTS495, Department of Genomic Medicine, GENYO - Centre for Genomics and Oncological Research – Pfizer, University of Granada, Junta de Andalucía, Andalusian Regional Government, PTS Granada, Avenida de la Ilustración, 114, Granada 18016, Spain; [b] Department of Otolaryngology, Instituto de Investigación Biosanitaria ibs. GRANADA, Hospital Universitario Virgen de las Nieves, Universidad de Granada, Granada, Spain; [c] Department of Surgery, Division of Otolaryngology, Universidad de Granada, Granada, Spain
* Corresponding author. Otology & Neurotology Group CTS495, GENYO. Centre for Genomics and Oncological Research: Pfizer, University of Granada, Andalusian Regional Government, PTS Granada, Avenida de la Ilustración, 114, Granada 18016, Spain.
E-mail address: antonio.lopezescamez@genyo.es
Twitter: @ALEscamez (J.A.L.-E.); @Sana_Amanat (S.A.)

Otolaryngol Clin N Am 53 (2020) 501–513
https://doi.org/10.1016/j.otc.2020.03.003
0030-6665/20/© 2020 Elsevier Inc. All rights reserved.

loss or anxiety, an association known as pleiotropic effect. The major limitation of most studies is that tinnitus has been considered as a single clinical condition, whereas there are several subtypes of patients with tinnitus that are likely to have different underlying mechanisms. For future genetic studies, it is essential to consider an appropriate selection of tinnitus phenotypes, including age of onset, severity of hearing loss, mechanism of hearing loss, and comorbidities to investigate the interaction among multiple variables.[1,3] To achieve this goal a European School on Tinnitus Research (https://esit.tinnitusresearch.net) has been established to provide training for doctoral candidates and set up the background work for tinnitus research in the European Union.[4] Furthermore, guidelines for biobanking samples for genetic studies in hearing and tinnitus research to promote personalized medicine have been published.[5]

PREVALENCE OF TINNITUS WORLDWIDE

There are several studies on the prevalence of tinnitus in the general population, in younger and older adults across different ethnic backgrounds including European ancestry (British, Sweden, Polish, Italy), non-Hispanic white population, Sub-Saharan (Egypt, Nigeria), and Asian (Japan, Taiwan).[6] These studies reported approximately the same prevalence of tinnitus, whereas one of the studies reported marginally a higher prevalence in non-Hispanic white population.[3] To investigate the effect of age in the prevalence of tinnitus, several studies have been conducted on different age groups; the prevalence of tinnitus was higher in adults older than 65 years, probably associated with the higher prevalence of hearing loss. In addition, to investigate the influence of tinnitus on daily life, a study was conducted comparing different regions in the United Kingdom; tinnitus was reported as an annoyance symptom in 5.3% of the population on average (**Tables 1** and **2**).[6]

TINNITUS PHENOTYPING STRATEGIES

The precise selection of tinnitus patients with a homogenous phenotype is the primary step to define tinnitus subtypes or profiles for genetic studies. Each form should also be classified based on co-occurring symptoms whether the tinnitus is isolated or non-isolated (eg, associated with other medical symptoms/signs as a syndromic condition). Inappropriate selection of tinnitus patients can produce a selection bias and nonsignificant results, false positives, or loss of statistical power. Furthermore, an inaccurate phenotype can produce the false association of gene variants with tinnitus subtypes, such as the *SLC6A4* gene, which was previously associated with depression.[7] Moreover, the use of standardized instruments or questionnaires to characterize tinnitus, hearing, and psychological profiles should be encouraged. These parameters are helpful to measure the heritability of tinnitus in concordance twins studies or the risk recurrence in siblings to estimate the familial aggregation in specific tinnitus subtypes.[3]

TINNITUS ASSOCIATION WITH OTHER DISORDERS

Many individuals report tinnitus in the general population and many syndromes and diseases have tinnitus as one of the core symptoms, making tinnitus research a challenge. Some of the associated conditions are psychological (anxiety, depression), neurologic (migraine, vestibular schwannoma), sleep disorders, metabolic, and Wilson disease, but the most remarkable condition is hearing loss, including high-frequency sensorineural hearing loss, presbycusis, and Meniere disease (MD).[6,8] Tinnitus and

Table 1
Prevalence of tinnitus across different populations and age groups

Reference	Region or Population	Sample (N)	Tinnitus Cases (N)	Other Conditions	Age Group (y)	Estimated Prevalence (%)
Hinchcliffe et al,[28] 1961	Wales, Scotland	400	—	—	55–64	39
					65–74	37
Hendrickx et al,[9] 2007	European Union 7 European centers	981	208	—	—	21
Lasisi et al,[29] 2010	Nigeria	1302	184	—	≥65	14
Khedr et al,[30] 2010	Egypt	8484	439	—	>60	18
Michikawa et al,[31] 2010	Japan	1320	245	—	≥65	19
Shargorodsky et al,[32] 2010	United States Non-Hispanic (white/black) Hispanic, others	14,178	—	—	60–69	14–31 [b]Non-Hispanic white
Dziendziel et al,[33] 2019	Polish	548	460	Otosclerosis patients	18–82	34 Tinnitus before hearing loss
Axelsson et al,[34] 1989	Sweden	3600	337	—	20–80	14
Gallus & Garavello,[35] 2015	Italy	2952	≈1724	—	45–64	6
					≥65	12
Lechowicz et al,[36] 2018	Polish	138	97	Hearing loss	—	23
Chang et al,[37] 2019	Taiwan	597	191	Dizziness (24%)	≥65	32

Table 2
Prevalence of self-reported tinnitus in young individuals based on epidemiologic studies

Data Reference	Epidemiologic Studies	Prevalence by Age (20–29)	Prevalence by Age (30–39)
Hoffmann & Reed,[38] 2004	United Kingdom National Study of Hearing (1980–1986)	5.7	7.4
	Gothenburg, Sweden (1989)	7.5	5.8
	US NHIS Hearing Supplement (1990)	5.1	6.0
	Disability Supplement (1994–1995)	1.4	2.0
	Nord-Trøndelag, Norway Hearing Loss Study (1996–1998)	9.8	9.6

hyperacusis also has an association with autism, but the information available in these patients is limited (**Fig. 1**).

EVIDENCE TO SUPPORT TINNITUS HERITABILITY
Familial Aggregation

Familial studies have seldom been carried out in tinnitus research and few of them have studied familial aggregation. A study on 198 families with tinnitus was conducted in seven European centers. In this study 208/981 individuals reported tinnitus using a question, "Nowadays, do you ever get noises in your head or ear (tinnitus), which usually last longer than 5 minutes." Unfortunately, the characterization of tinnitus or other comorbidities was not reported in detail. Familial aggregation was measured by three different methods: (1) mixed model approach, (2) the familial correlation, and (3) the estimated risk if someone else in the family is also affected by tinnitus. By using a Cox proportional model, familial aggregation was found and this clustering was independent of age, gender, hearing loss, and noise exposure. However, this "familial effect" observed could have either genetic or environmental origins, because families usually share the same environment.[9]

Another study on familial tinnitus was conducted in 2010, as part of the HUNT study.[10] For this study 51,574 subjects older than 18 years were recruited and self-

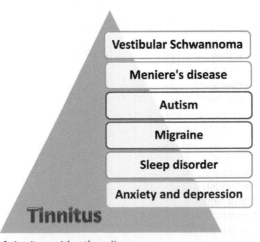

Fig. 1. Association of tinnitus with other diseases.

reported questionnaire data were used. To calculate the heritability three different patterns were used: (1) parents-offspring, (2) spouse, and (3) siblings. Amazingly, this study reported a low heritability of 0.11 for tinnitus in Norwegian families and found an association with environmental factors in male siblings. The major limitations of these studies are that tinnitus phenotyping was limited: age of onset, tinnitus pitch, and loudness were not measured; duration of tinnitus and its relationship with hearing loss were not reported. A selection bias is possible and persistent tinnitus should not be compared with occasional tinnitus lasting a few minutes, which is reported by many individuals.

Genetic Susceptibility to Bilateral Tinnitus

A stronger evidence to support heritability has been found in twin studies. A large cohort including 10,464 Swedish twin pairs was recruited to investigate the genetic susceptibility of self-reported tinnitus. The comparison of monozygotic with dizygotic twins showed a higher concordance in monozygotic twins with an estimated heritability of 0.27 and 0.56 for unilateral and bilateral tinnitus, respectively.[1,2] This study suggests that bilateral, but not unilateral tinnitus has a significant genetic contribution comparable with autism and higher than Alzheimer disease.[1]

Genetic Heritability and Environmental Factors

To identify the association of clinically significant tinnitus with environmental or genetic factors a parent-offspring study was performed in Swedish adoptees. Adoptive and biologic parents were recruited and the report showed that there were no environmental factors associated with the transmission of tinnitus; rather, a genetic contribution with an estimated heritability of 0.32 was found (**Fig. 2**).[11]

SEX-SPECIFIC EFFECTS ON TINNITUS HERITABILITY

To investigate the biologic sex-specific effect on tinnitus heritability, the large Swedish twin cohort extended their analysis for men and women. This study found a significant difference of heritability in both sexes. For bilateral tinnitus, the genetic heritability was 0.41 for females and 0.68 for males. However, when individuals younger than 40 years old were selected for further analysis, a significant increase in tinnitus heritability from 0.41 to 0.62[1] for women was observed (**Fig. 3**).

EVIDENCE FOR A GENETIC CONTRIBUTION TO TINNITUS

Genetic studies on tinnitus are still in their infancy, but are yet much needed to investigate the molecular neurobiology of tinnitus generation or maintenance.[2] These studies have found several candidate genes that could play an important role in the mechanisms involved in tinnitus. A genetic study on chronic tinnitus was performed on 240 white subjects and the tinnitus severity was measured using tinnitus questionnaire in a case-control study; however, no allele was found to be significantly associated, after correcting for multiple testing. However, multiple regression analysis found that the combined effect of *GDNF* and *BDNF* genotypes could play a role in predicting tinnitus severity in females ($P = .04$).[12]

A small study on a Turkish population with 52 subjects with chronic tinnitus and 42 control subjects without tinnitus did not find a significant association between *GDNF* gene variants and tinnitus.[13]

Another study investigated the role of common variants in the *KCNE1* gene in 201 chronic tinnitus subjects and 938 control subjects. Seven variants were investigated

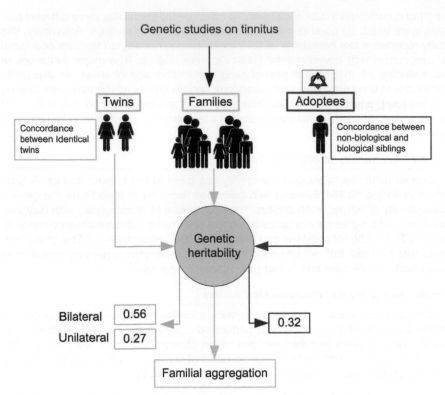

Fig. 2. Genetic heritability to tinnitus in families, twin cohorts, and adoptees.

in the *KCNE1* gene including five previously known and two novel variants. However, none of the variants was found to be associated with tinnitus severity.[14]

A group of 128 male tinnitus cases with occupational noise was recruited to investigate the contribution of potassium recycling pathway genes (*KCNE1* and *SLC12A2*) to the increase of tinnitus susceptibility. The variant rs915539 in the *KCNE1* gene was associated with tinnitus development independently of hearing loss.[15]

A large family with late-onset high-frequency hearing loss and two probands with tinnitus were considered for genome-wide linkage analysis. A large deletion in *COCH* gene was identified in this family and suggested the need to investigate the entire *COCH* gene instead of particular exon. The *COCH* gene causes monogenic nonsyndromic sensorineural hearing impairment (SNHL) with a variable vestibular dysfunction named DFNA9.[16] However, the 23 familial cases with autosomal-dominant SNHL and 20 MD cases from Japanese ancestry were selected to search for *COCH* mutation. In one subject affected with autosomal-dominant SNHL and tinnitus a novel mutation in *COCH* gene was found suggesting that allelic variation in *COCH* gene could influence the risk for the tinnitus development. However, no *COCH* mutation was found in patients with MD.[17] Unfortunately, the prevalence of tinnitus in monogenic SNHL has not been estimated and it is difficult to determine the effect of rare variants in tinnitus generation.

Additionally, the variants in *HTR7*,[18] *KCNE3*,[19,20] *KCTD12*,[21] ACE, ADD1,[22] and *NF2*[23] have been reported to be associated with tinnitus; however, most of these studies were underpowered and have not been replicated.

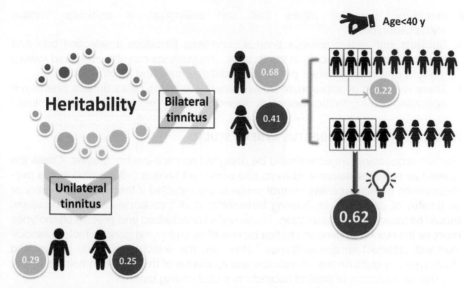

Fig. 3. Sex-differences in the genetic heritability to bilateral tinnitus.

In a pilot genome-wide association study in Belgium, 167 tinnitus cases and 749 control subjects were recruited with the age range of 55 to 65 years. In this study 4 million single-nucleotide polymorphisms were tested to search for an association with tinnitus. The study was underpowered and none of the single-nucleotide polymorphisms could reach the genome-wide significant threshold. However, gene enrichment analysis suggested several associated pathways including vascular smooth muscle contraction, nucleoside diphosphate kinase dynamin, coenzyme A biosynthesis and NRF2-mediated oxidative stress response, and endoplasmic reticulum overload response (**Table 3**).[24]

DESIGNING HUMAN GENETIC STUDIES TO INVESTIGATE TINNITUS

Human genetic variation is usually explained by single-nucleotide variation, copy number variants, and/or insertions or deletions in the primary sequence of DNA molecules. Several strategies are considered to design human genetic studies including:

1. Concordance studies in monozygotic/dizygotic twins or families with the same ethnic background to demonstrate the heritability.
2. Selection of genotyping or sequencing platforms to investigate common or rare variation, either in candidate genes or the human genome. Although to search for common variants genotyping is preferred, to define rare allelic variation exome (coding region or exon sequencing) genome (coding and noncoding regions) sequencing is the standard technology.[3,25]

SELECTING A HOMOGENOUS TINNITUS PHENOTYPE

There are several reasons for recruiting patients with homogenous tinnitus profiles:

1. Reducing genetic noise signals in the tinnitus cohort. This homogeneity is achieved by defining the clinical phenotype by a precise definition of the condition.

2. Identifying potential alleles that can distinguish a particular tinnitus endophenotype.
3. Subjects with heterogeneous tinnitus conditions introduce a selection bias and they can increase variability in the dataset. This variance can ultimately lead toward the loss of power to detect potential candidate genes and its effects.
4. There is a need of appropriate measurements to characterize tinnitus phenotype according to the condition being addressed (eg, noise- or stress-induced tinnitus).[3]

STRATEGIES TO DESIGN TINNITUS GENETIC STUDIES

Tinnitus sequencing projects should be designed as case-control studies. Cases are defined as subjects reporting chronic and persistent tinnitus (>3 months) with a psychoacoustic profile, whereas control subjects are selected if they have temporary or no tinnitus at all. However, hearing thresholds at all frequencies and comorbidities should be taken into consideration. These well-characterized and precise phenotypes improve the results of genetic studies by revealing underlying genetic factors associated with different tinnitus subtypes.[2] However, the selection of study groups and phenotype depends on the prevalence and incidence of the condition being studied; and the identification of control subjects is a challenging task.[3]

TINNITUS EXTREME PHENOTYPE APPROACH IN MENIERE DISEASE

The extreme phenotype approach is based on a case-control study design and it assumes that patients from both extremes of a particular phenotype (very high or very low) have an enrichment of rare variants in coding regions and they will target relevant genes, facilitating the identification of the underlying genetic causes for a particular condition. Using this approach, the sequencing of a small number of individuals could be enough to find a burden of rare missense variants in extremes of a quantitative phenotype. We have defined extreme tinnitus phenotype in patients with MD by selecting young patients with MD showing a fast progression of MD symptoms and with a Tinnitus Handicap Inventory (THI)[26] score greater than 56 points. We further divided this extreme group into two subgroups known as almost extreme (THI >56) and very extreme (THI >76). The selection of very extreme subjects is theoretically informative, but might be vulnerable to phenotype heterogeneity in a clinical spectrum.[27]

FUTURE DIRECTIONS

Tinnitus is a complex condition associated with several comorbidities and the selection of individuals is essential to reduce heterogeneity in clinical research. The design of future genetic studies should consider the following issues:

1. A careful selection of individuals with well-defined phenotype for tinnitus and the main associated conditions (hearing loss, anxiety, migraine, sleep disturbance).
2. The phenotype should include at least the age of onset, familial history, duration of tinnitus, assessment of functional impact by validated tools (ie, THI, tinnitus functional index), and tinnitus features (unilateral or bilateral, intermittent or persistent).
3. Use of standardized validated questionnaire (ie, to measure the prevalence of persistent tinnitus) and its association with the major comorbidities (hearing loss, migraine, sleep disorder, anxiety) rather asking a single and general question during survey.
4. Reproducibility: replication of genetic association in an independent population.

Table 3
Genetic studies on chronic tinnitus and associated conditions

Reference	Tinnitus Phenotype	Duration	Others	Tinnitus Questionnaire	Population	Tinnitus cases (N)	Sex F	Sex M	Age (Mean ± SD) or Years	Sequencing Method	Genetic Findings
Sand et al,[14] 2010	Chronic	>6 mo	—	TQ	German	201	49	152	49.9 ± 12.0	Genotyping	rs17173510, rs1805128, rs2070357, rs41314071, rs1805127, chr21: 35821347C > G, chr21: 35821794G > A
Sand et al,[20] 2011	Chronic	>6 mo	—	TQ	German	288	86	202	50.1 ± 12.6	Genotyping	rs2270676, rs17215437
Sand et al,[12] 2012	Chronic	>6 mo	—	TQ	German	240	69	171	50.3 ± 12.9	Genotyping	GDNF, BDNF
Sand et al,[21] 2012	Chronic	—	—	TQ	German	95	28	67	50.6 ± 12.1	Genotyping	rs34544607
Pawełczyk et al,[15] 2012	—	—	Susceptible or resistant to noise	"Do you suffer from tinnitus?"	Polish	128	—	128	42 mean years	Genotyping	rs915539
Gallant et al,[16] 2013	—	—	[a]BLSNHI	—	US	2 siblings	1	1	31 and 38 y	Genotyping	c.1196_1213del (18 bp in exon 11)

(continued on next page)

Table 3
(continued)

Reference	Tinnitus Phenotype	Duration	Others	Tinnitus Questionnaire	Population	Tinnitus cases (N)	Sex F	Sex M	Age (Mean ± SD) or Years	Sequencing Method	Genetic Findings
Yano et al,[39] 2014	—	—	Hearing loss	—	Japanese	≈59%	—	—	—	Whole mitochondrial genome screening	Mitochondrial mutation (C1494 T, A1555 G, A3243 G, T7511 C)
Orenay-Boyacioglu et al,[13] 2016	Chronic	>3 mo	—	THI	Turkish	52	19	33	18–55 y	Genotyping	rs3812047, rs884344
Yüce et al,[22] 2016	Severe chronic	>6 mo	—	STI, THI	Turkish	89	48	41	48.1 ± 13.5	Genotyping	ACE I/D rs1799752, ADD1 rs4961
Gilles et al,[24] 2017	—	—	Noise exposure	[b]Question	Belgium	167	67	100	61.2 ± 3.1	GWAS	Metabolic pathway
El Charif et al,[40] 2019	Moderate, severe	—	[c]Testicular cancer survivors	[d]Question	United States + Canada	154	—	154	>18–<55 y	GWAS	OTOS (rs7606353)

Abbreviations: GWAS, genome-wide association study; SD, standard deviation; STI, Strukturiertes Tinnitus-Interview; THI, tinnitus handicap inventory; TQ, tinnitus questionnaire.

[a] BLSNHI = late onset bilateral sensorineural hearing impairment.

[b] "Have you ever worked for more than a year in an environment where you had to shout to an individual standing at less than a meter from you" and "Nowadays, do you ever hear noises in your head or ear(s) (tinnitus) which usually last longer than 5 min?"

[c] Testicular cancer survivors following cisplatin-based chemotherapy.

[d] "Have you had in the last 4 wk: Ringing or buzzing in the ears?" and "Do you have: ringing and buzzing in the ears?"

5. Generation of genetic data to implement personalized medicine for treatment (eg, drug development).

SUMMARY

Tinnitus is the perception of sound in the absence of an external sound from the environment and it is reported by 15% of adult population. The prevalence of tinnitus across different age groups is different and a higher prevalence has been reported for adults older than 65 years. There are few studies on tinnitus heritability comparing both sexes; however, a significant heritability has been found in bilateral tinnitus in men compared with women (all age groups), but young females (<40 year old) with bilateral tinnitus also showed higher heritability than men.

Tinnitus is sometimes associated with psychological disorders including depression, anxiety, and suicide risk. There are several genetic studies on tinnitus and its associated disorders including MD and migraine. These studies were conducted on familial and sporadic cases to identify the genetic cause of the condition for better diagnosis and drug development. Several candidate genes and pathways have been involved in the pathophysiology of tinnitus, including *BDNF*, *GDNF*, voltage-gated potassium channels, and metabolic pathways, but the current evidence to support a genetic contribution to tinnitus is limited.

ACKNOWLEDGMENTS

This project is a part of European School of Interdisciplinary Tinnitus research and Sana Amanat is a PhD student in the Biomedicine Program at the University of Granada. This study was funded by grant H2020 MSC-ITN-2017–722046 and FEDER funds for Segovia Arana and a grant from ISCIII (JALE). The project leading to these results has received funding from "la Caixa" Foundation (ID 100010434), under agreement LCF/PR/DE18/52010002.

DISCLOSURE

The authors have nothing to disclose.

REFERENCES

1. Maas IL, Brüggemann P, Requena T, et al. Genetic susceptibility to bilateral tinnitus in a Swedish twin cohort. Genet Med 2017;19(9):1007–12.

2. Vona B, Nanda I, Shehata-Dieler W, et al. Genetics of tinnitus: still in its infancy. Front Neurosci 2017. https://doi.org/10.3389/fnins.2017.00236.

3. Lopez-Escamez JA, Bibas T, Cima RFF, et al. Genetics of tinnitus: an emerging area for molecular diagnosis and drug development. Front Neurosci 2016; 10:1–13.

4. Schlee W, Hall DA, Canlon B, et al. Innovations in doctoral training and research on tinnitus: the European School on Interdisciplinary Tinnitus Research (ESIT) perspective. Front Aging Neurosci 2018;9:447.

5. Szczepek AJ, Frejo L, Vona B, et al. Recommendations on collecting and storing samples for genetic studies in hearing and tinnitus research. Ear Hear 2019; 40(2):219–26.

6. Møller AR, Langguth B, DeRidder D, et al, editors. Textbook of tinnitus. New York: Springer Science & Business Media; 2010.

7. Arias B, Aguilera M, Moya J, et al. The role of genetic variability in the SLC6A4 , BDNF and GABRA6 genes in anxiety-related traits. Acta Psychiatr Scand 2012;194–202. https://doi.org/10.1111/j.1600-0447.2011.01764.x.

8. Langguth B, Hund V, Busch V, et al. Tinnitus and headache. Biomed Res Int 2015; 2015. https://doi.org/10.1155/2015/797416.

9. Hendrickx JJ, Huyghe JR, Demeester K, et al. Familial aggregation of tinnitus: a European multicentre study. B-ENT 2007;3:51–60.

10. Kvestad E, Czajkowski N, Engdahl B, et al. Low heritability of tinnitus: results from the second Nord-Trøndelag health study. Arch Otolaryngol Head Neck Surg 2010;136(2):178–82.

11. Cederroth CR, Pirouzifard M, Trpchevska N, et al. Association of genetic vs environmental factors in Swedish adoptees with clinically significant tinnitus. JAMA Otolaryngol Head Neck Surg 2019;145(3):222–9.

12. Sand PG, Langguth B, Schecklmann M, et al. GDNF and BDNF gene interplay in chronic tinnitus. Int J Mol Epidemiol Genet 2012;3(3):245–51.

13. Orenay-Boyacioglu S, Coskunoglu A, Caki Z, et al. Relationship between chronic tinnitus and glial cell line-derived neurotrophic factor gene rs3812047, rs1110149, and rs884344 polymorphisms in a Turkish population. Biochem Genet 2016;54(4):552–63.

14. Sand PG, Luettich A, Kleinjung T, et al. An examination of KCNE1 mutations and common variants in chronic tinnitus. Genes (Basel) 2010;1(1):23–37.

15. Pawełczyk M, Rajkowska E, Kotyło P, et al. Analysis of inner ear potassium recycling genes as potential factors associated with tinnitus. Int J Occup Med Environ Health 2012;25(4):356–64.

16. Gallant E, Francey L, Fetting H, et al. Novel COCH mutation in a family with autosomal dominant late onset sensorineural hearing impairment and tinnitus. Am J Otolaryngol 2013;34(3):230–5.

17. Usami S, Takahashi K, Yuge I, et al. Mutations in the COCH gene are a frequent cause of autosomal dominant progressive cochleo-vestibular dysfunction, but not Meniere's disease. Eur J Hum Genet 2003;5:744–8.

18. Gellynck E, Heyninck K, Andressen KW, et al. The serotonin 5-HT7 receptors: two decades of research. Exp Brain Res 2013;230(4):555–68.

19. Pawlak-Osińska K, Linkowska K, Grzybowski T. Genes important for otoneurological diagnostic purposes: current status and future prospects. Acta Otorhinolaryngol Ital 2018;38(3):242–50.

20. Sand PG, Langguth B, Kleinjung T. Deep resequencing of the voltage-gated potassium channel subunit KCNE3 gene in chronic tinnitus. Behav Brain Funct 2011;7(1):39.

21. Sand PG, Langguth B, Itzhacki J, et al. Resequencing of the auxiliary GABAB receptor subunit gene KCTD12 in chronic tinnitus. Front Syst Neurosci 2012;6:1–5.

22. Yüce S, Sancakdar E, Bağci G, et al. Angiotensin-converting enzyme (ACE) I/D and alpha-adducin (ADD1) G460W gene polymorphisms in Turkish patients with severe chronic tinnitus. J Int Adv Otol 2016;12(1):77–81.

23. Selvanathan SK, Shenton A, Ferner R, et al. Further genotype: phenotype correlations in neurofibromatosis 2. Clin Genet 2010;77(2):163–70.

24. Gilles A, Camp G, Van de Heyning P, et al. A pilot genome-wide association study identifies potential metabolic pathways involved in tinnitus. Front Neurosci 2017; 11:1–10.

25. Lohmann K, Klein C. Next generation sequencing and the future of genetic diagnosis. Neurotherapeutics 2014;11(4):699–707.

26. Newman CW, Jacobson GP, Spitzer JB, et al. Development of the tinnitus handicap inventory. Arch Otolaryngol Head Neck Surg 1996;122:143–8.

27. Li D, Lewinger JP, Gauderman WJ, et al. Using extreme phenotype sampling to identify the rare causal variants of quantitative traits in association studies. Genet Epidemiol 2011;35(8):790–9.

28. Hinchcliffe R. Prevalence of the commoner ear, nose, and throat conditions in the adult rural population of Great Britain: a study by direct examination of two random samples. Br J Prev Soc Med 1961;15(3):128–40.

29. Lasisi AO, Abiona T, Gureje O. Tinnitus in the elderly: profile, correlates, and impact in the Nigerian study of ageing. Otolaryngol Head Neck Surg 2010; 143(4):510–5.

30. Khedr EM, Ahmed MA, Shawky OA, et al. Epidemiological study of chronic tinnitus in Assiut, Egypt. Neuroepidemiology 2010;35(1):45–52.

31. Michikawa T, Nishiwaki Y, Kikuchi Y, et al. Prevalence and factors associated with tinnitus: a community-based study of Japanese elders. J Epidemiol 2010;20(4): 271–6.

32. Shargorodsky J, Curhan GC, Farwell WR. Prevalence and characteristics of tinnitus among US adults. Am J Med 2010;123(8):711–8.

33. Dziendziel B, Skarżyński PH, Rajchel JJ, et al. Prevalence and severity of tinnitus in Polish otosclerosis patients qualified for stapes surgery. Eur Arch Otorhinolaryngol 2019;276(6):1585–90.

34. Axelsson A, Ringdahl A. Tinnitus—a study of its prevalence and characteristics. Br J Audiol 1989 Jan 1;23(1):53–62.

35. Gallus S, Garavello W. Prevalence and determinants of tinnitus in the Italian adult population. Neuroepidemiology 2015;12–9. https://doi.org/10.1159/000431376.

36. Lechowicz U, Pollak A, Raj-Koziak D, et al. Tinnitus in patients with hearing loss due to mitochondrial DNA pathogenic variants. Eur Arch Otorhinolaryngol 2018; 275(8):1979–85.

37. Chang NC, Dai CY, Lin WY, et al. Prevalence of persistent tinnitus and dizziness in an elderly population in southern Taiwan. J Int Adv Otol 2019;15(1):99–105.

38. Hoffman HJ, Reed GW. Epidemiology of tinnitus. In: Snow JB, editor. Tinnitus: theory and management. Hamilton [Ont.]: BC Decker; Lewiston, NY: Sales and distribution, U.S., BC Decker, 2004;16:16–41.

39. Yano T, Nishio SY, Usami SI, et al. Frequency of mitochondrial mutations in nonsyndromic hearing loss as well as possibly responsible variants found by whole mitochondrial genome screening. J Hum Genet 2014;59(2):100–6.

40. El Charif O, Mapes B, Trendowski MR, et al. Clinical and genome-wide analysis of cisplatin-induced tinnitus implicates novel ototoxic mechanisms. Clin Cancer Res 2019;25(13):4104–16.

Classification of Tinnitus
Multiple Causes with the Same Name

Claudia Barros Coelho, MD, PhD[a,b,c,]*, Roberto Santos, MBBS[a],
Kadja Ferraz Campara, MBBS[a], Richard Tyler, PhD, MSc[c,d]

KEYWORDS

- Tinnitus causes • Tinnitus subtypes • Classification of tinnitus
- Hearing loss and tinnitus

KEY POINTS

- Tinnitus is associated with many different causes, likely many different mechanisms, and many different subtypes.
- Any change compromising the auditory system, in any location, can lead to tinnitus.
- This article focuses on identifying some of the different subtypes. One way to classify tinnitus is to parallel the way hearing loss is classified: conductive versus sensorineural.
- This article reviews a broad range of approaches to understand and demarcate different tinnitus subtypes based on hearing loss.
- Appreciating and understanding different subtypes will help lead the way to different treatments, and will be critical for exploring and finding cures for different subtypes.

TINNITUS: FROM PERCEPTION TO REACTIONS

Occasionally, after exposure to loud sounds such as concerts and parties, many people when in a quiet environment, such as a bedroom, perceive some hearing loss accompanied by tinnitus, a sound that is generated in the auditory system. In most cases, it disappears completely by the next morning. Almost any form of hearing loss, such as from ear wax, otitis, or even a foreign body in the ear canal, can cause transitory tinnitus.

Once the person recovers from the temporary hearing loss, tinnitus perception fades away. However, for some people, this noise in the ears or in the head does

[a] College of Medicine, University of Vale do Taquari-UNIVATES, Center of Medical Sciences, Rua Avelino Talini, 171 - Universitário, Lajeado - RS, 95914-014, Brazil; [b] Postgraduate Program in Medical Sciences, University of Vale do Taquari-UNIVATES, Center of Medical Sciences, Rua Avelino Talini, 171 - Universitário, Lajeado - RS, 95914-014, Brazil; [c] Department of Otolaryngology–Head & Neck Surgery, University of Iowa, 200 Hawkins Drive, 21151 Pomerantz Family Pavilion, Iowa City, IA 52242-1089, USA; [d] Department of Speech Pathology and Audiology, University of Iowa, The Wendell Johnson Speech and Hearing Center, 250 Hawkins Drive, Iowa City, IA 52242-1089, USA
* Corresponding author. Julio de Castilhos 966/207 Lajeado-RS - Brazil 95900-022
E-mail address: claudiabarroscoelho@gmail.com

Otolaryngol Clin N Am 53 (2020) 515–529
https://doi.org/10.1016/j.otc.2020.03.015
0030-6665/20/© 2020 Elsevier Inc. All rights reserved.
oto.theclinics.com

not disappear, and it becomes another dimension in their lives. It is present all the time and, even more, it interferes in thoughts, emotions, hearing, sleep, and concentration. It can cause intense suffering for a few.

In the first case, it is called tinnitus perception. In the second case it is it is called chronic tinnitus. This tinnitus can cause extreme distress in everyday life.

PERCEPTUAL CHARACTERISTICS OF THE TINNITUS

The tinnitus can be pulsatile, nonpulsatile, constant, or intermittent; it can be tonal, or sound like buzzing, whooshing, beeping, hissing, or ringing; and it can affect 1 or both ears.

It can be subjective (perceived only by the affected individual) or objective (also heard by an observer); constant or intermittent; perceived in 1 or both ears, or within the head; pulsatile (synchronous with the heart beat or asynchronous); loud or faint; and can manifest with a variety of pitches. Tinnitus can be acute (<3 months), sub-acute (3–6 months), or chronic (>12 months). The onset can be gradual or sudden, and can change characteristics over time.[1,2]

Tinnitus is associated with many different causes; this article provides an overview of clinical situations associated with tinnitus.

SUBTYPES OF PATIENTS WITH TINNITUS

One approach to classifying tinnitus is to parallel the way hearing loss is classified: conductive versus sensorineural. Conductive hearing loss results from obstruction or damage to the outer or middle ear, preventing sound from being conducted to the inner ear. Sensory hearing loss results from cochlea or the stria vascularis damage. Sensorineural hearing loss results from damage of the hair cells, cochlear synapses, spiral ganglion neurons, and/or more proximal auditory structures. Any change compromising the auditory system, in any location, can lead to tinnitus.

CONDUCTIVE TINNITUS

A change in blood flow, muscles, or physiology of the middle ear can lead to tinnitus.

Ear Infections

Any form of ear infection can be accompanied by tinnitus. Once the infection process is resolved, tinnitus disappears. However, some patients keep experiencing tinnitus. One possible explanation is what is called unmasking. Tinnitus was already present but without perception, and, during the temporary hearing loss, or its increase, the patient's attention to the symptom can increase and it can become noticeable.

Tympanic Membrane and Ossicular Chain

Middle ear disorders that disrupt sound energy passing from the tympanic membrane to the inner ear can cause conductive hearing loss and tinnitus, such as tympanic membrane perforation; disruption or fixation of the ossicular chain resulting from infections, trauma, otosclerosis, or Paget disease; chronic otitis media and cholesteatoma; and eustachian tube dysfunctions.

Glomic Tumors

Glomus tympanicum tumors, or tympanic paraganglioma, are the most common benign tumors of the middle ear. Derived from the neural crest, the proliferation of paraganglion cells is highly vascularized. They are rare, hypervascularized, benign neoplasms, but locally invasive.

Paraganglioma of the temporal bone originates from the tympanic plexus of the Arnold and Jacobson nerves (glomus tympanicum) or the adventitia layer of the jugular bulb (glomus jugular). Glomic tumors usually affect middle-aged women. Clinical manifestations are secondary to the tumor invasion on surrounding structures and include hearing loss (conductive and/or sensory), tinnitus (neurosensorial or pulsatile), dizziness, facial palsy, dysphagia, hoarseness, and pain. The otoscopic examination shows a red, pulsatile mass of the middle ear that can blanch during pneumatic otoscopy, the so-called Brown sign.[3]

Myoclonus

Middle ear myoclonus is defined as a rhythmic movement of the tympanic membrane secondary to repetitive contraction of the tensor tympani and stapedial muscles.[4] Tinnitus is usually unilateral, and the sound characteristic might give about a clue to the myoclonus's location. When the source is the tympanic tensor muscle, tinnitus sounds like a click and a butterfly, whereas, when produced by the stapedius muscle, it sounds like a buzzing noise.[5,6] The cause remains unknown, but has been associated with facial paralysis, trauma, vascular conditions, infections, demyelinating disorders, anxiety, and tumors.[4] Occasionally, rhythmic movements of the tympanic membrane can be visualized on otoscopic examination.

A clear mechanism for this rare subtype of tinnitus is not well understood but it is likely to be caused by the propagation of the muscle contraction noise, vibration of the tympanic membrane during contraction of these muscles, and alteration of cochlear microphony.[6]

Palatal myoclonus caused by the tensor veli palatini and levator veli palatini can also cause tinnitus. Tinnitus is heard in both ears and presents as clicks, resembling the noise made by the snapping together of 2 fingers.[7] The cause is unknown but could be associated with many clinical conditions, such as vascular lesions, trauma, infection, multiple sclerosis, or psychogenic, or it could be idiopathic. Palatal myoclonus can be diagnosed on direct oral cavity examination.[5]

The tinnitus sound could be a result of the eustachian tube snapping open or from the breaking of surface tension as the walls of the eustachian tube open under the action of peritubal muscles.[7]

Tonic Tensor Tympani Syndrome

Tinnitus is one of the symptoms of the tonic tensor tympani syndrome, initially described by Klochoff[8] as the tonic tensor phenomenon. Other complaints include ear fullness, tinnitus, dysacusis, tension headache, dizziness, and disequilibrium.

The tensor tympani muscle is 2.0 cm long, inserts in the neck of the malleus and the cartilage portion of the eustachian tube, and is innervated by the mandibular branch of the trigeminal nerve. Contraction of the tensor tympani muscle pulls the eardrum membrane inward and displaces the stapes into the scala vestibuli.

Clinically, the tonic tensor tympani syndrome is associated with acoustic shock injury, neck harm caused by whiplash, and temporomandibular disorders.[9] Myofascial disorders (trigger points) of masticatory muscles (eg, masseter and medial pterygoid, which are also innervated by the mandibular branch of trigeminal nerve) are also prevalent.

When the tensor tympani remains in a tonic contraction (fixed), it decreases tympanic compliance, causing attenuation of low-frequency acoustic energy transmission through the middle ear. The audiometric signature of this syndrome is (1) a decrease of the acoustic tympanometry static peak compliance,[10,11] (2) low-frequency conductive hearing loss, and possibly (3) a small low-frequency sensorineural hearing loss.[11,12]

SENSORINEURAL TINNITUS

Sensorineural tinnitus is when the sensory or nervous system initiate the tinnitus. This initiation could take place in the cochlea, the auditory nerve, the temporal lobe, or perhaps even other parts of the neural system throughout the brain.

Sensorineural tinnitus is almost always accompanied by a sensorineural hearing loss, which is the most common type of tinnitus. It is important to remember how audiometric zero and normal hearing were established. After examining thousands of attendees of 1939 World's Fair in New York and San Francisco, the average hearing of 19-year-olds at 1 kHz was set to be 0 dB hearing loss. This level was considered to be the audiometric zero; the minimum sound pressure that the average young human with normal hearing could detect.[13] Normal hearing refers to a range about the average value. If someone had hearing thresholds at age 19 years of −10 dB hearing loss, and if that person's thresholds are now 0 dB hearing loss, they have a hearing loss. Even small changes on hearing thresholds can cause tinnitus. It is important to remember that human hearing extends up to 20 kHz, whereas hearing is typically tested only up to 8 kHz.

Patients with tinnitus may present normal audiometric thresholds but complain of difficulty hearing sounds when there is background noise.

Presbycusis Tinnitus

As people age, they lose their hearing gradually. Age-related hearing loss (presbycusis) is the number 1 communication disorder and is one of the top three chronic health conditions of the elderly. It reduces the capacity to understand speech, resulting in social isolation. For some, this might also include tinnitus as a result of the natural aging process, which might be difficult to distinguish from other unknown causes. Establishing presbycusis tinnitus is likely to require an insidious onset of a high-frequency sensorineural hearing loss, usually bilateral and symmetric, originating after some age (eg, 60 years or even 70 years), and a progression of loss over time, with no other likely causes. Physiologic changes in hearing with aging are associated with the damage of the cochlear sensory hair cells and morphologic changes of the stria vascularis leading to deficiency in the circulation and perfusion of the cochlea.[14]

Metabolic Tinnitus

The auditory system requires glucose and high energy availability to function. Maintenance of inner ear fluid homeostasis depends on the supply of oxygen and glucose by the stria vascularis. Changes in blood flow or metabolites cause impairment to the inner ear function, damaging the auditory system and possibly causing hearing disorders, including tinnitus. Some clinical situations that might affect inner ear homeostasis are discussed here.

Diabetes type II

The cochlea is a target of hyperglycemia. Abnormal blood glucose levels, even for short periods of time, might result in subclinical pathologic changes such as microangiopathy in the stria vascularis, damaging the cochlea and auditory neuropathy and causing hearing loss and tinnitus. Hearing evaluation among diabetics shows low-frequency hearing loss, associated or not with midfrequency and high-frequency hearing loss,[15] and most pronounced in the right ear.[16]

Hypothyroidism

Hypothyroidism, a common endocrinological disorder, results from reduced thyroid hormone actions at the peripheral tissues, slowing down the whole-body functions. It can also present in a subclinical form in patients with thyroid peroxidase antibodies and thyroid-stimulating hormone values in the upper normal range. Chances to develop hypothyroidism increases with age, and it is 10 times more common in women than in men.[17] Decrease of cerebral blood flow and glucose metabolism in hypothyroidism might affect the stria vascularis causing damage to the cochlea, hearing loss, and tinnitus. Hearing loss is usually bilateral mild to moderate, with a flat audiogram.[18]

Dyslipidemia

High serum low-density lipoprotein level is a vascular risk factor; in the inner ear it damages the cochlear microcirculation, causing hearing impairment and tinnitus.[19] Low high-density lipoprotein level increases the chances to develop low frequency/mid frequency hearing loss.[15]

Anemia

Anemia (low hemoglobin level) harms the cochlea because of deficiency of oxygen delivery, resulting in sensorineural hearing loss tinnitus.[20–22]

Vitamin and mineral deficiencies

Several reports have linked vitamin and mineral deficiencies to hearing loss and tinnitus, including vitamin B_{12},[23,24] B_1,[24] D_3,[25] folate,[26] zinc,[27–29] and magnesium.[30]

Causes include malabsorption syndromes, continuous use of proton-pump inhibitors, bariatric surgery, and vegetarianism.

Noise-Induced Tinnitus

Noise exposure is one of the most common causes of tinnitus. Focusing on it as subtype could therefore be important for many patients. Noise-induced hearing loss (NIHL) is accompanied by a notched audiogram, worse hearing at 3 to 6 kHz, and then an improvement at 8 kHz as an example. Subgrouping noise-induced tinnitus could require a history of noise exposure. It might also be helpful to distinguish between several years of noise exposure, versus a sudden NIHL, perhaps resulting from an impulse noise; for example, a gunshot. Air bag explosions can also result in impulsive noise-induced tinnitus but may also include head trauma, so that would have to be excluded in the subgrouping. If the noise-induced tinnitus affected only 1 ear, this would allow an important within-subject control. In addition, with a sudden-onset noise-induced tinnitus (eg, following an explosion or gunshot), it would be possible to distinguish immediate effects related to tinnitus, in contrast with long-term noise effects, which could include many parts of the nervous system.

Noise-induced hearing loss

NIHL is typically from long-term, continuous exposure to noise. The extent of the damage to the inner ear depends on the degree of sound intensity, the duration of the exposure, and genetic susceptibility. Tinnitus is usually bilateral, continuous, and high-pitched.[31,32]

Acoustic trauma

Acoustic trauma hearing loss results from a single or repeated sudden intense noise exposure, such as firearm shooting, car airbag release, and recreational music. It has been reported to immediately cause tinnitus.[33]

Acoustic shock

Acoustic shock injury (ASI) results from of a brief exposure to sudden unexpected loud sounds causing tinnitus, ear pain, ear pressure, hyperacusis/phonophobia, and vertigo. Nonotological symptoms include insomnia, headaches, and disorientation. High levels of emotional trauma and anxiety may be present. Usually, symptoms are temporary and disappear within hours to days following exposure. ASI has been described mostly among call center staff using a telephone headset or handset.[34–37] Clinical examination and audiometric testing are usually normal. The proposed neurophysiologic mechanism is an exaggerated startle response with contraction of the tensor tympani muscle.[35]

Sudden Sensorial Hearing Loss and Tinnitus

Sudden sensorineural hearing loss (SSHL) is defined as a loss of hearing of 30 dB or more in 3 consecutive frequencies in 1 or both ears that occurs within 72 hours. Tinnitus associated with SSHL is usually unilateral with an abrupt onset. As a comorbidity, it may become chronic and become the patient's primary concern.[38]

Viral inflammation, vascular occlusion, and immune diseases are possible causes, causing damage to the inner ear, the cochlea, or auditory pathways.[39] Some causes require urgent diagnosis, such as vestibular schwannoma (acoustic neuroma), stroke, malignancy, noise, and ototoxic medication, which may present as SSHL.[38] Although the presence of tinnitus causes greater emotional reactions in these patients,[40] its presence is a positive outcome factor for hearing recovery.[41]

Rapidly Progressive Bilateral Sensorineural Hearing Loss and Tinnitus

Rapidly progressive bilateral sensorineural hearing loss is defined as a shift of 15 dB or more at any frequency or 10 dB or more at 2 or more consecutive frequencies, or a significant change in discrimination score that occurs within 3 months or more apart.[42] Tinnitus is usually associated with the sensorineural hearing loss and is more frequent among women 30 to 60 years old. If the patient presents a positive response to steroid therapy, hearing loss is classified as immune mediated. In about 15% to 30% of cases, there is an association with autoimmune diseases such as systemic lupus erythematosus, rheumatoid arthritis, ankylosing spondylitis, multiple sclerosis, ulcerative colitis, and Cogan syndrome. Pathophysiologic findings include cochlear inflammation, noninflammatory vasculopathy, and type II to IV hypersensitivity reactions.[43]

Ototoxicity

Ototoxic drugs and chemicals might damage the auditory system, causing functional harm to the cochlear hair cells. As a consequence, they might cause tinnitus and hearing loss. The symptoms develop during or after the end of use. Audiometry shows neurosensory bilateral hearing loss, symmetric or asymmetric with 1 ear being affected later. At present, more than 150 drugs are known to be ototoxic.[44] The most common drugs are aminoglycosides (irreversible), vancomycin (irreversible), macrolide antibiotics (reversible), platinum-based anticancer drugs (irreversible), loop diuretics (reversible), and quinine (reversible). Of interest is the widespread use of salicylate as a pain medication. It might induce mild to moderate hearing loss when used in high doses. Hearing loss is usually bilateral and symmetric and is associated with tinnitus; both the hearing loss and the tinnitus usually disappear within 24 to 72 hours after cessation of the drug.

Auditory Neuropathy Spectrum Disorder

Auditory neuropathy spectrum disorder (ANSD) is a retrocochlear hearing condition in which the patient has normal functioning outer hair cells (expressed by normal otoacoustic emission response) or cochlear microphonics, absent middle ear muscle reflexes, and an absent/abnormal auditory brainstem response.[45]

Clinically, ANSD is manifested by poor speech recognition severely affected by background noise, which does not correspond with pure tone thresholds. Bilateral low-pitched tinnitus (<1000 Hz) is a common complaint and can be severe enough to affect the quality of life of these individuals.[46] Mechanisms include injury to the inner hair cells and their synapses, the synaptic transmission to spiral ganglion, and neural signal transmission from the auditory nerve to the brainstem. Causal factors in adults include noise exposure, aging,[45] and genetic causes. There are at least 13 genes that affect the synaptic transmission or central auditory signaling pathway, including presynaptic (inner hair cell), postsynaptic spiral ganglion, and the auditory nerve spiral ganglion cell bodies and proximal axons.[47]

Vestibular Schwannomas

Vestibular schwannomas (VSs) are benign slow-growing intracranial tumors of Schwann cells of the vestibulocochlear nerve originating from the internal auditory canal or the cerebellopontine angle. VS has a prevalence of 8% among all intracranial tumors and 90% among cerebellopontine angle and internal auditory canal neoplasms.[48] They are classified in 2 physiologically distinct types: sporadic VS and neurofibromatosis type 2.

Sporadic VSs (90%) are unilateral, usually manifest around age 50 to 55 years, without gender predilection. Patients have progressive unilateral hearing loss and tinnitus that might be associated with facial numbness and facial paralysis, balance problems, and vertigo. Sudden hearing loss is the first clinical presentation in some cases.[49]

Neurofibromatosis type 2 is an autosomal-dominant inherited disorder, which predisposes affected individuals to develop a multiple neoplasm syndrome. It results from mutations in the *NF2* tumor suppressor gene located on chromosome 22q. It mostly occurs in young adulthood (age 20–30 years), with bilateral vestibular nerve schwannomas associated with other tumors of the nervous system, visual problems, skin tumors, and peripheral neuropathy. Initially, hearing loss is often unilateral, and is associated with or preceded by tinnitus. Dizziness and imbalance problems, facial paresthesia, and facial nerve palsy can also occur.[50,51]

Tinnitus and hearing loss are likely caused by compression of the auditory nerve, secondary to spasm or occlusion of the labyrinthine artery and potentially toxic substances secreted by the tumor to the inner ear or the cochlear nerve.[49]

Ménière's Disease

Tinnitus is a cardinal symptom in Ménière's disease (MD), a disorder of the inner ear. A typical clinical picture of MD presents as intermittent episodes of vertigo lasting from minutes to hours, fluctuating hearing loss, tinnitus, and aural fullness.[52] MD is more common among women aged 40 to 50 years. The symptoms are usually unilateral but can become bilateral over time.

Multifactorial factors such as genetics, metabolism, allergies, autoimmune reactions, and stress are associated with the cause of MD. Excessive endolymph accumulation in the cochlea, vestibule, and semicircular canals leads to endolymphatic hydrops, causing damage to the ganglion cells,[53] which causes hearing loss and tinnitus. Usually, tinnitus sounds like low-pitched buzzing.[31,32]

The audiometric curve is characteristic, an up-sloping low-frequency sensorineural hearing loss with better hearing at 2000 Hz and worse hearing at frequencies greater than 2000 Hz. Fluctuations may lead to a flat sensorineural hearing loss.[52]

Vascular Conflict of Cranial Nerve VIII: Typewriter Tinnitus

This characteristic unilateral intermittent tinnitus is a form of tinnitus that occurs when a blood vessel (anterior-inferior cerebellar artery) is in close contact with the auditory nerve at its entrance into the brainstem. Tinnitus is described as sounding like a type-writer, Morse code, or machine-gun. Hearing loss usually manifests at tinnitus frequencies. If the vascular conflict affects the facial and/or the vestibular nerve, associated ipsilateral hemifacial spasms, otalgia, or vertiginous spells might occur.[54] Because typewriter tinnitus responds very well to carbamazepine,[55] the medication response is proposed to be used as diagnostic tool.[56] Tinnitus probably results from hyperactivity in the cochlear nerve generated by the conflict with the artery.[57]

VISUAL SNOW SYNDROME

Visual snow syndrome (VSS) is the perception of continuous television-static–like tiny flickering dots in the entire visual field. Visual snow has been called the tinnitus of the eyes.

Clinical criteria for the definition of VSS have recently been proposed[58]:

1. Visual snow: dynamic, continuous, tiny dots in the entire visual field lasting more than 3 months.
2. Presence of at least 2 additional visual symptoms of the 4 following categories: (1) palinopsia (persistent recurrence of a visual image after the stimulus has been removed); (2) enhanced entoptic phenomena (images produced by the eye's own structures); (3) photophobia; (4) nyctalopia (night blindness).
3. Symptoms are not consistent with typical migraine visual aura.
4. Symptoms are not better explained by another disorder.

There is a high prevalence of bilateral persistent tinnitus among patients with VSS (>60%). Possibly, both disorders share a common pathophysiologic mechanism that could involve thalamocortical loops secondary to dysfunctional neuronal excitability and impaired habituation response.[59]

Other symptoms include migraines, tremors, balance problems, vertigo, and fatigue.[60]

TINNITUS AND THE VESTIBULAR SYSTEM
Vestibular Migraine and Tinnitus

Tinnitus is present in about 46% to 68% of cases of vestibular migraine.[61]

The diagnosis of vestibular migraine is based on an association of recurrent vestibular symptoms that precede, occurs with, or occur after migraine. Symptoms include headache, visual aura, and/or photophobia and phonophobia in at least 50% of the episodes, in the absence of another diagnosis.[62] Vestibular migraine attacks can last from minutes to days.[63]

Fluctuating hearing loss and aural fullness can also be part of the clinical history, with a mild sensorineural hearing loss on the audiogram. Vestibular migraines occur at any time in life, but middle-aged women are the most commonly affected. Episodes might be triggered by stress, lack of sleep, dehydration, certain foods, and physical activity.[61] Among women of childbearing age, attacks are associated with the menstrual cycle.[63] One possible explanation for the presence of tinnitus is that migraine may cause damage in the inner ear secondary to release of neuropeptides such as calcitonin gene–related peptide.[63]

Benign Paroxysmal Positional Vertigo and Tinnitus

Benign paroxysmal positional vertigo (BPPV) is a common peripheral vestibular disorder of the semicircular canals elicited by specific head movements causing recurrent sudden brief vertigo episodes. Most cases result from abnormally displaced otoconia into the semicircular canals producing a false sense of head rotation and nystagmus. The diagnosis is made using provocative maneuvers leading to a distinctive pattern of nystagmus observed in the plane of the affected canal. In general, BPPV is a self-limited condition but it can interfere with daily activities and contribute to the risk of falls in elderly patients.[64]

Tinnitus is associated with the onset of positional vertigo in about 19% of patients affected by BPPV. Tinnitus is intermittent, slightly intense, mostly unilateral, and localized in the same ear as the BPPV, which disappears or decreases immediately or shortly after the repositioning maneuver.[65,66] A possible explanation for this finding was proposed by Barozzi and colleagues[66] in 2013 based on Gussen's[67] previous work. She examined human temporal bones with cochlea-vascular degeneration related to heredity, aging, or viral causes. Otoconial displacement was observed within the ductus reuniens and cochlear duct as far as the basal turn of the cochlear spiral. Tinnitus in BPPV can be triggered by cochlear changes secondary to the presence of displaced otoconia.

SOMATOSENSORY MODULATION OF TINNITUS
Cross-Modal Interaction Among the Sensory Cortex

In their natural environments, humans and animals receive multimodal sensory stimuli. The sensation of external stimuli in the environment is taken to the brain by specialized sensory organs such as the eyes, the ears, or the skin. These inputs are processed in primary sensory cortices, such as the primary auditory cortex, the primary somatosensory cortex, or the visual cortex. Anatomic connections suggest that there is a multimodal functional interaction among sensory cortical regions, which means that they all interact in the brain in order to acquire a faster perception of the external world and its stimuli.

The deprivation of a sensory modality is likely to induce compensatory changes, named cross-modal plasticity.[68] For example, congenitally deaf individuals have superior visual abilities, and blind individuals present better auditory perception. Neurons from the deprived cortex are recruited from another sensory modalities. It has been shown that the auditory cortex can be activated by visual stimuli in deaf individuals. Cross-modal interaction in the presence of sensory deprivation of 1 of the senses is a plastic phenomenon in which the brain often compensates for loss with supranormal performance in 1 or more of the intact sensory systems.

Tinnitus Modulation

A subgroup of patients with tinnitus are able to change their tinnitus perception, intensity pitch, and location as a result of some trigger activity. These changes are mainly evoked with head, jaw, and eye movements or by applying pressure to a muscle in the head, neck, jaws, or a limb,[69,70] and trigger-point palpation.[71] These findings provide more evidence of interactions among the somatosensory and the auditory pathway.

The changes on tinnitus central percept are defined as tinnitus somatosensory modulation and are common among people with tinnitus.

Somatosensory Tinnitus

Somatosensory tinnitus should be suspected when the patient can modulate the loudness or intensity of the tinnitus with eye movements; cutaneous stimulation of skin on the hand region; through movements of the head, neck, and limb; and passive palpation of myofascial trigger points.[69–73]

Somatosensory tinnitus affects people of any age and is not necessarily related to hearing loss and degree of tinnitus severity.[74] Tinnitus can be pulsatile or nonpulsatile and the localization is often associated with the ear ipsilateral to the somatic disorder.[75]

Clinical criteria suggesting the presence of somatic tinnitus have recently been reported,[76] taking into account tinnitus characteristics and associated clinical symptoms. They include:

1. Tinnitus modulation: if movement of the head, neck, jaw, or eyes activates tinnitus modulation, use somatic maneuvers and digital pressure on myofascial trigger point.
2. Tinnitus characteristics: simultaneous appearance or intensification of tinnitus with neck or jaw complaints/pain, trauma, and bad posture.
3. Associated symptoms and signs, such as frequent pain in the cervical spine, head, or shoulder girdle; myofascial trigger points; muscle tension in the suboccipital muscles and extensor muscles of the cervical spine; temporomandibular disorders; bruxism and dental diseases.

Specific maneuvers performed using forceful movements of the head and neck, and eye movements, have been used to evaluate the presence of tinnitus modulation, but their absence does not exclude somatosensory tinnitus.

VASCULAR TINNITUS

Tinnitus associated with vascular structures has a characteristic sound synchronized to the heartbeat, which is produced by the turbulence of blood flow transmitted to the cochlea. The examiner in same cases can also hear it. Changes in tinnitus can be observed during head rotation and on compression of the internal jugular vein. The prevalence of this type of tinnitus is about 4% among people with tinnitus. Tinnitus may be caused by vascular anomalies or variants and is classified according to the site of generation. Some of them are described here; for a comprehensive review, see Sismanis[77] (2003).

Arterial Tinnitus

Atherosclerotic carotid artery disease

Pulsatile tinnitus may be the first manifestation of carotid artery occlusive disease; tinnitus is secondary to bruits produced by the turbulence of the blood flow in the compromised artery. Carotid artery occlusion may result in stroke, neurologic disability, or loss of life. Carotid atherosclerosis is an inflammatory disease that progresses to an eventual rupture of the atherosclerotic plaque. It is more frequent in men more than 50 years old. Risk factors include arterial hypertension, diabetes mellitus, dyslipidemia, cigarette smoking, and hyperhomocysteinemia. It is possible to auscultate a bruit on the carotid during the physical examination; its presence increases the risk of stroke and transient ischemic attacks.[78]

Arteriovenous Tinnitus

Pulsatile tinnitus can also be a clinical manifestation of arteriovenous malformations (AVMs) of the brain, an abnormal tangle of blood vessels connecting arteries and veins, and disrupting normal blood flow and oxygen circulation. Patients with these congenital lesions, which may enlarge over time, are at risk of serious intracerebral hemorrhage, stroke, or brain damage, depending on size and vascular anatomy location. Symptomatic presentation is most commonly intracerebral hemorrhage, focal seizures, neurologic deficits, and headaches. Aggressive therapy is used in most patients with AVMs, even if discovered incidentally.[79]

Depending on the localization, a bruit can also be heard when performing an auscultation on the scalp.

Venous Blood Flow Tinnitus

Idiopathic intracranial hypertension

Idiopathic intracranial hypertension is a syndrome characterized by increased intracranial pressure of unknown cause in the absence of clinical and radiological evidence of intracranial disorder. The mechanism responsible has been suggested to be a dysfunction of the cerebrospinal fluid dynamics caused by various hormonal and metabolic medical conditions and the use of certain medications.[78] Symptoms associated with a pulse beat–synchronous tinnitus include headaches, visual dysfunctions, hearing loss (often low-frequency sensorineural hearing loss), dizziness, aural fullness, and papilledema.[77]

Venous hum

This term is used to describe pulsatile tinnitus of unclear cause. Diagnosis of this condition should be made only after appropriate evaluation and elimination of other disorders.

GENETICS OF TINNITUS

The identification of genetic factors implicated in tinnitus will represent an important development. Candidate genes responsible for tinnitus may provide insights into the pathogenesis, novel gene-based diagnostic approaches, and therapy development.

However, because of the complexity and heterogeneity of tinnitus, genetic research is still in its infancy. As suggested by Lopez-Escamez and colleagues[80] in 2016, a possible methodological approach to advance tinnitus genetic subtyping is to cluster a few variables that could configure a phenotype. For example, a recent twin-cohort study has provided initial evidence that bilateral tinnitus is likely to be influenced by genetic factors and might constitute a genetic subtype.[81]

So far, no specific genetic locus has been identified; tinnitus is probably a polygenic condition. A recent genome-wide association study has identified potential metabolic pathways and has provided new insights into moderate genetic influences for tinnitus.[81,82]

SUMMARY

It is clear that there is not one single type of tinnitus. There are many causes and many different mechanisms. Appreciating and understanding different subtypes will lead to different treatments. This article focuses on identifying some of the different subtypes. It is hoped that clinical trials can focus on specific subtypes, which should increase the likelihood that treatments can be found for some patients with tinnitus.

REFERENCES

1. Tyler RS, Aran JM, Dauman R. Recent advances in tinnitus. Am J Audiol 1992; 1(4):36–44. https://doi.org/10.1044/1059-0889.0104.36.
2. Dauman R, Tyler RS. Some considerations on the classification of tinnitus. In: Aran JM, Dauman R, editors. Proceedings of the fourth international tinnitus seminar. Amsterdam: Kugler Publications; 1992. p. 225–9.
3. Sweeney AD, Carlson ML, Wanna GB, et al. Glomus tympanicum tumors. Otolaryngol Clin North Am 2015;48(2):293–304.
4. Golz A, Fradis M, Netzer A, et al. Stapedius muscle myoclonus. Ann Otol Rhinol Laryngol 2003;112(6):522–4.
5. Fox GN, Baer MT. Palatal myoclonus and tinnitus in children. West J Med 1991; 154(1):98–102.
6. Zipfel TE, Kaza SR, Greene JS. Middle-ear myoclonus. J Laryngol Otol 2000; 114(3):207–9.
7. Pulec JL, Simonton KM. Palatal myoclonus: a report of two cases. Laryngoscope 1961;71(6):668–71.
8. Klochoff I. Impedance fluctuation and a "tensor tympani syndrome." Proceedings of the 4th International Symposium on Acoustic Measurements. Lisbon, September 25-28,1979, Universidad Nova de Lisboa Ed Penha & Pizarro. 69–76.
9. Noreña AJ, Fournier P, Londero A, et al. An integrative model accounting for the symptom cluster triggered after an acoustic shock. Trends Hear 2018;22. 2331216518801725.
10. Pau HW, Punke C, Zehlicke T, et al. Tonic contractions of the tensor tympani muscle: a key to some non-specific middle ear symptoms? Hypothesis and data from temporal bone experiments. Acta Otolaryngol 2005;125(11):1168–75.
11. Bance M, Makki FM, Garland P, et al. Effects of tensor tympani muscle contraction on the middle ear and markers of a contracted muscle. Laryngoscope 2013; 123(4):1021–7.
12. Wickens B, Floyd D, Bance M. Audiometric findings with voluntary tensor tympani contraction. J Otolaryngol Head Neck Surg 2017;46(1):2.
13. Houser DS, Yost W, Burkard R, et al. A review of the history, development and application of auditory weighting functions in humans and marine mammals. J Acoust Soc Am 2017;141(3):1371.
14. Kurata N, Schachern PA, Paparella MM, et al. Histopathologic evaluation of vascular findings in the cochlea in patients with presbycusis. JAMA Otolaryngol Neck Surg 2016;142(2):173–8.
15. Bainbridge KE, Hoffman HJ, Cowie CC. Risk factors for hearing impairment among U.S. adults with diabetes: National Health and Nutrition Examination Survey 1999-2004. Diabetes Care 2011;34(7):1540–5.
16. Frisina ST, Mapes F, Kim S, et al. Characterization of hearing loss in aged type II diabetics. Hear Res 2006;211(1):103–13.
17. Devdhar M, Ousman YH, Burman KD. Hypothyroidism. Endocrinol Metab Clin North Am 2007;36(3):595–615, v.
18. Bhatia PL, Gupta OP, Agrawal MK, et al. Audiological and vestibular function tests in hypothyroidism. Laryngoscope 1977;87(12):2082–9.
19. Olzowy B, Canis M, Hempel J-M, et al. Effect of atorvastatin on progression of sensorineural hearing loss and tinnitus in the elderly: results of a prospective, randomized, double-blind clinical trial. Otol Neurotol 2007;28(4):455–8.
20. Broadway-Duren JB, Klaassen H. Anemias. Crit Care Nurs Clin North Am 2013; 25(4):411–26.

21. Sunwoo W, Lee DY, Lee JY, et al. Characteristics of tinnitus found in anemia patients and analysis of population-based survey. Auris Nasus Larynx 2018;45(6):1152–8.
22. Schieffer KM, Chuang CH, Connor J, et al. Association of iron deficiency anemia with hearing loss in US adults. JAMA Otolaryngol Neck Surg 2017;143(4):350–4.
23. Shemesh Z, Attias J, Ornan M, et al. Vitamin B12 deficiency in patients with chronic-tinnitus and noise-induced hearing loss. Am J Otolaryngol 1993;14(2):94–9.
24. Houston DK, Johnson MA, Nozza RJ, et al. Age-related hearing loss, vitamin B-12, and folate in elderly women. Am J Clin Nutr 1999;69(3):564–71.
25. Ikeda K, Kobayashi T, Itoh Z, et al. Evaluation of vitamin D metabolism in patients with bilateral sensorineural hearing loss. Am J Otol 1989;10(1):11–3.
26. Lasisi AO, Fehintola FA, Yusuf OB. Age-related hearing loss, vitamin B12, and folate in the elderly. Otolaryngol Head Neck Surg 2010;143(6):826–30.
27. Ochi K, Kinoshita H, Kenmochi M, et al. Zinc deficiency and tinnitus. Auris Nasus Larynx 2003;30(Suppl):S25–8.
28. Coelho C, Witt SA, Ji H, et al. Zinc to treat tinnitus in the elderly: a randomized placebo controlled crossover trial. Otol Neurotol 2013;34(6):1146–54.
29. Berkiten G, Kumral TL, Yıldırım G, et al. Effects of serum zinc level on tinnitus. Am J Otolaryngol 2015;36(2):230–4.
30. Uluyol S, Kılıçaslan S, Yağız Ö. Relationship between serum magnesium level and subjective tinnitus. Kulak Burun Bogaz Ihtis Derg 2016;26(4):225–7.
31. Nicolas-Puel C, Faulconbridge RL, Guitton M, et al. Characteristics of tinnitus and etiology of associated hearing loss: a study of 123 patients. Int Tinnitus J 2002;8(1):37–44.
32. Pan T, Tyler RS, Ji H, et al. The relationship between tinnitus pitch and the audiogram. Int J Audiol 2009;48(5):277–94.
33. Noreña AJ, Eggermont JJ. Changes in spontaneous neural activity immediately after an acoustic trauma: implications for neural correlates of tinnitus. Hear Res 2003;183(1):137–53.
34. Lawton BW. Audiometric findings in call centre workers exposed to acoustic shock. Proc Inst Acoust 2003;25:10.
35. Westcott M. Acoustic shock injury (ASI). Acta Otolaryngol 2006;126(sup556):54–8.
36. McFerran DJ, Baguley DM. Acoustic shock. J Laryngol Otol 2007;121(4):301–5.
37. Hooper RE. Acoustic shock controversies. J Laryngol Otol 2014;128(Suppl 2):S2–9.
38. Chandrasekhar SS, Tsai Do BS, Schwartz SR, et al. Clinical practice guideline: sudden hearing loss (update). Otolaryngol Neck Surg 2019;161(1_suppl):S1–45.
39. Schuknecht HF, Donovan ED. The pathology of idiopathic sudden sensorineural hearing loss. Arch Otorhinolaryngol 1986;243(1):1–15.
40. Chen J, Liang J, Ou J, et al. Mental health in adults with sudden sensorineural hearing loss: an assessment of depressive symptoms and its correlates. J Psychosom Res 2013;75(1):72–4.
41. Danino J, Joachims HZ, Eliachar I, et al. Tinnitus as a prognostic factor in sudden deafness. Am J Otolaryngol 1984;5(6):394–6.
42. Rauch SD. Clinical management of immune-mediated inner-ear disease. Ann N Y Acad Sci 1997;830(1):203–10.
43. George DL, Pradhan S. Idiopathic sensorineural hearing disorders in adults–a pragmatic approach. Nat Rev Rheumatol 2009;5(9):505–12.
44. Lanvers Kaminsky C, Zehnhoff Dinnesen A, Parfitt R, et al. Drug-induced ototoxicity: mechanisms, pharmacogenetics, and protective strategies. Clinical

pharmacology & therapeutics. 2017. Available at: https://ascpt.onlinelibrary. wiley.com/doi/abs/10.1002/cpt.603. Accessed November 10, 2019.

45. Moser T, Starr A. Auditory neuropathy — neural and synaptic mechanisms. Nat Rev Neurol 2016;12(3):135–49.

46. Prabhu P. Is tinnitus a major concern in individuals with auditory neuropathy spectrum disorder? – Questionnaire based study. World J Otorhinolaryngol Head Neck Surg 2019;5(1):1–5.

47. Shearer AE, Hansen MR. Auditory synaptopathy, auditory neuropathy, and cochlear implantation. Laryngoscope Investig Otolaryngol 2019;4(4):429–40.

48. Carlson ML, Link MJ, Wanna GB, et al. Management of sporadic vestibular schwannoma. Otolaryngol Clin North Am 2015;48(3):407–22.

49. Kaul V, Cosetti MK. Management of vestibular schwannoma (Including NF2): facial nerve considerations. Otolaryngol Clin North Am 2018;51(6):1193–212.

50. Evans DGR. Chapter 5 - neurofibromatosis type 2. In: Islam MP, Roach ES, editors. Handbook of clinical neurology, vol. 132. Waltham (MA): Elsevier; 2015. p. 87–96.

51. Asthagiri AR, Parry DM, Butman JA, et al. Neurofibromatosis type 2. Lancet 2009; 373(9679):1974–86.

52. Sajjadi H, Paparella MM. Meniere's disease. Lancet 2008;372(9636):406–14.

53. Nakashima T, Pyykkö I, Arroll MA, et al. Meniere's disease. Nat Rev Dis Primers 2016;2:16028.

54. De Ridder D, Heijneman K, Haarman B, et al. Tinnitus in vascular conflict of the eighth cranial nerve: a surgical pathophysiological approach to ABR changes. Prog Brain Res 2007;166:401–11.

55. Levine RA. Typewriter tinnitus: a carbamazepine-responsive syndrome related to auditory nerve vascular compression. ORL J Otorhinolaryngol Relat Spec 2006; 68(1):43–6 [discussion: 46–7].

56. Sunwoo W, Jeon YJ, Bae YJ, et al. Typewriter tinnitus revisited: The typical symptoms and the initial response to carbamazepine are the most reliable diagnostic clues. Sci Rep 2017;7(1):10615.

57. De Ridder D, Vanneste S, Adriaensens I, et al. Vascular compression of the cochlear nerve and tinnitus: a pathophysiological investigation. Acta Neurochir (Wien) 2012;154(5):807–13.

58. Puledda F, Schankin C, Goadsby PJ. Visual snow syndrome: a clinical and phenotypical description of 1,100 cases. Neurology 2020. https://doi.org/10. 1212/WNL.0000000000008909.

59. Lauschke JL, Plant GT, Fraser CL. Visual snow: a thalamocortical dysrhythmia of the visual pathway? J Clin Neurosci 2016;28:123–7.

60. Bou Ghannam A, Pelak VS. Visual snow: a potential cortical hyperexcitability syndrome. Curr Treat Options Neurol 2017;19(3):9.

61. Abouzari M, Goshtasbi K, Moshtaghi O, et al. Association between vestibular migraine and migraine headache: yet to explore. Otol Neurotol 2019. https:// doi.org/10.1097/MAO.0000000000002528.

62. Lempert T, Olesen J, Furman J, et al. Vestibular migraine: diagnostic criteria. J Vestib Res 2012;22(4):167–72.

63. Furman JM, Balaban CD. Vestibular migraine. Ann N Y Acad Sci 2015; 1343(1):90–6.

64. Bhattacharyya N, Gubbels SP, Schwartz SR, et al. Clinical practice guideline: benign paroxysmal positional vertigo (update) executive summary. Otolaryngol Neck Surg 2017;156(3):403–16.

65. Gavalas GJ, Passou EM, Vathilakis JM. Tinnitus of vestibular origin. Scand Audiol Suppl 2001;(52):185–6.
66. Barozzi S, Socci M, Ginocchio D, et al. Benign paroxysmal positional vertigo and tinnitus. Int Tinnitus J 2013;18(1):16–9.
67. Gussen R. Saccule otoconia displacement into cochlea in cochleosaccular degeneration. Arch Otolaryngol 1980;106(3):161–6.
68. Bavelier D, Neville HJ. Cross-modal plasticity: where and how? Nat Rev Neurosci 2002;3(6):443–52.
69. Cacace AT, Lovely TJ, McFarland DJ, et al. Anomalous cross-modal plasticity following posterior fossa surgery: some speculations on gaze-evoked tinnitus. Hear Res 1994;81(1–2):22–32.
70. Levine RA. Somatic (craniocervical) tinnitus and the dorsal cochlear nucleus hypothesis. Am J Otolaryngol 1999;20(6):351–62.
71. Rocha CACB, Sanchez TG, de Siqueira JTT. Myofascial trigger point: a possible way of modulating tinnitus. Audiol Neurotol 2008;13(3):153–60.
72. Simmons R, Dambra C, Lobarinas E, et al. Head, neck, and eye movements that modulate tinnitus. Semin Hear 2008;29(4):361–70.
73. Sanchez TG, Kii MA. Modulating tinnitus with visual, muscular, and tactile stimulation. Semin Hear 2008;29(04):350–60.
74. Ward J, Vella C, Hoare DJ, et al. Subtyping somatic tinnitus: a cross-sectional UK cohort study of demographic, clinical and audiological characteristics. PLoS One 2015;10(5):e0126254.
75. Levine RA, Nam E-C, Melcher J. Somatosensory pulsatile tinnitus syndrome: somatic testing identifies a pulsatile tinnitus subtype that implicates the somatosensory system. Trends Amplif 2008;12(3):242–53.
76. Michiels S, Ganz Sanchez T, Oron Y, et al. Diagnostic criteria for somatosensory tinnitus: a delphi process and face-to-face meeting to establish consensus. Trends Hear 2018;22. 2331216518796403.
77. Sismanis A. Pulsatile tinnitus. Otolaryngol Clin North Am 2003;36(2):389–402.
78. Bhattacharya P, Chaturvedi S. Chapter 80 - carotid artery disease. In: Caplan LR, Biller J, Leary MC, et al, editors. Primer on cerebrovascular diseases. 2nd edition. San Diego (CA): Academic Press; 2017. p. 388–92. https://doi.org/10.1016/B978-0-12-803058-5.00080-1.
79. Graham GD. Arteriovenous malformations in the brain. Curr Treat Options Neurol 2002;4(6):435–44.
80. Lopez-Escamez JA, Bibas T, Cima RFF, et al. Genetics of tinnitus: an emerging area for molecular diagnosis and drug development. Front Neurosci 2016;10. https://doi.org/10.3389/fnins.2016.00377.
81. Maas IL, Brüggemann P, Requena T, et al. Genetic susceptibility to bilateral tinnitus in a Swedish twin cohort. Genet Med 2017;19(9):1007–12.
82. Bogo R, Farah A, Karlsson KK, et al. Prevalence, incidence proportion, and heritability for tinnitus: a longitudinal twin study. Ear Hear 2017;38(3):292–300.

Noise
Acoustic Trauma to the Inner Ear

Ronna Hertzano, MD, PhD[a,b,c], Erika L. Lipford, BSc[a],
Didier Depireux, PhD[a,d],*

KEYWORDS

- Tinnitus • Noise trauma • Hearing loss • Hidden hearing loss
- Temporary threshold shift • Permanent threshold shift

KEY POINTS

- There are different types of hearing loss: temporary, hidden, and permanent hearing loss.
- All types of hearing loss are associated with tinnitus. It is likely that all tinnitus are associated with some form of hearing loss.
- Predicting the severity of noise-induced hearing loss from the noise exposure (whether sudden or lifelong) is complex.
- Furthermore, the relationship between the tinnitus perceived by the patient and the characteristics of the hearing loss is currently poorly understood.

INTRODUCTION
Hearing Loss and Tinnitus are Closely Associated

(Subjective) Tinnitus is a symptom of many possible underlying causes (Claudia Barros Coelho and colleagues' article, "Classification of Tinnitus: Multiple Etiologies with the Same Name," in this issue), with the generative source of tinnitus (if there is a localized one) serving as an active topic of fundamental animal research.[1] In humans, particularly those with distressing tinnitus, the heterogeneity observed indicates that in all likelihood, there are a variety of mechanisms that give rise to the percept of tinnitus.[2,3] Indeed, multiple mechanisms are likely at work within one individual, and if a specific event such as trauma led to tinnitus, it is plausible that the mechanisms giving rise to the tinnitus acutely following the initial traumatic event differ from the ones responsible for the chronic percept of tinnitus.[4]

Tinnitus itself is not a disease but rather a symptom of an underlying condition that can be classified into subtypes based on its many causes. For nonchemically induced

[a] Department of Otorhinolaryngology Head and Neck Surgery, University of Maryland School of Medicine, Baltimore, MD, USA; [b] Anatomy and Neurobiology, University of Maryland School of Medicine, Baltimore, MD, USA; [c] Institute for Genome Sciences, University of Maryland School of Medicine, Baltimore, MD, USA; [d] R&D OtolithLabs, Washington, DC, USA
* Corresponding author. 1875 Connecticut Avenue Northwest, Washington, DC20009.
E-mail address: depireux@gmail.com

Otolaryngol Clin N Am 53 (2020) 531–542
https://doi.org/10.1016/j.otc.2020.03.008
0030-6665/20/© 2020 Elsevier Inc. All rights reserved.

tinnitus associated with exposure to loud noises, blast wave injury, Ménière disease, or simply aging, sensorineural hearing loss is a common denominator. Tinnitus is also often associated with conductive hearing loss resulting from recurrent ear infections, chronic serous otitis media, otosclerosis, perforated tympanic membranes, or even cerumen impaction (ear wax build-up). Less commonly, tinnitus develops following head injury, circulatory system changes such as anemia and high blood pressure, vestibular schwannoma, diabetes, thyroid disorders, and many other conditions.

Chemical induction is equally prevalent, with tinnitus being the most commonly reported side effect mentioned in response to prescribed medicine, arising when patients start (eg, nonsteroidal anti-inflammatory drugs) or even stop taking a medication (benzodiazepines). In cases of particularly ototoxic medications such as cisplatin, more than 90% of patients will acquire hearing loss over some frequency range (typically the higher frequencies) and develop the associated tinnitus by the third round of chemotherapy treatment.[5–8] As detailed in a later article (Fatima T. Husain's article, "Perception of, and Reaction to, Tinnitus: The depression factor," in this issue), certain factors such as stress and anxiety negatively enhance the reaction to the tinnitus, with this tinnitus reaction being exacerbated by exposure to certain medications, head injury, and particularly in those with depression.[9]

In this article, the authors focus primarily on trauma-induced tinnitus, and in particular noise-induced tinnitus, whether acute or chronic. Indeed, "tinnitus induction by acoustic trauma is most likely the most common form observed in the human patient."[10] As the presence of tinnitus is associated with hearing loss, with age being the main predictor of its prevalence in the adult population in the United States,[11] age-related hearing loss and tinnitus go hand-in-hand. The earliest well-established theory considers tinnitus to be the perceptual consequence of neuronal hyperactivity in the central auditory system, emerging after loss of the neural input from the ear to the brain that would be expected from a healthy inner ear.

Although we do not yet understand the neural origins of tinnitus, it is clear that tinnitus often develops in multiple phases. In the case of trauma to the inner ear resulting from noise exposure, the early phase of tinnitus may be directly related to damage sustained by the structures of the inner ear itself, whereas over a period of a few days, the main correlate of the tinnitus might shift to a locus in the central nervous system (CNS).[12–15] In animals, evidence for changes in neural activity associated with tinnitus immediately following noise trauma can be seen within an hour of trauma in cats[3] and a few hours in hamsters.[16]

Therapeutic developments for tinnitus would greatly benefit from a comprehensive understanding of the neural origins and pathologic evolution of tinnitus. However, this goal has been confounded by evidence suggesting that patients could have tinnitus in the absence of hearing deficits as measured by standard audiogram.[17,18] This challenges the widely accepted view of tinnitus as being initiated via impairment in cochlear function, which leads to hyperactivity in the relevant CNS structures.[19–22] Because cochlear damage is usually thought to result in an initial elevation of hearing thresholds, as measured through the standard audiogram, absence of any clear deficit in cochlear function was believed to indicate that hearing loss of peripheral origin and tinnitus, while often comorbid, could arise independently from each other.[17,18] More recent research has indicated that in fact, all subjective tinnitus are likely associated with hearing loss, although not always apparent from the standard audiogram. Data have shown that normal hearing thresholds do not necessarily indicate absence of cochlear damage. Following mild acoustic trauma, mice can exhibit only a temporary threshold shift in hearing together with a permanent deafferentation of approximately 50% of the auditory nerve fibers (albeit in the high-frequency region of the cochlea[23]).

Thus, if a sufficient population of low-threshold auditory nerve fibers remains responsive to sound, the audiogram can present as normal, even when hearing is not. Conversely, impaired function of efferent fibers (from brainstem to cochlea) can still be associated with normal thresholds.[24,25]

Further investigation by Schaette and McAlpine showed that humans with tinnitus and otherwise normal audiograms, extended to 16 kHz, indeed had a deficit in auditory nerve function manifested as a reduction in nerve output at high sound levels, indicating deafferentation of high-threshold auditory nerve fibers.[26] This deficit seems to be compensated for at the level of the brainstem, supporting the view that tinnitus is promoted by homeostatic mechanisms that act to normalize levels of neural activity in the central auditory system.

DIFFERENT TYPES OF HEARING LOSS

Mounting evidence implicates tinnitus as an indicator of underlying auditory deficits, however mild these deficits might be. It has become appreciated that certain types of hearing deficits not revealed by a standard audiogram might be compensated for by a maladaptive mechanism within the central auditory pathways leading to the perception of tinnitus.[27,28] This takes us from the former concept of "some form of hearing loss is associated with tinnitus" to a picture in which "tinnitus is a symptom of a form of hearing loss." As such, the authors briefly summarize their understanding of hearing loss, in particular noise-induced hearing loss (NIHL), the most commonly studied form of hearing loss in animal models.

In animals, NIHL presents as a continuum of 3 main forms of damage with escalating severity, where the transition from one type to another can depend on relatively small changes in the duration and the intensity of the sound exposure, as well as the structure of the sound (eg, gaussian vs nongaussian).

- The mildest form of NIHL is defined by a temporary decrease in the sensitivity to sound, referred to as temporary threshold shift (TTS). In TTS, the sensitivity to sound is initially impaired within a day, and by definition, returns to baseline within a week from exposure. Research on animal models indicates this type of hearing loss does not result in a loss of the sensory hair cells of the inner ear, although its exact molecular underpinnings are only partially understood.[29,30]
- Next on the continuum is hidden hearing loss (HHL). HHL, in addition to the temporary loss of hearing sensitivity seen in TTS, is characterized by a permanent loss of neural connections from a subgroup of afferent (sensory) neurons located in the center of the cochlea called spiral ganglion type I sensory neurons, which carry information from the inner hair cells to the cochlear nucleus of the brainstem.[31] Although type I sensory neurons relay information from the inner hair cells to the cochlear nucleus, they are divided into at least 3 subgroups based on their spontaneous rate and relative sensitivity to sound (designated as type Ia–Ic). The neurons presumed to be involved in HHL consist primarily of type Ic afferent neurons, characterized by a high threshold of response to sounds and a low spontaneous rate of activity. Noise exposure causes retraction of the neural processes of these neurons from their associated hair cells. In consequence, their loss, while leaving hearing thresholds unchanged, results in significant functional impairment that manifests as a decreased ability to resolve speech in the presence of competing noise, hence the name "hidden" hearing loss.[32] By convention, at least in animal models, no loss of hair cells is seen in noise exposures that result in TTS/HHL. The situation is likely the same in humans, with

evidence of deafferentation of the human inner hair cells, in temporal bones, with aging and noise.[33–35]

- At the end of the NIHL continuum is the permanent threshold shift (PTS)-inducing noise exposure, which results in both the loss of neuronal connections as well as a permanent loss of sensitivity to sound.[29,36] Depending on the severity and structure of the noise exposure, the damage in the cochlea following a PTS-inducing noise exposure may vary considerably, from loss of outer hair cells, to significant disruption in the integrity of the organ of Corti.[37,38]

Note that in addition to the loss of neural connections mentioned earlier, which can result in a reduced transmission of information from the cochlea to the brain, it has been shown that in rats, there can be up to 30% damage to the outer hair cells before any hearing loss is detectable using compound action potential threshold.[39]

NOISE PARAMETERS DO NOT ALWAYS PREDICT PATTERN OF HEARING DEFICITS

The type and severity of the NIHL (TTS/HHL/PTS) depends on a combination of extrinsic and intrinsic factors. Extrinsic factors principally depend on the intensity, frequency, and duration of the exposure to sound, although other poorly understood factors such as sound statistics likely have an impact. Intrinsic factors are more complex and include circadian changes to gene expression,[40] cortisol levels,[41] genetic factors,[42] and sex hormones among others.[36,43,44] Small changes in intrinsic or extrinsic factors can dramatically influence the outcomes of a noise exposure. For example, a difference of 2 dB in the intensity of a long duration sound exposure can determine whether a subject will sustain HHL or PTS (a change of 2 dB corresponds roughly to an increase of sound power by 60%).

It is also worth noting that different areas within the cochlea may sustain different types of damage from a single traumatic noise exposure. For example, a midfrequency high-intensity noise exposure can result in a PTS in the midfrequencies, HHL in the high frequencies, and only a TTS in the lower frequencies. It is therefore impossible to anticipate the type of damage and the associated tinnitus that will result from noise exposure and trauma, as a patient can exhibit a combination of all 3 types of hearing impairment. Thus, any treatment, pharmacologic or otherwise, will need to mitigate the hearing threshold shifts in all forms of NIHL, as well as reverse or prevent the loss of synapses in both HHL and PTS. It is possible that this dual pattern of hearing loss (midfrequencies and high frequencies in response to a midfrequency noise exposure) is at play in aging and partially accounts for the universal loss of high-frequency hearing in all humans' experience.

HYPERACUSIS AND RECRUITMENT

Both hyperacusis and recruitment are often associated with tinnitus and must be considered when developing therapeutic strategies.[45–47] Hyperacusis is defined by a lowered threshold to discomfort from sound, wherein sounds perceived as loud by normal hearing persons are instead perceived as painfully loud by the hyperacusis patient. The comorbidity of tinnitus and hyperacusis seems somewhat paradoxial at first glance, as the patient typically does not perceive the constant subjective tinnitus sound to be painful. However, sounds perceived as tinnitus and the pain related to hyperacusis likely arise from separate pathways,[48] with the perception of pain carried by a small subset of neurons in the auditory nerve.[49]

In contrast, recruitment is characterized as a rapid growth in the perceived loudness of sound that is incongruent with the relatively small increase in sound level that actually occurs. Although the physiologic correlate of these two distinct conditions is unclear, the resulting hypersensitivity to sounds can lead to a challenge in alleviating the associated tinnitus, particularly for patients whose tinnitus is reduced by sound stimulation such as hearing aids or devices that offer different levels of sound therapy (LaGuinn P. Sherlock and David J. Eisenman's article, "Current Device-Based Clinical Treatments for Tinnitus," in this issue) Patients with hyperacusis, recruitment, or other forms of sound sensitivity may encounter some discomfort when using sound amplifying devices.

SYNAPTOPATHY, ENDOCOCHLEAR POTENTIAL LOSS, AND OTHER UNMEASURED DEFICITS

The endocochlear potential is a positive electrical potential present in the central part of the cochlear duct called the scala media. The value of this potential, measured in the endolymphatic fluid that fills the scala media, varies between +80 mV and +120 mV along the length of the cochlear duct. It is an essential driving force within the cochlea, allowing for the initial transduction of the acoustic signals into an electrical/neural signal, via a driving force that generates an electrical gradient between the positive potential of the fluid that bathes the stereociliae of the hair cells (+80 to +120 mV) and the negative potential inside the apical part of the hair cells (−45 mV). The physical acoustic signal propagating along the cochlear duct leads to mechanical oscillations of the stereociliae, which lead to the opening and closing of ionic channels in the stereociliae. The large electric potential across the boundary between endolymph and the inside of the hair cells drives rapid ionic fluxes into the hair cells, eventually leading to the "mechanotransduction" of sounds into neural signals via the hair cells.

Although there is no directly measured correlation between a change in endocochlear potential and the emergence of tinnitus, it is thought that large variations in endocochlear potential might be an important contributing factor: in the healthy inner ear, the highly positive endocochlear potential is achieved by maintaining a high endolymph concentration of potassium (K+), which is associated with higher auditory nerve spontaneous activity.[50] The outer hair cells of the cochlea can modify the endocochlear potential via mechanoelectrical transduction channel opening. Acute noise trauma reduces the opening probability of these channels, leading to a temporary increase in the endocochlear potential.[51,52] The associated increase in endocochlear potential can depolarize the inner hair cells and, through a somewhat complicated cascade of events, cause a fusion of the synaptic ribbon to the plasmatic membrane, an increased release of glutamate, and depolarization of the associated nerve fibers.[53] This may lead to a subsequent increase in the spontaneous rate of activity of the corresponding auditory nerve fibers lasting a few days. Conversely, a decrease of the endocochlear potential, such as the decrease that may occur weeks after cochlear injury, results in a decreased electromotive driving force and therefore a hearing threshold shift. In PTS, these shifts are associated with chronic tinnitus.

As mentioned earlier, there are indications that tinnitus is always associated with a hearing loss, although in some cases it is an HHL. Noise exposure or aging can lead to a permanent loss of some synapses between the hair cells and the cochlear nerve fibers.[54,55] Following even a relatively mild noise trauma then, a rapid and excessive release of the neurotransmitter glutamate from ribbon synapses in the inner hair cells causes a partial disconnection/retraction of the afferent neurons to the inner hair cells.

Although some neural terminals can re-form a functional connection with the hair cells, thus restoring hearing to a level corresponding to individuals' recovering hearing thresholds[56] and tinnitus disappearing in the days following a comparatively higher level sound exposure, sometimes it is thought that the neural reconnection is incomplete. As mentioned in the description of the different types of hearing loss (particularly HHL), this mechanism seems to preferentially affect low spontaneous rate auditory nerve fibers, which are the neurons responsible for coding moderate-to-high sound levels.[31] Another possible mechanism includes the loss of the Schwann cells closest to the synapse, impairing the early part of the transmission of the neural signal from the cochlea to the brain.[57] In either case, this incomplete reconnection or damage to the synapse or reduced transmission of neural information to the brain may result in tinnitus, even in patients with a normal audiogram.

PARAMETERS

In the United States, guidelines have been designed to determine a safe daily exposure to noise to minimize the risks for hearing loss over a lifetime. Exposure is estimated on a daily exposure basis, averaged using a time-weighted method (TWA) detailed on the Websites of the cognizant agency. It is measured on a dBA scale. This "A-weighting" is a frequency-dependent curve that is applied to the physical sound pressure levels (SPL) measured to mimic the effects of human hearing, for instance the fact that our hearing is poor above 70 Hz and is nonexistent above 20 kHz. The US Department of Labor's Occupational Safety and Health Administration (OSHA) guidelines set legal limits on noise exposure in the workplace. OSHA's "Permissible Exposure Limit" is 90 dBA for all workers based on a worker's TWA over an 8-hour day, whereas the Center for Disease Control and Prevention's National Institute for Occupational Safety and Health "Recommended Exposure Limit" for occupational noise exposure is 85 dBA, as an 8-hour TWA. Exposures at or greater than this level are considered hazardous to hearing.

However, no such guidelines exist to predict lifetime noise exposures that might lead to tinnitus. A few experiments were conducted in humans, exposing small groups of volunteers to what is now considered traumatic sounds. Exposure to a 1/3 octave, 110 dB SPL for 5 minutes noise band, induced tinnitus in 75% of (previously) normal-hearing subjects.[58,59] Impulse noise from assault rifles,[60,61] from airbag deployment,[62] or associated with sudden sensorineural hearing loss were also shown to be strongly associated with tinnitus.[63]

Although the noise exposure is generally well controlled in animal studies (although this is not necessarily the case in the animal facilities where animals are often assumed to be recovering in quiet, a likely confounding factor in many studies[64]), the parameters used to induce behavioral evidence of tinnitus through acoustic trauma are quite variable. Typically, a high-level noise stimulus is applied for 1 to 2 hours, under anesthesia or not, either to one or both ears. Focusing on the rat, a typical stimulation paradigm consists of an octave-band noise with a peak intensity of 116 dB SPL centered at 16 kHz for 1 hour.[65] However, sound level (80 dB SPL –130 dB SPL), duration (2 min–7 hours), frequency (2 kHz –22 kHz), and frequency range (pure tones to broadband noise) vary significantly between studies. Given the large variability, no clear rule of thumb emerges as to which *combination* of parameters consistently leads to tinnitus, and in the case of blast-wave–induced tinnitus, parameters might be even harder to quantify. Despite uncertainty on the exact parameters, these studies indicate that the reliable emergence of noise-induced tinnitus will depend on a yet-to-be-determined function of intensity, spectrum, duration, and statistics of the traumatic stimulus.

Additional "modulators" of this function will include sex or gender and stressor factors.[36,43]

If the characteristics of the noise exposure (intensity, spectrum, duration) can be used to predict the pattern of the resulting audiologic threshold shifts, then it should be possible to predict the patients' tinnitus percept ("What does your tinnitus sound like?") that would correspond to the shifted audiogram. In several early human experiments previously mentioned, some rules were consistently observed, such as the fact that when subjected to pure tone trauma, the participants' tinnitus was half an octave greater than the frequency of trauma.[66] Unfortunately, more general rules regarding the relationship between hearing deficits as measured by an audiogram and the tinnitus percept, even for stable losses associated with PTS, are ambiguous and rarely linear. This is no doubt due in part to the fact that high-frequency (human) audiometric data are usually very sparse above 4 kHz. If subjects have a perception of pitch to their tinnitus, about three-quarters of these subjects report it as being greater than 8 kHz, limiting the actual scope of many studies that never measured the audiogram densely enough, if at all, around the tinnitus frequency. The consistent finding is that tinnitus pitch, if it is perceived, generally falls within the area of hearing loss, with the strongest predictor of tinnitus pitch being the degree of hearing loss or location along the frequency axis of deepest hearing loss.[67,68] However, it should be noted that other researchers have found a "lack of reliability," with the pitch match to a pure tone being quite variable on repeated measures, often spanning a range of 2 to 3 octaves.[69]

CENTRAL ISSUES ASSOCIATED WITH HEARING LOSS

It is likely that an acute trauma to the cochlea leads to hearing loss, decreasing the neural input to the CNS. For instance, it is known that even normal hearing volunteers who wore silicone earplugs for 7 days to simulate a temporary hearing loss developed tinnitus in that short timescale, although the tinnitus resolved after removing the earplug.[70] It is thought that a sudden reduction in part of the cochlear output may be compensated for by a change in the neural gain of neurons along the auditory pathway, resulting in increased spontaneous neural activity. Thus, localized cochlear injury/trauma manifested as synaptopathy, hair cell loss/dysfunction, or a significant change of endocochlear potential results in a location- or frequency-specific decrease in the activity of part of the auditory nerve. Upregulation of activity in the central auditory pathway is a compensatory effort to counteract the lack of signals in that particular frequency region. This, possibly coupled with other factors such as increased synchrony across neighboring auditory nerve fibers, may underlie the initial induction of tinnitus. This gain increase leads to the perception of a continuous sound and may also underlie the hyperacusis often associated with chronic noise-induced tinnitus.[71,72]

It might be helpful to think of the frequently used analogy between the pathophysiology of tinnitus and that of pain and phantom limb perception.[73] It has been noted that[74] (1) pain and tinnitus can arise from a great variety of lesions; (2) there is no one specific mechanism for pain perception; (3) pain is a subjective phenomenon that is difficult to quantify; and (4) treatment of pain symptoms is difficult and often ineffective. The analogy between chronic pain and tinnitus is particularly apt with respect to their acute peripheral generation and their chronic central persistence once the acute injury has resolved or at least stabilized. Chronic pain is often a consequence of peripheral injury, in which the initial injury does not typically account for the sustained nature of the pain. Similarly, although tinnitus is often associated with peripheral cochlear dysfunction, that dysfunction may not account for the sustained and distressing tinnitus perception. The consequent large variation between individual experiences of pain makes the development of effective therapy difficult.

Although, in this article, for lack of space, the authors have not touched on the importance of the interactions between the somatosensory system and tinnitus, they briefly mention that in an important segment of the tinnitus population, nonauditory networks also involved in chronic pain (perception, salience, distress) are implicated.[75] These networks might be involved in the maintenance of the perception of tinnitus even once the initial tinnitus triggering event has resolved.[76] Phantom pain and phantom sound perception might share the same basic underlying mechanisms, wherein the maladaptive cortical activity in the auditory cortex becomes a conscious percept by the larger brain networks located in the frontal and parietal areas of cortex, such as "self-awareness" and "salience network." The latter network intersects with the central autonomic control system and affects the limbic–auditory and somatosensory interactions, which are indispensable for consciously maintaining the phantom perception. This perception may become associated with distress, simultaneously activating distress networks located in anterior cingulate cortex, anterior insula, and amygdala.[75,76]

SUMMARY

There are many types of hearing loss; the broad categories being conductive hearing loss, sensorineural hearing loss (itself divided into temporary, hidden, and permanent), and hearing loss of central origin. All indications are that tinnitus, when not caused directly by a CNS issue (eg, stroke), is always associated with one or more forms of hearing loss. On the one hand, this strong comorbidity indicates that, although medical treatment of tinnitus might exist, it is unlikely there will a cure for tinnitus independently of a cure for hearing loss. On the other hand, it points to tinnitus potentially being an early symptom of an underlying auditory injury before measurable audiometric changes.

Be that as it may, the relationship between the characteristics of the hearing loss (for instance the shape of the audiogram) and the tinnitus percept (its pitch if any and its perceived spectrum and localization) does not follow any clear rules. Also, although tinnitus is intimately linked with peripheral cochlear dysfunction, cochlear damage does not account for the sustained and sometimes distressing nature of tinnitus perception, and in particular it does not account for the reaction of the patient to the tinnitus.

A lot of progress has been made in understanding the events that lead to hearing loss and its associated tinnitus from noise exposure, whether sudden and traumatic or resulting from a lifelong exposure to noise, but much more has yet to be observed, learned, and understood before we can hope to have a cure for hearing loss in all its forms and the associated tinnitus.

DISCLOSURE

This work was supported by grants from NIDCD (R01DC013817 to R.H.) and from CDMRP (602MR130240 to R.H. and D.D.).

REFERENCES

1. Brozoski TJ, Bauer CA. Animal models of tinnitus. Hear Res 2016;338:88--97.

2. Eggermont JJ. The auditory cortex and tinnitus - a review of animal and human studies. Eur J Neurosci 2015;41(5):665–76.

3. Eggermont JJ. Animal models of spontaneous activity in the healthy and impaired auditory system. Front NeuralCircuits 2015;9:19.

4. Turner JG, Larsen D. Effects of noise exposure on development of tinnitus and hyperacusis: Prevalence rates 12 months after exposure in middle-aged rats. Hear Res 2016;334:30–6.

5. Kopelman J, Budnick AS, Sessions RB, et al. Ototoxicity of high-dose cisplatin by bolus administration in patients with advanced cancers and normal hearing. Laryngoscope 1988;98(8 Pt 1):858–64.

6. McKeage MJ. Comparative adverse effect profiles of platinum drugs. DrugSaf 1995;13(4):228–44.

7. Malgonde MS, Nagpure PS, Kumar M. Audiometric patterns in ototoxicity after radiotherapy and chemotherapy in patients of head and neck cancers. Indian J PalliatCare 2015;21(2):164–7.

8. Bokemeyer C, Berger CC, Hartmann JT, et al. Analysis of risk factors for cisplatin-induced ototoxicity in patients with testicular cancer. Br J Cancer 1998;77(8): 1355–62.

9. Baguley D, McFerran D, Hall D. Tinnitus. Lancet 2013;382(9904):1600–7.

10. Eggermont JJ, Roberts LE. The neuroscience of tinnitus. TrendsNeurosci 2004; 27(11):676–82.

11. Gopinath B, McMahon CM, Rochtchina E, et al. Incidence, persistence, and progression of tinnitus symptoms in older adults: the Blue Mountains Hearing Study. Ear Hear 2010;31(3):407–12.

12. Kaltenbach JA, Godfrey DA. The Cochlear Nucleus as a Generator of Tinnitus-Related Signals. In: Kandler K, editor. The Oxford handbook of the auditory brainstem. New York: Oxford University Press; 2018. p. 189–221.

13. Kaltenbach JA, Afman CE. Hyperactivity in the dorsal cochlear nucleus after intense sound exposure and its resemblance to tone-evoked activity: a physiological model for tinnitus. Hear Res 2000;140(1–2):165–72.

14. Kaltenbach JA, Godfrey DA, Neumann JB, et al. Changes in spontaneous neural activity in the dorsal cochlear nucleus following exposure to intense sound: relation to threshold shift. Hear Res 1998;124(1–2):78–84.

15. Saunders JC. The role of central nervous system plasticity in tinnitus. J CommunDisord 2007;40(4):313–34.

16. Heffner HE, Koay G. Tinnitus and hearing loss in hamsters (Mesocricetusauratus) exposed to loud sound. BehavNeurosci 2005;119(3):734–42.

17. Barnea G, Attias J, Gold S, et al. Tinnitus with normal hearing sensitivity: extended high-frequency audiometry and auditory-nerve brain-stem-evoked responses. Audiology 1990;29(1):36–45.

18. Sanchez TG, Medeiros IR, Levy CP, et al. Tinnitus in normally hearing patients: clinical aspects and repercussions. Braz J Otorhinolaryngol 2005;71(4):427–31.

19. Schaette R, Kempter R. Development of tinnitus-related neuronal hyperactivity through homeostatic plasticity after hearing loss: a computational model. Eur J Neurosci 2006;23(11):3124–38.

20. Parra LC, Pearlmutter BA. Illusory percepts from auditory adaptation. J AcoustSoc Am 2007;121(3):1632–41.

21. Roberts LE, Eggermont JJ, Caspary DM, et al. Ringing ears: the neuroscience of tinnitus. J Neurosci 2010;30(45):14972–9.

22. Rauschecker JP, Leaver AM, Muhlau M. Tuning out the noise: limbic-auditory interactions in tinnitus. Neuron 2010;66(6):819–26.

23. Kujawa SG, Liberman MC. Adding insult to injury: cochlear nerve degeneration after "temporary" noise-induced hearing loss. J Neurosci 2009;29(45):14077–85.

24. Jacobson M, Kim S, Romney J, et al. Contralateral suppression of distortion-product otoacoustic emissions declines with age: a comparison of findings in CBA mice with human listeners. Laryngoscope 2003;113(10):1707–13.

25. Zhu X, Vasilyeva ON, Kim S, et al. Auditory efferent feedback system deficits precede age-related hearing loss: contralateral suppression of otoacoustic emissions in mice. J Comp Neurol 2007;503(5):593–604.

26. Schaette R, McAlpine D. Tinnitus with a normal audiogram: physiological evidence for hidden hearing loss and computational model. J Neurosci 2011; 31(38):13452–7.

27. Eggermont JJ, Tass PA. Maladaptive neural synchrony in tinnitus: origin and restoration. Front Neurol 2015;6:29.

28. Shore SE, Roberts LE, Langguth B. Maladaptive plasticity in tinnitus–triggers, mechanisms and treatment. Nat Rev Neurol 2016;12(3):150–60.

29. Ryan AF, Kujawa SG, Hammill T, et al. Temporary and permanent noise-induced threshold shifts: a review of basic and clinical observations. OtolNeurotol 2016; 37(8):e271–5.

30. Henderson D, Bielefeld EC, Harris KC, et al. The role of oxidative stress in noise-induced hearing loss. Ear Hear 2006;27(1):1–19.

31. Furman AC, Kujawa SG, Liberman MC. Noise-induced cochlear neuropathy is selective for fibers with low spontaneous rates. J Neurophysiol 2013;110(3): 577–86.

32. Plack CJ, Barker D, Prendergast G. Perceptual consequences of "hidden" hearing loss. TrendsHear 2014;18.

33. Wu PZ, Liberman LD, Bennett K, et al. Primary neural degeneration in the human cochlea: evidence for hidden hearing loss in the aging ear. Neuroscience 2019; 407:8–20.

34. Kujawa SG, Liberman MC. Translating animal models to human therapeutics in noise-induced and age-related hearing loss. Hear Res 2019;377:44–52.

35. Valero MD, Burton JA, Hauser SN, et al. Noise-induced cochlear synaptopathy in rhesus monkeys (Macacamulatta). Hear Res 2017;353:213–23.

36. Milon B, Mitra S, Song Y, et al. The impact of biological sex on the response to noise and otoprotective therapies against acoustic injury in mice. Biol Sex Differ 2018;9(1):12.

37. Spoendlin H, Brun JP. Relation of structural damage to exposure time and intensity in acoustic trauma. ActaOtolaryngol 1973;75(2):220–6.

38. Canlon B. The effect of acoustic trauma on the tectorial membrane, stereocilia, and hearing sensitivity: possible mechanisms underlying damage, recovery, and protection. ScandAudiolSuppl 1988;27:1–45.

39. Chen GD, Fechter LD. The relationship between noise-induced hearing loss and hair cell loss in rats. Hear Res 2003;177(1–2):81–90.

40. Meltser I, Cederroth CR, Basinou V, et al. TrkB-mediated protection against circadian sensitivity to noise trauma in the murine cochlea. CurrBiol 2014;24(6): 658–63.

41. Tahera Y, Meltser I, Johansson P, et al. Glucocorticoid receptor and nuclear factor-kappa B interactions in restraint stress-mediated protection against acoustic trauma. Endocrinology 2006;147(9):4430–7.

42. Ohlemiller KK, Gagnon PM. Genetic dependence of cochlear cells and structures injured by noise. Hear Res 2007;224(1–2):34–50.

43. Shuster BZ, Depireux DA, Mong JA, et al. Sex differences in hearing: probing the role of estrogen signaling. J AcoustSoc Am 2019;145(6):3656.
44. Villavisanis DF, Berson ER, Lauer AM, et al. Sex-based differences in hearing loss: perspectives from non-clinical research to clinical outcomess. OtolNeurotol 2020;41(3):290-8.
45. Baguley DM, Hoare DJ. Hyperacusis: major research questions. HNO 2018; 66(5):358-63.
46. Dauman R, Bouscau-Faure F. Assessment and amelioration of hyperacusis in tinnitus patients. ActaOtolaryngol 2005;125(5):503-9.
47. Chen G, Lee C, Sandridge SA, et al. Behavioral evidence for possible simultaneous induction of hyperacusis and tinnitus following intense sound exposure. J Assoc Res Otolaryngol 2013;14(3):413-24.
48. Flores EN, Duggan A, Madathany T, et al. A non-canonical pathway from cochlea to brain signals tissue-damaging noise. CurrBiol 2015;25(5):606-12.
49. Liu C, Glowatzki E, Fuchs PA. Unmyelinated type II afferent neurons report cochlear damage. ProcNatlAcadSciUS A 2015;112(47):14723-7.
50. Mittal R, Aranke M, Debs LH, et al. Indispensable role of ion channels and transporters in the auditory system. JCellPhysiol 2017;232(4):743-58.
51. Patuzzi R. Non-linear aspects of outer hair cell transduction and the temporary threshold shifts after acoustic trauma. AudiolNeurootol 2002;7(1):17-20.
52. Norena AJ. Revisiting the cochlear and central mechanisms of tinnitus and therapeutic approaches. AudiolNeurootol 2015;20(Suppl 1):53-9.
53. Moser T, Neef A, Khimich D. Mechanisms underlying the temporal precision of sound coding at the inner hair cell ribbon synapse. J Physiol 2006;576(Pt 1): 55-62.
54. Kujawa SG, Liberman MC. Synaptopathy in the noise-exposed and aging cochlea: primary neural degeneration in acquired sensorineural hearing loss. Hear Res 2015;330(Pt B):191-9.
55. Sergeyenko Y, Lall K, Liberman MC, et al. Age-related cochlear synaptopathy: an early-onset contributor to auditory functional decline. J Neurosci 2013;33(34): 13686-94.
56. Pujol R, Puel JL. Excitotoxicity, synaptic repair, and functional recovery in the mammalian cochlea: a review of recent findings. Ann N YAcadSci 1999;884: 249-54.
57. Wan G, Corfas G. Transient auditory nerve demyelination as a new mechanism for hidden hearing loss. Nat Commun 2017;8:14487.
58. Atherley GR, Hempstock TI, Noble WG. Study of tinnitus induced temporarily by noise. J AcoustSoc Am 1968;44(6):1503-6.
59. Loeb M, Smith RP. Relation of induced tinnitus to physical characteristics of the inducing stimuli. J AcoustSoc Am 1967;42(2):453-5.
60. Mrena R, Savolainen S, Pirvola U, et al. Characteristics of acute acoustical trauma in the Finnish Defence Forces. Int J Audiol 2004;43(3):177-81.
61. Buchler M, Kompis M, Hotz MA. Extended frequency range hearing thresholds and otoacoustic emissions in acute acoustic trauma. OtolNeurotol 2012;33(8): 1315-22.
62. McFeely WJ Jr, Bojrab DI, Davis KG, et al. Otologic injuries caused by airbag deployment. OtolaryngolHeadNeckSurg 1999;121(4):367-73.
63. Schreiber BE, Agrup C, Haskard DO, et al. Sudden sensorineural hearing loss. Lancet 2010;375(9721):1203-11.
64. Turner JG, Bauer CA, Rybak LP. Noise in animal facilities: why it matters. J Am Assoc Lab AnimSci 2007;46(1):10-3.

65. von der Behrens W. Animal models of subjective tinnitus. NeuralPlast 2014;2014: 741452.
66. Davis H, Morgan CT, Hawkin JE Jr, et al. Temporary deafness following exposure to loud tones and noise. Laryngoscope 1946;56:19–21.
67. Sereda M, Edmondson-Jones M, Hall DA. Relationship between tinnitus pitch and edge of hearing loss in individuals with a narrow tinnitus bandwidth. Int J Audiol 2015;54(4):249–56.
68. Sereda M, Hall DA, Bosnyak DJ, et al. Re-examining the relationship between audiometric profile and tinnitus pitch. Int J Audiol 2011;50(5):303–12.
69. Henry JA. "Measurement" of Tinnitus. OtolNeurotol 2016;37(8):e276–85.
70. Schaette R, Turtle C, Munro KJ. Reversible induction of phantom auditory sensations through simulated unilateral hearing loss. PLoS One 2012;7(6):e35238.
71. Baguley DM, Andersson G. Hyperacusis: mechanisms, diagnosis, and therapies. Oxford (UK): Plural Publishing; 2007.
72. Formby C, Gold SL, Keaser ML, et al. Secondary benefits from tinnitus retraining therapy (TRT): clinically significant increases in loudness discomfort level and in the auditory dynamic range. SeminHear 2007;28(4):227–60.
73. Goodhill V. The management of tinnitus. Laryngoscope 1950;60(5):442–50.
74. Baguley DM. Mechanisms of tinnitus. Br Med Bull 2002;63:195–212.
75. Haider HF, Bojic T, Ribeiro SF, et al. Pathophysiology of subjective tinnitus: triggers and maintenance. Front Neurosci 2018;12:866.
76. De Ridder D, Vanneste S, Weisz N, et al. An integrative model of auditory phantom perception: tinnitus as a unified percept of interacting separable subnetworks. NeurosciBiobehav Rev 2014;44:16–32.

Noise
Acoustic Trauma and Tinnitus, the US Military Experience

Sarah M. Theodoroff, PhD[a,b,]*, Dawn Konrad-Martin, PhD[a,b]

KEYWORDS

- Tinnitus • Noise • Ototoxicity • Hearing disorders • Hyperacusis

KEY POINTS

- Military Service Members and Veterans often have a history of high noise exposure and experience tinnitus and other auditory complaints at higher rates compared with the general population.
- Tinnitus is a perceptual consequence of noise exposure and may be an early indicator of underlying auditory injury that can manifest before changes detected audiometrically.
- When combined with an ototoxic agent (eg, ionizing radiation, platinum-based chemotherapy, certain aminoglycoside antibiotics, loop diuretics, macrolides), noise exposure results in more severe auditory impairment than expected from either source independently, warranting the monitoring of patients receiving these therapies for development or exacerbation of tinnitus and hearing loss.

INTRODUCTION

It is well established that noise exposure is a risk factor for military personnel, Veterans, and civilians to develop tinnitus.[1,2] In 2010, the US Department of Health and Human Services announced an initiative called Healthy People 2020, which aims to improve the overall health of individuals living in the United States by the year 2020.[3] One of the goals of Healthy People 2020 is to reduce the prevalence and severity of auditory disorders. In their midcourse review, it was noteworthy that compared with data from 2005 to 2006, adolescents' (aged 12–19) use of hearing protection when exposed to loud noise in 2009 to 2010 had worsened. The midcourse review also highlighted that compared with 2007, which revealed 44.5% of adults (aged ≥18) sought advice from a doctor about their tinnitus, in 2014 the percentage had increased to 48.5%. Additionally, in 2014, 61.8% of adults (compared with 45.8% in

[a] VA RR&D National Center for Rehabilitative Auditory Research, Veterans Affairs Portland Health Care System, Portland, OR, USA; [b] Department of Otolaryngology/Head & Neck Surgery, Oregon Health & Science University, Portland, OR, USA
* Corresponding author. 3710 Southwest US Veterans Hospital Road (NCRAR – P5), Portland, OR 97239.
E-mail address: sarah.theodoroff@va.gov

Otolaryngol Clin N Am 53 (2020) 543–553
https://doi.org/10.1016/j.otc.2020.03.004
0030-6665/20/Published by Elsevier Inc.

2007) reported tinnitus severe enough in the last 5 years to have seen an otolaryngologist or audiologist. Unfortunately, only 14.7% of the 45.8% of adults in 2007 who sought medical advice for bothersome tinnitus, reported trying any form of treatment. Overall, these data suggest that it is necessary to improve outreach efforts to inform as many individuals and groups as possible about the extent of noise-induced damage to the auditory system and the importance of taking preventative measures.

The purpose of this article is to increase the medical community's awareness of the multifaceted nature of noise-induced tinnitus, focusing on the experience of military personnel and Veterans, and to provide a clinical decision-making guide that can support effective referrals and resources to help patients manage their tinnitus. A related goal is to increase awareness that military, occupational, or recreational exposures to high noise levels, particularly firearm use, can exacerbate auditory injury from commonly used ototoxic drug therapies, further increasing the risk of incident tinnitus and hearing loss resulting from independent exposure to either of these damaging agents.

Noise exposure is a major public health concern that negatively impacts numerous health systems resulting in auditory deficits (hearing loss, tinnitus) and nonauditory consequences (sleep disturbances, annoyance, cardiovascular disease[4]). A recently published article by Kerns and colleagues[5] found noisy work conditions were associated with high blood pressure, high cholesterol, and hearing difficulty. In general, "noise" refers to unwanted sound and "noise exposure" typically refers to exposure to hazardous levels of any type of sound that can result in hearing loss.[4]

The National Institute for Occupational Safety and Health has published standards for permissible occupational noise exposure for an 8-hour workday not to exceed 85 to 90 dBA.[6] A limitation of current industrial standards is that they severely underestimate the effect of exposure to short-duration sounds. For example, the output of military weapons far exceeds these permissible levels and are approximately 150% higher than published acceptable standards.[7] Noise-induced hearing loss is preventable, and yet to date, has remained a major health burden in the United States and worldwide affecting billions of individuals.[8–10]

Military personnel and Veterans are exposed in training and during their military service to levels of noise that results in hearing loss and tinnitus.[1,11,12] Noise-induced tinnitus and hearing loss are so pervasive they have remained the top two service-connected disabilities for Veterans receiving compensation for more than a decade.[13] The perception of tinnitus is often associated with elevated hearing thresholds, but an important caveat is that noise-induced tinnitus can occur in the absence of hearing loss measured through conventional pure-tone audiometry and by itself, is suggestive of pathologic injury to the auditory system.[14] Studies in humans have demonstrated important relationships between tinnitus and reduced auditory nerve activity as assessed using auditory brainstem response wave I,[15] or the acoustic reflex,[16] after statistically adjusting for variations in outer hair cell function using otoacoustic emissions. This is broadly consistent with results in animal models of tinnitus that demonstrate reduced peripheral input causes enhanced neural activity in the central auditory system, that is, increased central gain,[17] which can occur in response to damage at the level of the inner hair cells and auditory nerve.[18,19]

In general, Veterans are twice as likely to have tinnitus compared with non-Veterans and exposure to loud sounds during their military service is a major contributing factor to this outcome.[20] Data regarding the prevalence and impact of tinnitus on military Service Members are less known. This gap in knowledge was recently addressed by Henry and colleagues[21] who showed that 34% of Service Members (n = 182) had constant tinnitus and 44% of Veterans (n = 246) had constant tinnitus. Service

Members with tinnitus reported negative consequences similar to Veterans, such as difficulty with concentration, job performance, sleep, and emotional well-being.[21]

Additionally, previously identified risk factors for tinnitus in Service Members and Veterans include age; sex; blast exposure; and co-occurring mental health conditions, such as post-traumatic stress disorder (PTSD).[1] Of note, Veterans who served in Iraq and Afghanistan (Operations Iraqi and Enduring Freedom/New Dawn, respectively) are at increased risk for major depression, anxiety disorders, and PTSD.[22]

The adverse functional and psychosocial impacts of tinnitus and the benefit of treatment are illustrated in the video case example found on the National Center for Rehabilitative Auditory Research's Web site (https://www.ncrar.research.va.gov/PatientVoices/Index.asp). The video introduces you to Brian, a 40-year-old Veteran with bothersome tinnitus that he describes as "hell," an "invisible disability" that "affects [his] well-being and way of life." He was interested in participating in tinnitus research to learn ways to cope with his tinnitus. He reported a history of high noise exposure including from weapons fire and aircraft engines, having spent most of his 4-year military tour aboard aircraft carriers.

As a first step, he received a comprehensive audiologic evaluation, and substantial hearing loss was found. He learned that whenever tinnitus and hearing loss co-occur, it is important to address both conditions. The audiologic and tinnitus counseling he received prompted him to try amplification, a sound-based approach to help him with his tinnitus and improve his ability to communicate. In the video, he describes experiencing substantial relief from his tinnitus by using hearing aids. He also receives benefit from cognitive behavioral therapy and meditation to manage his reactions to his tinnitus. He also describes major improvements in his spousal relationship because of improved communication, which he had no idea had been the source of many "fights" that had created stress in the relationship. Sadly, Brian struggled with tinnitus and hearing loss for years without a proper health care referral.

Clinical Practice Guidelines

From the foregoing, it should be clear that Service Members and Veterans often have a history of high noise exposure and PTSD, and therefore are likely to experience bothersome tinnitus and other auditory complaints that require appropriate health care. In addition to PTSD, there are many comorbid conditions that can exacerbate tinnitus symptom severity, which is why it is essential to perform a thorough medical evaluation on all patients with tinnitus. Unfortunately, many health care providers are either not familiar with clinical practice guidelines for tinnitus or choose not to follow their recommendations for other reasons.[2] Tunkel and colleagues[23] published a comprehensive clinical practice guideline for tinnitus and provide an evidence-based framework with suggested recommendations for tinnitus assessment and management, which are endorsed by the American Academy of Otolaryngology–Head and Neck Surgery Foundation (AAO-HNS), American Academy of Audiology, and American Speech-Language-Hearing Association.

The AAO-HNS clinical practice guideline for tinnitus strongly recommends all patients with tinnitus receive a targeted history and physical examination. These initial assessment procedures are essential to identify the tinnitus patients' primary complaint and inform the selection of appropriate follow-up testing, procedures, and referrals. When a patient reports tinnitus, in addition to questions to determine its type (ie, primary vs secondary), it is helpful to determine if it is bothersome and if the patient experiences any triggers that exacerbate the condition. Sometimes patients are not aware of triggers that result in their tinnitus perception fluctuating. Therefore, asking specific follow-up questions (eg, "Does the loudness of your tinnitus change from time to time?" and "Does your tinnitus change when you move your jaw or clench your teeth?") is helpful to screen for potential somatic components to the tinnitus and aid in the clinical decision-making process.

Somatosensory Tinnitus

When patients' report history of head injury, it is helpful to determine if the tinnitus perception is modulated by head and neck maneuvers and/or started after the injury. When attributes of the tinnitus percept, such as pitch or loudness, change immediately following certain head, neck, and/or jaw maneuvers, forceful muscle contractions, or eye movements, somatosensory tinnitus is suspected and suggests an interaction between the somatosensory and auditory systems.[24–27] Numerous studies have revealed that tinnitus is somatically modulated in many people[26] and could be attributed to cortical neuroplasticity initiated by subcortical changes occurring at the auditory brainstem level.[25,28]

When somatic manipulations directly influence the tinnitus perception, it suggests the possibility of an underlying musculoskeletal deficit of the head or neck and warrants taking a nontraditional approach to tinnitus management.[29] Tinnitus and musculoskeletal disabilities involving the head and neck (eg, cervical strain) are commonly reported by Veterans receiving care at VA facilities[13]; therefore, it is logical to postulate that many Veterans will have clinical features suggestive of somatosensory tinnitus, but the prevalence of somatosensory tinnitus in Veterans is unknown. Although limited research has been done investigating the effectiveness of various treatments for somatosensory tinnitus, what has been published related to physiotherapy is promising.[29–32]

Hyperacusis

From a clinical perspective, all patients with tinnitus, regardless of the type of tinnitus, should be screened for hyperacusis. Estimates vary and are as high as 60% to 79% of patients with tinnitus have comorbid hyperacusis.[33,34] Hyperacusis is defined as an intolerance of sounds at low-to-moderate intensity levels that results in physical discomfort and can increase stress and anxiety.[35] When patients report any degree of decreased sound tolerance (DST), whether it be hyperacusis or another type of sound intolerance, it is paramount to address the issue clinically because it can negatively impact every aspect of daily functioning.[36]

Patients with severe DST often change their daily activities to avoid exposure to the "noise" of everyday life, which in turn leads to social isolation, worsening of symptoms, and reduced quality of life.[37] Clinical evidence suggests long-term avoidance and deprivation of sound counterintuitively results in increasing one's sensitivity, rather than contributing to any degree of symptom reduction.[38] Many people who initially have a minimal degree of DST begin to use hearing protection in quiet environments with the intention of improving their condition, or preventing it from worsening. However, the act of depriving the ear and brain from processing sounds at normal everyday levels ultimately increases the auditory system's responsiveness to sound and, in turn, increases the severity of their DST.

Often patients have a difficult time articulating their complaints and DST is defined differently among patients. Current clinical test procedures are not adequate to characterize the auditory-neurobehavioral phenomenon of DST and future research is needed to address these gaps in knowledge. When patients with tinnitus present with comorbid DST, asking for concrete examples of situations that evoke the response can assist in determining if the sound intolerance is related to the perceived loudness or some other aspect of the sound environment. Asking clarifying questions also assists in determining if the patient's complaint is a different problem entirely, such as difficulty understanding speech in noise.

Ototoxic Medications

Also, critically important is to screen patients with tinnitus for use of ototoxic medications. Tinnitus is a common side effect of ototoxic medications and can occur in the absence of hearing loss with medications, such as anticonvulsants, diuretics, tricyclic antidepressants, vasodilators, organic solvents, and more.[39] When combined with an ototoxic agent, noise exposure results in more severe auditory damage than expected from either source independently.[40] This synergistic interaction between noise and ototoxic medications has been shown to result in more extensive damage to cochlear hair cells and supporting cells than would be caused by either one independently.[41–43] This combined effect is especially important to consider for patients who are prescribed the more potent ototoxic medications, such as certain aminoglycosides and antineoplastic agents that cause hearing loss and tinnitus at high rates.[44,45] Encouraging patients to use of hearing protection when exposed to noise is critical, but for these patients, it is recommended to take extra time to explain that they are far more vulnerable to the negative effects of being around moderate to high levels of noise.

When patients are taking highly ototoxic medications (eg, head and neck patients receiving adjuvant chemotherapy with a platinum-based drug), it is recommended to monitor these patients prospectively for the development of, or exacerbation of, tinnitus and self-perceived hearing difficulties.[46] These perceptual consequences are indicators of changes in the auditory status of the patient, and yet may go unnoticed because of the multitude of other medical concerns that need to be addressed when providing complex medical care. Additional considerations regarding patient-specific susceptibility for developing chemoradiotherapy-induced tinnitus and/or hearing loss include age, concomitant administration of ototoxic medications (nonsteroidal anti-inflammatory drugs, diuretics, aminoglycosides), and cumulative dose.[47] It has also been shown in animal models that cisplatin-induced ototoxicity can compound noise-induced auditory injury months following completion of the chemotherapeutic agent, suggesting a lasting effect in the form of increased susceptibility to damage.[48] This is consistent with recent results showing platinum compounds accumulate in the stria vascularis where they are not readily cleared.[49] When extrapolated to humans using evidence from human temporal bones, results in animal models of cisplatin ototoxicity indicate that the drug may reside indefinitely in the cochlea consistent with development of late effects and long-term vulnerability to damage from noise.

When seeing patients who have a primary complaint of tinnitus, consider asking, "In the last 6 months, have you been exposed to loud noises where you had to shout to be heard?" Any affirmative responses would prompt the follow-up question: "Afterward, did you experience any ear pain, tinnitus, trouble understanding speech in noisy environments, or changes in your tinnitus or hearing?" Asking questions about exposure to noise in a general sense is a good opportunity to learn about your patient's noise exposure history from a variety of sources (military, occupational, and recreational activities), and to have an honest conversation about hearing protection use (**Box 1**). There are many beneficial ways to help patients manage tinnitus-related problems, but until a cure is found, preventative measures remain the best option.

The most effective means to reduce the risk of noise-induced tinnitus is by using hearing protection. Earplugs and earmuffs come in a variety of styles; many patients and health care providers are not familiar with how to select appropriate hearing protection devices (HPDs) or verify they are being worn correctly to receive the most benefit. Providing instruction and making sure individuals receive the necessary

---

Box 1
Suggested noise-exposure questions to include as part of assessment

In the last 3 to 6 months, have you been exposed to loud noises where you had to shout to be heard?
Yes, Sometimes, No

If Yes or Sometimes:
  After the event, did you experience any (circle all that apply):
    Ear pain, Tinnitus, Trouble understanding speech in noisy environments, Change in tinnitus, Change in hearing

How often did or does your job cause you to be exposed to loud noises where you had to shout to be heard?
Never, Rarely, Sometimes, Usually, Always

If Sometimes-Always: Were you wearing hearing protection when this occurred?
Never, Rarely, Sometimes, Usually, Always
When you were exposed to loud noises, did you experience tinnitus?
Yes, Sometimes, No

How often did or do recreational activities cause you to be exposed to loud noises where you had to shout to be heard (eg, music concerts, power tools, motorcycles, hunting, target shooting)?
Never, Rarely, Sometimes, Usually, Always

If Sometimes-Always: Were you wearing hearing protection when this occurred?
Never, Rarely, Sometimes, Usually, Always
When you were exposed to loud noises, did you experience tinnitus?
Yes, Sometimes, No

---

training, including how to properly insert earplugs, are methods used in hearing conservation programs as strategies that have been shown to be successful in improving the use of HPDs effectively.[50]

Other factors to be aware of and discuss with patients include: (1) overall comfort when wearing HPDs, a variable that strongly influences how consistently HPDs are used; (2) personal health beliefs related to perceived risk (or lack of perceived risk); and (3) motivation to protect their hearing, including protection against developing auditory conditions, such as tinnitus and hyperacusis. The National Hearing Conservation Association has resources for interested health care professionals who want to learn more about best practice for promoting use of HPDs on their Web site: www.hearingconversation.org.

SUMMARY

Because of repeated exposures to noise, military Service Members and Veterans are more likely to have tinnitus compared with civilians, and those who have comorbid mental health diagnoses are more likely to have increased tinnitus symptom severity.[51] Accumulating evidence suggests that tinnitus developed as a perceptual consequence of noise exposure may be an indicator of underlying auditory injury and maladaptive compensatory mechanisms within the central auditory pathways.[52] The prevailing view that "tinnitus is a symptom of hearing loss" is therefore misleading and does not tell the whole story.

It is critical for health care providers to know what can be done to help patients with tinnitus so that the phrase "nothing can be done" will cease being said. Not only is that statement inaccurate, hearing it reduces patients' confidence in the ability of health

Table 1
Definitions of key concepts addressed in this article and recommendations for consideration

Finding	Definition	Recommendation
Primary tinnitus (with or without measurable hearing loss)*	Perception of sound in the absence of an external source that is idiopathic and may or may not be associated with sensorineural hearing loss*	Follow standard AAO-HNS Clinical Practice Guidelines and have patient be seen by an audiologist who is knowledgeable about tinnitus
Primary tinnitus + ototoxic medication	Ototoxic agents that result in damaging auditory/vestibular end organs and possible damage to subcortical and cortical structures	Perform prospective ototoxicity monitoring and encourage use of hearing protection when exposed to noise
Somatosensory tinnitus	Changes in tinnitus percept (pitch, loudness, timber) following head and neck maneuvers, forceful muscle contractions, eye movements, or jaw movements	Consider referrals to neurologist and physical therapist for additional work-up to rule out comorbid musculoskeletal head/neck deficit triggering or exacerbating the tinnitus
Hyperacusis	Intolerance of sounds at low-to-moderate intensity levels that results in physical discomfort (and may result in negative reactions)	Referral to audiologist who specializes in assessment and management of tinnitus and hyperacusis (modified test battery recommended so as not to exacerbate the condition); important to identify if tinnitus and/or hyperacusis is exacerbated by acoustic stimulation
History of noise exposure (occupational and/or recreational)	Exposure to intensity levels that can damage auditory function (eg, operating light or heavy machinery, manufacturing/factory work, lawn equipment, shooting range, attending sporting events, music concerts, mass transportation)	Review proper use of hearing protection devices and the different types available; discuss any barriers that exist to wearing hearing protection

*Definition from Tunkel DE, Bauer CA, Sun GH, et al. Clinical practice guidelines: Tinnitus. Otolaryngol Head Neck Surg 2014;151(2 Suppl):S1-40.

care providers to help them and can lead patients to explore unhealthy options for short-term relief.

When patients present in the clinic with tinnitus, it is essential to determine what type of tinnitus the patient has and if it is bothersome or not. Being familiar with current clinical practice guidelines on tinnitus assessment and management not only promotes best practices, it aids clinicians in their decision-making process. Evaluating patients with tinnitus is nuanced and careful consideration should be paid to auditory and nonauditory comorbidities. Although there is no "cure," there are many cost-effective management approaches available to help treatment-seeking patients with bothersome tinnitus. **Table 1** is a miniguide that can be used as a reference for the major topics addressed in this article. The recommendations in **Table 1** are not exhaustive; because of individual differences related to how tinnitus manifests and what is considered bothersome about it, tinnitus assessment and management should take a stepped-care approach, including consideration of the patient's preferences along with a discussion of realistic goals and expectations, to best meet their needs.

There is a lot of misinformation and false claims about tinnitus on the Internet[53,54]; that, plus lack of guidance, can result in patients feeling overwhelmed and unsure of what to do. At a minimum, providing patients a handout with community resources, and/or a list of credible Web sites to obtain additional information (eg, American Tinnitus Association [www.ata.org], Dangerous Decibels [http://dangerousdecibels.org], Noisy Planet [www.noisyplanet.nidcd.nih.gov]) helps patients be informed consumers. Ultimately, incorporating these elements into the care of patients with tinnitus will lead to improved health care outcomes and patient satisfaction.

ACKNOWLEDGMENTS

This work was supported by a VA RR&D Small Projects in Rehabilitation Research Award (SPiRE; #C3181-P PI-Theodoroff) and a Merit Review Award (#C3127-R PI-Konrad-Martin). This material is the result of work supported with resources and the use of facilities at the VA Rehabilitation Research and Development, National Center for Rehabilitative Auditory Research (Center Award #C9230C; PIs-Feeney and Konrad-Martin) at the VA Portland Health Care System in Portland, Oregon. These contents do not necessarily represent the views of the US Department of Veterans Affairs, Department of Defense, or the United States Government.

DISCLOSURE

The authors declare no competing interests, neither financial or nonfinancial.

REFERENCES

1. Theodoroff SM, Lewis MS, Folmer RL, et al. Hearing impairment and tinnitus: prevalence, risk factors, and outcomes in US Service members and Veterans deployed to the Iraq and Afghanistan wars. Epidemiol Rev 2015;37:71–85.

2. Bhatt JM, Lin HW, Bhattachayya N. Prevalence, severity, exposures, and treatment patterns of tinnitus in the United States. JAMA Otolaryngol Head Neck Surg 2016;142(10):959–65.

3. National Center for Health Statistics. Chapter 20: Hearing and other sensory or communication disorders. Healthy people 2020 midcourse review 2016. Hyattsville (MD).

4. Basner M, Babisch W, Davis A, et al. Auditory and non-auditory effects of noise on health. Lancet 2014;383:1325–32.

5. Kerns E, Masterson EA, Themann CL, et al. Cardiovascular conditions, hearing difficulty, and occupational noise exposure within US industries and occupations. Am J Ind Med 2018;61(6):477–91.

6. Occupational Safety and Health Administration. Hearing Conservation Program. US Dept. Labor; Occupational Noise Exposure. Available at: http://www.osha.gov/SLTC/noisehearingconservation/index.html. Accessed May 2, 2019.

7. Dancer A, Buck K. Noise: a limiting factor for the use of modern weapon systems? In new directions for improving audio effectiveness (pp. KN1-1 – KN1-14). Meeting Proceedings RTO-MP-HFM-123, 2005, Keynote 1. Neuilly-sur-Seine, France: RTO, April 1, 2005. Available at: http://www.rto.nato.int/abstracts.aps.

8. Martinez LF. Can you hear me now? Occupational hearing loss, 2004-2012. Monthly labor review. U.S. Bureau of Labor Statistics; 2012. Available at: http://www.bls.gov/opub/mlr/2012/07/art4full.pdf.

9. Nelson JT, Swan AA, Swiger B, et al. Hearing testing in the US Department of Defense: potential impact on Veterans Affairs hearing loss disability awards. Hear Res 2017;349:13–20.

10. Salosom JA, Haagsma JA, Davis A, et al. Global burden of disease study. Lancet 2015;3:e712–23.

11. Helfer TM, Jordan NN, Lee RB, et al. Noise-induced hearing injury and comorbidities among postdeployment US Army Soldiers: April 2003-June 2009. Am J Audiol 2011;20(1):33–41.

12. Eggermont JJ, Roberts LE. The neuroscience of tinnitus: understanding abnormal and normal auditory perception. Front Syst Neurosci 2012;6:53.

13. Veterans Benefits Administration, US Department of Veterans Affairs. Annual benefits report for fiscal year 2018. Available at: https://www.benefits.va.gov/REPORTS/. Accessed October 23, 2019.

14. Shaheen LA, Liberman MC. Cochlear synaptopathy changes sound-evoked activity without changing spontaneous discharge in the mouse inferior colliculus. Front Syst Neurosci 2018;12:59.

15. Bramhall N, Beach EF, Epp B, et al. The search for noise-induced cochlear synaptopathy in humans: mission impossible? Hear Res 2019;377:88–103.

16. Wojtczak M, Beim JA, Oxenham AJ. Weak middle-ear-muscle reflex in humans with noise-induced tinnitus and normal hearing may reflect cochlear synaptopathy. eNeuro 2017;4(6) [pii:ENEURO.0363-17.2017].

17. Jastreboff PJ. Phantom auditory perception (tinnitus): mechanisms of generation and perception. Neurosci Res 1990;8(4):221–54.

18. Auerbach BD, Rodrigues PV, Salvi RJ. Central gain control in tinnitus and hyperacusis. Front Neurol 2014;5:206.

19. Brotherton H, Plack CJ, Maslin M, et al. Pump up the volume: could excessive neural gain explain tinnitus and hyperacusis? Audiol Neurootol 2015;20(4):273–82.

20. Folmer RL, McMillan GP, Austin DF, et al. Audiometric thresholds and prevalence of tinnitus among male Veterans in the United States: data from the National Health and Nutrition Examination Survey, 1999-2006. J Rehabil Res Dev 2011;48(5):503–16.

21. Henry JA, Griest SE, Blankenship C, et al. Impact of tinnitus on military service members. Mil Med 2019;184(Suppl 1):604–14.

22. Greer N, Ackland P, Sayer N. Relationship of deployment-related mild traumatic brain injury to posttraumatic stress disorder, depressive disorders, substance use disorders, suicidal ideation, and anxiety disorders: a systematic review. Washington (DC): Evidence Synthesis Program, Health Services Research and Development Service, Office of Research and Development, Department of Veterans Affairs; 2019. VA ESP Project #09-009. Available at: https://www.hsrd.research.va.gov/publications/esp/reports.cfm.

23. Tunkel DE, Bauer CA, Sun GH, et al. Clinical practice guidelines: tinnitus. Otolaryngol Head Neck Surg 2014;151(2 Suppl):S1–40.

24. Levine RA. Somatic (craniocervical) tinnitus and the dorsal cochlear nucleus hypothesis. Am J Otolaryngol 1999;20:351–62.

25. Shore SE. Plasticity of somatosensory inputs to the cochlear nucleus: implications for tinnitus. Hear Res 2011;281:38–46.

26. Ralli M, Greco A, Turchetta R, et al. Somatosensory tinnitus: current evidence and future perspectives. J Int Med Res 2017;45(3):933–47.

27. Marks KL, Martel DT, Wu C, et al. Auditory-somatosensory bimodal stimulation desynchronizes brain circuitry to reduce tinnitus in guinea pigs and humans. Sci Transl Med 2018;10(422).

28. Theodoroff SM, Kaltenbach JA. The role of the brainstem in generating and modulating tinnitus. Am J Audiol 2019;28(1S):225–38.

29. Sanchez TG, Rocha CB. Diagnosis and management of somatosensory tinnitus: review article. Clinics (Sau Paulo) 2011;66(6):1089–94.

30. Cherian K, Cherian N, Cook C, et al. Improving tinnitus with mechanical treatment of the cervical spine and jaw. J Am Acad Audiol 2013;24:544–55.

31. Michiels S, Van de Heyning P, Truijen S, et al. Does multi-modal cervical physical therapy improve tinnitus in patients with cervicogenic somatic tinnitus? Man Ther 2016;26:125–31.

32. Cote C, Baril I, Morency C, et al. Long-term effects of a multimodal physiotherapy program on the severity of somatosensory tinnitus and identification of clinical indicators for predicting favorable outcomes of the program. J Am Acad Audiol 2019;30:720–30.

33. Andersson G, Vretblad P, Larsen HC, et al. Longitudinal follow-up of tinnitus complaints. Arch Otolaryngol Head Neck Surg 2001;127(2):175–9.

34. Dauman R, Bouscau-Faure F. Assessment and amelioration of hyperacusis in tinnitus patients. Acta Otolaryngol 2005;125(5):503–9.

35. Aazh H, Moore BCJ, Lammaing K, et al. Tinnitus and hyperacusis therapy in a UK National Health Service audiology department: patients' evaluations of the effectiveness of treatments. Int J Audiol 2016;55(9):514–22.

36. Theodoroff SM, Reavis KM, Griest SE, et al. Decreased sound tolerance associated with blast exposure. Sci Rep 2019;9:10204.

37. Landon J, Shepherd D, Stuart S, et al. Hearing every footstep: noise sensitivity in individuals following traumatic brain injury. Neuropsychol Rehabil 2012;22(3):391–407.

38. Formby C, Sherlock LP, Gold SL. Adaptive plasticity of loudness induced by chronic attenuation and enhancement of the acoustic background. J Acoust Soc Am 2003;114(1):55–8.

39. Brown RD, Penny JE, Henley CM, et al. Ototoxic drugs and noise. Ciba Found Symp 1981;85:151–71.

40. Bhattacharyya TK, Dayal VS. Ototoxicity and noise-drug interaction. J Otolaryngol 1984;13(6):361–6.

41. Gratton MA, Salvi RJ, Kamen BA, et al. Interaction of cisplatin and noise on the peripheral auditory system. Hear Res 1990;50(1–2):211–23.
42. Fetoni AR, Rolesi R, Paciello F. Styrene enhances the noise induced oxidative stress in the cochlea and affects differently mechanosensory and supporting cells. Free Radic Biol Med 2016;101:211–25.
43. Hammill TL, McKenna E, Hecht Q, et al. I'm wearing my hearing protection – am I still at risk for hearing loss? Lurking ototoxins in the military environment. Mil Med 2019;184:615–20.
44. Fligor BJ. Pediatric ototoxicity: current trends and management. Semin Hear 2019;40(2):154–61.
45. El Charif O, Mapes B, Trendowski MR, et al. Clinical and genome-wide analysis of cisplatin-induced tinnitus implicates novel ototoxic mechanisms. Clin Cancer Res 2019;25(13):4104–16.
46. Schmitt NC, Page BR. Chemoradiation-induced hearing loss remains a major concern for head and neck cancer patients. Int J Audiol 2018;57(sup4):S49–54.
47. Theunissen EA, Bosma SC, Zuur CL, et al. Sensorineural hearing loss in patients with head and neck cancer after chemoradiotherapy and radiotherapy: a systematic review of the literature. Head Neck 2015;37(2):281–92.
48. DeBacker JR, Harrison RT, Bielefelt EC. Long-term synergistic interaction of cisplatin- and noise-induced hearing losses. Ear Hear 2017;38:282–91.
49. Francis SP, Cunningham LL. Non-autonomous cellular response to ototoxic drug-induced stress and death. Front Cell Neurosci 2017;11:252.
50. Smith PS, Monaco BA, Lusk SL. Attitudes towards use of hearing protection devices and effects of an intervention on fit-testing results. Workplace Health Saf 2014;62(12):491–9.
51. Carlson KF, Gilbert TA, O'Neil ME, et al. Health care utilization and mental health diagnoses among Veterans with tinnitus. Am J Audiol 2019;28:181–90.
52. Shore SE, Roberts LE, Langguth B. Maladaptive plasticity in tinnitus-triggers, mechanisms and treatment. Nat Rev Neurol 2016;12(3):150–60.
53. Deshpande AK, Deshpande SB, O'Brien C. A study of social medial utilization by individuals with tinnitus. Am J Audiol 2018;27(4):559–69.
54. Kieran SM, Skinner LJ, Donnelly M, et al. A critical evaluation of Web sites offering patient information on tinnitus. Ear Nose Throat J 2010;89(1):E11–4.

Perception of, and Reaction to, Tinnitus

The Depression Factor

Fatima T. Husain, PhD

KEYWORDS

• Tinnitus • Depression • Counseling • Cognitive behavior therapy • Antidepressants

KEY POINTS

- Although most adults reporting chronic tinnitus learn to habituate to the condition, a minority find it bothersome or "severe," adversely affecting concentration, communication, sleep, and emotion processing.
- Depression often co-occurs with severe tinnitus.
- Similar neural networks may be engaged in the conditions of depression and bothersome tinnitus.
- Cognitive behavior therapy, which has shown to help with chronic depression, also seems to help with tinnitus.
- Antidepressants may help with the depression co-occurring with tinnitus in some cases, but their routine use to treat tinnitus-related distress is not necessary.

INTRODUCTION

It may be obvious that tinnitus and depression are linked, but as any clinician treating patients with tinnitus knows it is also obvious that most individuals presenting with tinnitus do not report symptoms of depression. This article reviews evidence on the interactive association between depression and tinnitus severity and evidence that typical treatments for depression may reduce symptoms of tinnitus severity.

In the context of this review, it is useful to define subjective tinnitus as both the perception of a sound in the absence of an external source, and the psychological reaction to the sound itself. The sound or sounds range from tonal or narrow-band with a defined pitch, to hissing, to whooshing, to sounding like cicadas. The psychological reaction to the tinnitus sound, ranging from communication difficulties, sleep problems, challenges with concentration, to affective disorders, is collectively termed tinnitus-related distress or severity. The great majority of those who report tinnitus, have subjective tinnitus, that is, it can only be perceived by

Department of Speech and Hearing Science, The Neuroscience Program, The Beckman Institute for Advanced Science and Technology, University of Illinois at Urbana-Champaign, 901 South Sixth Street, Champaign, IL 61820, USA
E-mail address: husainf@illinois.edu

Otolaryngol Clin N Am 53 (2020) 555–561
https://doi.org/10.1016/j.otc.2020.03.005
0030-6665/20/© 2020 Elsevier Inc. All rights reserved.

oto.theclinics.com

them and the clinician relies on self-report from the patient. In contrast, a minority of tinnitus is classified as objective, meaning it can also be perceived by others, but this population is not the focus of this paper. As acute tinnitus becomes chronic, 70% to 80% of those with chronic subjective tinnitus habituate to it,[1,2] with the typical time period of such habituation being around 6 months.[3] A minority (20%–30%) will exhibit distressing reactions related to tinnitus, making sleep difficult and making intellectual work challenging, which can lead to depression or anxiety.[1,2] One factor that may exacerbate tinnitus severity after onset is depression, with a subgroup with a certain level of depression reporting worse symptoms at 6 months than at onset.[3]

Tinnitus severity is captured by many psychometrically validated questionnaires often used in the clinic or the laboratory, for example, the Tinnitus Handicap Inventory (THI)[4], the Tinnitus Functional Index (TFI)[5], and the Tinnitus Primary Function Questionnaire (TPFQ).[6] These questionnaires probe the patient's reaction along the various dimensions of tinnitus distress, with the responses often weighted as to the severity of the impact of these dimensions. A composite score, ranging from 0 to 100, is generated, which serves as an index of tinnitus severity. The developers of such questionnaires have also divided these scores into clinically relevant categories, ranging from mild to most bothersome, with the intention that those scoring in the more bothersome categories require the most medical assistance. Apart from probing various dimensions of tinnitus, the questionnaires ask some questions about depressive symptoms in general (eg, TFI and THI), or as related specifically to tinnitus (eg, TPFQ). However, these are not comparable with full-fledged questionnaires, such as the Beck Depression Inventory[7] or the Hospital Anxiety and Depression Scale.[8] When assessing depression in individuals with tinnitus, depression-specific questionnaires are often used concurrently with tinnitus severity measures, as discussed in the next section.

PREVALENCE OF DEPRESSIVE SYMPTOMS IN INDIVIDUALS REPORTING TINNITUS

It has been known for some time that individuals with tinnitus often report anxiety and depressive symptoms.[9] One of the first large-scale studies to investigate their comorbidity was Bartels and colleagues,[10] who assessed tinnitus severity, anxiety, depression, coping style, and quality of life in 265 individuals reporting having tinnitus. Although the authors did not find a significant effect of either anxiety or depression alone, they observed an additive effect of both on the quality of life in those with tinnitus. Bhatt and colleagues[11] found a greater prevalence of both anxiety and depression in the tinnitus population (26.1% and 25.6%, respectively), compared with the general population (9.2% and 9.1%, respectively). A recent study[12] explored gender differences in psychiatric distress and tinnitus severity. Of the 134 female and 114 male patients who had accessed care at an otology outpatient clinic in Seoul, tinnitus severity, as measured by the THI, did not significantly differ between the 2 groups. However, further statistical testing revealed that depressive symptoms (as measured by the Beck Depression Inventory), stress within the past month (measured by the Korean version of the Brief Encounter Psychosocial Instrument[13]), and the effect on life (as measured by a Likert or visual analog scale) were significantly associated with tinnitus severity in men, whereas only depressive symptoms and tinnitus annoyance (assessed using a visual analog scale) were related to tinnitus severity in female patients.

The aforementioned studies help us better understand the prevalence of anxiety and depression in the tinnitus population. Both appear to show similar levels of prevalence, but their additive effect needs to be clinically addressed. Furthermore, although the Han and colleagues[12] study incorporated hearing loss in their statistical models (they did not find a differential impact of it on the two genders), other studies have not considered the effect of comorbid hearing loss, which may also contribute to feelings of depression and anxiety.[3]

Suicidal ideation has been reported in patients who have severe tinnitus accompanied by different psychiatric comorbidities, including severe anxiety or depression; such patients require prompt identification and intervention. A recent article[14] reviewed 10 publications (of the 22 that were initially identified) that reported on expressed suicidal behavior and ideation in adults with tinnitus. Whereas depression and suicidal ideation were reported at higher rates in the tinnitus population in several of these studies, the authors could not unequivocally identify an association between suicidal ideation and tinnitus. This was primarily because of methodological differences in the various studies, differences in the reported comorbid factors (eg, inclusion of patients with posttraumatic stress disorder), and as yet unknown relationship between tinnitus, stress, and psychiatric disorders (eg, differing cortisol levels).

Prevalence studies have also noted common personality factors between tinnitus and depression,[15] with a consistent pattern of those seeking more help with tinnitus also suffering from depression and other mood disorders.[16] In the study by Langguth and colleagues,[15] agreeableness negatively correlated with tinnitus severity as measured by THI and the anxiety trait of neuroticism correlated both with depressive symptomatology and tinnitus handicap, as measured by the Tinnitus Questionnaire,[17,18] but not with THI. In another study,[19] the authors focused on parsing the impact of type D personality (a framework used to study personality in depression) on both health-related quality of life and tinnitus distress. They found that those who had type D personality tended to be more anxious and depressed, with low health-related quality of life and higher tinnitus severity. This impact was mediated both by anxiety and depressive symptomology and by a direct influence on the outcomes.

NEURAL NETWORKS OF DEPRESSION AND TINNITUS

There are parallels in the pathophysiology of depression and tinnitus—similar neural networks appear to be affected in both conditions[20] when compared with age-matched healthy controls. Some of these networks are more evident in individuals reporting bothersome or severe tinnitus and include, default mode, attention, salience, and emotion-processing networks.[21–23] Similarly, altered functional connectivity of the default mode, salience networks, emotion processing, and cognitive control (part of attention processing) networks[24,25] are implicated in major depressive disorder. However, it is unclear if this constitutes a genuine overlap between 2 different traits or whether depression is part of the tinnitus condition. It should be further noted that, like depression, the psychological impact of tinnitus is along a continuum and it may be difficult to completely describe the overlap or to completely dissociate the 2 conditions. One major difference in the brain imaging results is the role played by the auditory cortex. Whereas activation patterns of the auditory cortex and its connectivity have been noted in most brain imaging studies of tinnitus (eg, Husain[21]), it has not been similarly reported in the brain imaging literature on depression.

PHARMACOLOGIC TREATMENTS OF DEPRESSION AND TINNITUS

Given the greater prevalence of anxiety and depression in the tinnitus population, it may not be surprising to see greater use of antianxiety and antidepression medications in this group. Yet, Tunkel and colleagues[26] do not recommend routine use of antidepressants, among other pharmaceutical agents that are sometimes used to treat symptoms of tinnitus. To make this determination, they relied on the outcome of randomized-controlled trials, in particular the meta-review from the Agency for Health-care Research and Quality,[27] which analyzed 13 published studies. They concluded that, given the potential for some antidepressants to worsen tinnitus, the small effect sizes and studies with small sample sizes, the injurious side-effects and the cost for such medications, the harm far outweighed any benefits at the group level.

In a 2012 Cochrane review,[28] Baldo and colleagues[28] reviewed 6 trials that had enrolled 610 patients with tinnitus. They found the trial quality to be generally low, primarily because of high attrition rates, suboptimal outcome measures, and, interestingly enough, a "failure to separate the effects on tinnitus from the effects on symptoms of anxiety and depression". However, a trial using a selective serotonin re-uptake inhibitor in a group of 120 patients, found significant effects in a subgroup of patients, suggesting a deeper investigation into its effects is needed.[28]

Do some antidepressants make tinnitus worse? Certainly there are several reported side-effects of antidepressants that affect quality of life (eg, sexual dysfunction, drowsiness), which may in turn affect tinnitus-related distress. Tinnitus itself is commonly reported as a rare side effect of all available antidepressants,[26,29] but more research needs to be conducted in determining which type of antidepressants has more of a detrimental effect on tinnitus relative to others.

PSYCHOLOGY-BASED TREATMENTS OF DEPRESSION AND TINNITUS

Given the high prevalence of depressive symptoms in those reporting severe tinnitus, it is not surprising that cognitive behavior therapy (CBT)[30,31] has gained popularity as a successful management strategy for bothersome tinnitus. In fact, CBT is currently the only treatment option to have the highest degree of evidence (ie, grade A, based on multiple systematic reviews of randomized-controlled trials) among all tinnitus management strategies, including drugs.[26,32] Although CBT consists of 4 general principles,[30] when adapted to tinnitus[31] it has been modified to include 3 tiers: (1) cognitive restructuring; (2) attentional control training, and (3) relaxation training.

In recent years, CBT has been successfully implemented, both via in-person guidance and via online classes. In one of the earliest large-scale studies,[33] CBT was shown to have better outcomes in terms of reducing tinnitus severity in 245 patients compared with 247 patients who underwent usual care. These improvements seemed to persist at 12 months, roughly eight months after end of treatment.

Internet-based CBT has also shown promise and it may be the treatment of choice for some patients. A recent randomized-controlled trial did not find significant difference between Internet-based CBT and two-to-three, in-person, individualized meetings in the clinic.[34] The ameliorating effects of being exposed to CBT seem to persist even a year after cessation of treatment.[35] Some caveats to consider include that dropout rates for treatment are fairly high (see Andersson[36]) and that some patients may need additional monitoring. Plausible risk factors for the attrition have not been worked out yet.

CBT is not the only counseling-based therapy to show success with managing tinnitus distress. Other therapies include mindfulness-based stress reduction,[37,38] mindfulness-based cognitive therapy,[39–41] and acceptance and commitment therapy.[42] Of these, more evidence has been collected for the mindfulness-based therapies. Acceptance and commitment therapy, although only recently being applied to tinnitus, has shown promise in ameliorating tinnitus-related distress.[43,44]

Counseling, whether using the tenets of CBT or not, plays a central role in comprehensive tinnitus management programs, such as tinnitus retraining therapy,[45] progressive tinnitus management,[46] and tinnitus activities treatment.[47] These comprehensive programs incorporate assessment of tinnitus severity and tailored treatment strategies based on individual severity, including sound devices (hearing aids, sound generators) and a variety of counseling techniques from information (present in all management strategies), to directive (in tinnitus retraining therapy), to collaborative (in tinnitus activities treatment), to applying principles of CBT (in progressive tinnitus management).

In essence, these tinnitus management frameworks seek to improve self-efficacy in patients with tinnitus allowing them to control their reactions to the chronic internal sound and thereby habituate better. For the purposes of its relation to tinnitus, self-efficacy can be considered the extent to which patients believe they are in control of factors affecting their life.[48,49] Low self-efficacy is seen to be associated with increased levels of depression and anxiety regardless of tinnitus status. Treatments that seek to improve self-efficacy in patients with tinnitus facilitate habituation and improve quality of life.

CAVEATS AND FUTURE DIRECTIONS

It is imperative that any tinnitus patient reporting a high-level of distress and bothersome symptoms is identified and provided with immediate care. Furthermore, those not reporting severe-enough symptoms may yet benefit from psychology-based therapies or tinnitus management plans. This article reviewed one aspect of tinnitus severity, manifesting as clinically defined depression. However, depression is not the only mental health concern noted in patients with tinnitus. Anxiety typically also co-occurs with depression. Recently, tinnitus has also been noted as a common symptom of traumatic brain injury and posttraumatic stress disorder, especially in the military and veteran population.[50,51] Future studies should parse out the overlap between tinnitus and several mental health conditions and specifically, the contribution of tinnitus itself to the severity of these conditions and vice-versa. This is important both for the optimal, individualized treatment of patients with tinnitus and to improve our understanding of the neural mechanisms of the disorder. In the clinic, those who report severe or bothersome tinnitus, as classified by one of the tinnitus questionnaires (eg, TFI), should be further screened for anxiety and depression and appropriate treatment plans should be initiated, if warranted.

REFERENCES

1. Hallam RS. Tinnitus: living with the ringing in your ears. London: Harper Collins Publishing; 1989.
2. Davis A, Rafaie EA. Epidemiology of tinnitus. In: Tyler RS, editor. Tinnitus handbook. San Diego (CA): Singular; 2000. p. 1–24.
3. Wallhäusser-Franke E, D'Amelio R, Glauner A, et al. Transition from acute to chronic tinnitus: predictors for the development of chronic distressing tinnitus. Front Neurol 2017;8:605.
4. Newman CW, Jacobson GP, Spitzer JB. Development of the tinnitus handicap inventory. Arch Otolaryngol Head Neck Surg 1996;122(2):143–8.
5. Meikle MB, Henry JA, Griest SE, et al. The tinnitus functional index: development of a new clinical measure for chronic, intrusive tinnitus. Ear Hear 2012;33(2):153–76.
6. Tyler R, Ji H, Perreau A, et al. Development and validation of the Tinnitus Primary Function Questionnaire. Am J Audiol 2014;23(3):260–72.
7. Beck AT, Steer RA, Garbin MG. Psychometric properties of the Beck Depression Inventory—25 years of evaluation. Clin Psychol Rev 1988;8(1):77–100.
8. Zigmond AS, Snaith RP. The hospital anxiety and depression scale. Acta Psychiatr Scand 1983;67(6):361–70.

9. Dobie RA. Overview: suffering from tinnitus. In: Snow J, editor. Tinnitus: theory and management. Hamilton (Canada): BC Decker, Inc.; 2004. p. 1–7.

10. Bartels H, Middel BL, van der Laan BF, et al. The additive effect of co-occurring anxiety and depression on health status, quality of life and coping strategies in help-seeking tinnitus sufferers. Ear Hear 2008;29(6):947–56.

11. Bhatt JM, Bhattacharyya N, Lin HW. Relationships between tinnitus and the prevalence of anxiety and depression. Laryngoscope 2017;127(2):466–9.

12. Han TS, Jeong J-E, Park S-N, et al. Gender differences affecting psychiatric distress and tinnitus severity. Clin Psychopharmacol Neurosci 2019;17(1):113.

13. Yim J, Bae J, Choi S, et al. The validity of modified Korean-translated BEPSI (Brief Encounter Psychosocial Instrument) as instrument of stress measurement in outpatient clinic. J Korean Acad Fam Med 1996;17(1):42–53.

14. Szibor A, Mäkitie A, Aarnisalo AA. Tinnitus and suicide: an unresolved relation. Audiol Res 2019;9(1):222.

15. Langguth B, Kleinjung T, Fischer B, et al. Tinnitus severity, depression, and the big five personality traits. Prog Brain Res 2007;166:221–5.

16. Durai M, Searchfield G. Anxiety and depression, personality traits relevant to tinnitus: a scoping review. Int J Audiol 2016;55(11):605–15.

17. Goebel G, Hiller W. The tinnitus questionnaire. A standard instrument for grading the degree of tinnitus. Results of a multicenter study with the tinnitus questionnaire. HNO 1994;42(3):166–72 [in German].

18. Hallam R. TQ—Manual of the Tinnitus Questionnaire, revised and updated, 2008. London: Polpresa; 2009.

19. Bartels H, Pedersen SS, van der Laan BF, et al. The impact of Type D personality on health-related quality of life in tinnitus patients is mainly mediated by anxiety and depression. Otol Neurotol 2010;31(1):11–8.

20. Langguth B, Landgrebe M, Kleinjung T, et al. Tinnitus and depression. World J Biol Psychiatry 2011;12(7):489–500.

21. Husain FT. Neural networks of tinnitus in humans: elucidating severity and habituation. Hear Res 2016;334:37–48.

22. Elgoyhen AB, Langguth B, De Ridder D, et al. Tinnitus: perspectives from human neuroimaging. Nat Rev Neurosci 2015;16(10):632–42.

23. Shahsavarani S, Khan RA, Husain FT. Tinnitus and the brain: a review of functional and anatomical magnetic resonance imaging studies. Perspect ASHA Spec Interest Groups 2019;4(5):896–909.

24. Mulders PC, van Eijndhoven PF, Schene AH, et al. Resting-state functional connectivity in major depressive disorder: a review. Neurosci Biobehav Rev 2015;56:330–44.

25. Dutta A, McKie S, Deakin JW. Resting state networks in major depressive disorder. Psychiatry Res 2014;224(3):139–51.

26. Tunkel DE, Bauer CA, Sun GH, et al. Clinical practice guideline: tinnitus. Otolaryngol Head Neck Surg 2014;151(2 Suppl):S1–40.

27. Pichora-Fuller MK, Santaguida P, Hammill A, et al. Evaluation and treatment of tinnitus: comparative effectiveness. Rockville (MD): Agency for Healthcare Research and Quality (US); 2013.

28. Baldo P, Doree C, Molin P, et al. Antidepressants for patients with tinnitus. Cochrane Database Syst Rev 2012;(9):CD003853.

29. Miller CW. Development of tinnitus at a low dose of sertraline: clinical course and proposed mechanisms. Case Rep Psychiatry 2016;2016:1790692.

30. Andrews G. The essential psychotherapies. Br J Psychiatry 1993;162:447–51.

31. Henry JL, Wilson PH. The psychological management of chronic tinnitus: a cognitive-behavioral approach. Boston (MA): Allyn & Bacon; 2000.
32. Martinez-Devesa P, Perera R, Theodoulou M, et al. Cognitive behavioural therapy for tinnitus. Cochrane Database Syst Rev 2010;(9):CD005233.
33. Cima RF, Maes IH, Joore MA, et al. Specialised treatment based on cognitive behaviour therapy versus usual care for tinnitus: a randomised controlled trial. Lancet 2012;379(9830):1951–9.
34. Beukes EW, Andersson G, Allen PM, et al. Effectiveness of guided internet-based cognitive behavioral therapy vs face-to-face clinical care for treatment of tinnitus: a randomized clinical trial. JAMA Otolaryngol Head Neck Surg 2018;144(12):1126–33.
35. Beukes EW, Allen PM, Baguley DM, et al. Long-term efficacy of audiologist-guided Internet-based cognitive behavior therapy for tinnitus. Am J Audiol 2018;27(3S):431–47.
36. Andersson G. Clinician-supported internet-delivered psychological treatment of tinnitus. Am J Audiol 2015;24(3):299–301.
37. Bishop SR. What do we really know about mindfulness-based stress reduction? Psychosom Med 2002;64(1):71–83.
38. Roland LT, Lenze EJ, Hardin FM, et al. Effects of mindfulness based stress reduction therapy on subjective bother and neural connectivity in chronic tinnitus. Otolaryngol Head Neck Surg 2015;152(5):919–26.
39. Teasdale JD, Williams JMG, Segal ZV. The mindful way workbook: an 8-week program to free yourself from depression and emotional distress. New York: Guilford Publications; 2014.
40. Zimmerman BJ, Finnegan MK, Paul S, et al. Functional brain changes during mindfulness-based cognitive therapy associated with tinnitus severity. Front Neurosci 2019;13:747.
41. McKenna L, Marks EM, Vogt F. Mindfulness-based cognitive therapy for chronic tinnitus: evaluation of benefits in a large sample of patients attending a tinnitus clinic. Ear Hear 2018;39(2):359–66.
42. Hayes SC, Luoma JB, Bond FW, et al. Acceptance and commitment therapy: model, processes and outcomes. Behav Res Ther 2006;44(1):1–25.
43. Hesser H, Gustafsson T, Lundén C, et al. A randomized controlled trial of internet-delivered cognitive behavior therapy and acceptance and commitment therapy in the treatment of tinnitus. J Consult Clin Psychol 2012;80(4):649.
44. Zetterqvist Westin V, Schulin M, Hesser H, et al. Acceptance and commitment therapy versus tinnitus retraining therapy in the treatment of tinnitus: a randomised controlled trial. Behav Res Ther 2011;49(11):737–47.
45. Jastreboff PJ. Tinnitus retraining therapy. Prog Brain Res 2007;166:415–23.
46. Griest S. Development of a progressive audiologic tinnitus management program for veterans with tinnitus. J Rehabil Res Dev 2014;51(4):609.
47. Tyler RS, Gogel SA, Gehringer AK. Tinnitus activities treatment. Prog Brain Res 2007;166:425–34.
48. Bandura A. Self-efficacy: toward a unifying theory of behavioral change. Psychol Rev 1977;84(2):191.
49. Fagelson MA, Smith SL. Tinnitus self-efficacy and other tinnitus self-report variables in patients with and without post-traumatic stress disorder. Ear Hear 2016;37(5):541–6.
50. Moring JC, Peterson AL, Kanzler KE. Tinnitus, traumatic brain injury, and post-traumatic stress disorder in the military. Int J Behav Med 2018;25(3):312–21.
51. Fagelson MA. The association between tinnitus and posttraumatic stress disorder. Am J Audiol 2007;16(2):107–17.

Does Tinnitus Fill in the Gap Using Electrophysiology? A Scoping Review

Victoria Duda, MScS, PhD[a], Olivia Scully, BSc[a],
Marie-Sarah Baillargeon[a], Sylvie Hébert, PhD[a,b],*

KEYWORDS

- Tinnitus • Gap-prepulse inhibition of the startle reflex • GPIAS • Electrophysiology
- Gap detection • Review

KEY POINTS

- Gap-induced auditory evoked potentials (EPs) are used to objectively determine the presence of tinnitus.
- A scoping review of studies that examined the effectiveness of electroencephalograms evoked by gapped stimuli, more specifically gaps in noise, in determining the presence of tinnitus of experiments has yielded 8 studies.
- The results show a trend of increased postgap amplitudes and reduced gap salience.
- Conclusions are limited due to the small number of studies found, the differences in methods used, and confounding variables, such as the contribution of attention, tinnitus frequency, and hearing loss.

INTRODUCTION

Tinnitus is a phenomenon in which a sound is heard by an individual without the presence of external acoustic stimulation. Its origin is still a subject of much debate as there is currently no consensus on an objective measure of tinnitus in patient populations. Within the clinical setting, tinnitus is evaluated using questionnaires and psychometric assessments where its intensity and pitch can be matched to a stimulus. The issue with the current clinical method is that it is still a subjective method with problematic reliability[1] and cannot be tested among prelingual children and populations with low-functioning behavioral abilities or cognition. The lack of a standardized assessment of tinnitus leads to issues of poorly defined populations that are highly

[a] École d'orthophonie et d'audiologie, Faculty of Medicine, Université de Montréal, Pavillon 7077, Parc, C.P. 6128, Succ. Centre-ville, Montreal H3C 3J7, Canada; [b] International Laboratory for Brain, Music and Sound Research (BRAMS), Outremont, Quebec, Canada
* Corresponding author. École d'orthophonie et d'audiologie, Faculty of medicine, Université de Montréal, Pavillon 7077, Parc, C.P. 6128, Succ. Centre-ville, Montreal H3C 3J7, Canada.
E-mail address: sylvie.hebert@umontreal.ca

Otolaryngol Clin N Am 53 (2020) 563–582
https://doi.org/10.1016/j.otc.2020.03.006
0030-6665/20/© 2020 Elsevier Inc. All rights reserved.

heterogeneous. For instance, tinnitus can be reported in those without any signs of hearing loss and can occur with other comorbidities, such as anxiety or depression.

In the effort to produce a gold standard technique that could translate the findings of animal research to the human literature, a gap detection protocol was proposed known as the gap-prepulse inhibition of the startle reflex (GPIAS). The GPIAS reflex is elicited by the presentation of a loud startling sound following an interval of silence embedded in a background noise. The silent gap serves as a preindication of the oncoming loud stimulus (a "prepulse") so that the startle could be inhibited. The seminal study by Turner and colleagues[2] on rats with salicylate-induced tinnitus showed little inhibition of the startle reflex, implying that they did not hear the preceding gap. In particular, this effect occurred when the background noise was matched to a frequency presumably close to the tinnitus. This was unlike normal rats in which the gap increases inhibition of the startle reflex.[2] These findings led to the hypothesis that tinnitus may be filling in the gap. As such, the GPIAS paradigm has since been used as an objective measure of tinnitus in many other studies on both rats and mice.[2–12]

To determine whether these findings were applicable in humans, Fournier and Hébert[13] adapted the GPIAS for use in humans using the eye-blink startle reflex. They demonstrated that participants with high-frequency tinnitus showed an impaired inhibition of the startle reflex when a gap was used as a prestimulus within a background noise. These results were similar to Turner and colleagues,[2] although the stimuli were not matched to the frequency of the tinnitus and an effect was found in both high-frequency and low-frequency background noises. This finding cast doubt as to whether or not tinnitus contributes to the impaired startle reflex. Other potential confounds when testing gap detection or the GPIAS reflex in those with tinnitus are sensory gating deficits[14] and attention bias for particular auditory stimuli.[15] Furthermore, given that the neural circuitry controlling GPIAS is not fully understood, the role of the auditory cortex in those findings remains unclear.

One technique that can mitigate these potential confounds is measuring the synchronized activity of the eighth peripheral nerve of the cochlear nucleus up to the auditory cortex using electroencephalograms (EEGs). Auditory evoked potentials are averaged EEGs that reflect the changes in the electrical activity of the brain elicited by an external auditory stimulus or internal event. Evoked potentials are a series of positive and negative deflections that are believed to be associated with various aspects of information processing. They can be used to monitor the processing of a gap within a long-duration stimulus.[16] The advantage of evoked potentials is that the data are objective because certain components can occur in the absence of attention and thus can be recorded passively.[17–19]

This article presents a scoping review of experiments that examined the effectiveness of EEGs evoked by gapped stimuli, more specifically gaps in noise, in determining the presence of tinnitus. The research questions were whether tinnitus alters the activity of the EEG elicited by gaps, and whether the activation is different for short-latency (ie, subcortical) compared with long-latency (ie, cortical) potentials in the tinnitus population.

METHODS

The search was conducted June 20, 2019, by one of the authors (VD). The databases that were reviewed were PubMed, Ovid, CINAHL, and PsychINFO. The outcome of interest was the gap-elicited auditory evoked potentials in patients with tinnitus with and without hearing loss. Gaps were defined as silent periods embedded within a sound in which the evoked potential is elicited by either the offset of the gap or the onset of a sound following the gap. The keywords were chosen based on a previous scoping review that was conducted on a similar topic.[20] The search terms, and their variations, used alone or in combination were (1) tinnitus, ear, buzz, ring, roar, click, pulsate, or pulse; (2) electroencephalography, EEG, N1, P1, evoked potentials, brainstem response, ABR, BAER, or BSER; and (3) gaps, temporal resolution, intermittent, gap in noise (GIN), or silent interval. Mesh terms were searched when available. Only studies written in English or French were included; however, no articles were rejected based on language, as the entire final yield were articles written in English (**Table 1**).

Articles were included if there was mention of a tinnitus population, use of any form of auditory evoked potential, and a gapped stimulus. Both animal and human populations were considered. Articles were excluded if the participants had a history of ontological conditions, such as hypertension, tumors, demyelination, auditory neuropathy, or otitis media or externa. Articles reporting on individuals with cochlear implants, central auditory processing disorder, head trauma, psychological disorders, and sudden hearing loss were also excluded. Any non–peer-reviewed literature was excluded at the screening level, such as a magazines, conference proceedings, editorials, and manuals. Doctoral theses initially searched in the ProQuest Dissertations and Theses Global and Conference Papers Index, were deemed redundant to the articles found in the scientific databases and thus not included in this review.

A team approach was used to conduct the screening of the literature.[21] Two independent reviewers (OS and M-SB) independently analyzed all the articles for eligibility.[22] Any disagreement between the 2 parties was resolved by a third member (VD) until a consensus was reached. All results were compiled in Covidence Online Software (https://www.covidence.org). During the first level of screening, the adherence to the eligibility criteria was based on the title and abstract. Subsequently, a second level of screening was conducted in which the articles were eliminated based on a reading of the full text. The remaining articles were analyzed for content and organized in a table according to population characteristics (hearing loss, species, tinnitus etiology, use of a control group), techniques used (ie, gap onset or offset, gap salience, gap sizes used, stimulus frequencies), and outcomes measured.

RESULTS

A total of 1356 articles were imported from the databases. After removing all duplicates, 1257 articles were screened by title and abstract and 56 of those articles were analyzed by reading the full text. Forty-eight articles were excluded in the full-text review because the study did not use gapped stimuli (n = 24), the population did not have tinnitus as described in the eligibility criteria (n = 12), or the outcome measure was a frequency analysis of the EEG (n = 7). See **Fig. 1** for more details. Of the remaining articles, 8 were extracted for a narrative synthesis.[23–29] The objective for these extracted studies was to investigate amplitude changes in the EEG of tinnitus groups compared with those without tinnitus (n = 4), after tinnitus treatment (n = 1), or before tinnitus induction (n = 3).

POPULATION CHARACTERISTICS

The population characteristics for the extracted data from the 8 studies are shown in **Table 2**, grouped by etiology (eg, noise-induced, salicylate-induced, or idiopathic). Humans were tested in 5 studies and the remaining 3 studies tested guinea pigs (n = 2) and CBA/CaJ mice (n = 1). All but 1 study[27] had a control group. The mean

Table 1
The search terms used for searching 4 databases

PubMed	Ovid	CINAHL	PsychINFO
((ERP*) OR (electroencephalograph*) OR (N1*) OR (P1*) OR (ERP*) OR (evoked potentials, auditory, brain stem[MeSH Terms]) OR (brainstem response*) OR (brainstem potential*) OR (brain stem response*) OR (brain stem potential*) OR (ABR*) OR (BAER*) OR (BSER*)) AND ((tinnit*) OR (ear* AND (buzz* OR ring* OR roar* OR click* OR pulsat* OR pulse*)) OR Tinnitus[MESH] AND ((gap*) OR (temporal resolution) OR (intermittent*) OR (gaps in noise, GIN))	1 (Tinnitus or tinnit* or (ear* and (buzz* or ring* or roar* or click* or pulsat* or pulse*))).af. (91,360) 2 (Gap* in noise or gap* or temporal resolution* or intermittent* or GIN* or silent interval*).af. (626914) 3 (ERP or encephalo* or N1 or P1 or N2 or P2 or P3a or P3b or P300 or EEG or ABR or evoked brain stem auditory response or brain stem response or evoked brain stem response).af. (492381) 4 1 and 2 and 3 (308)	((MM "Tinnitus") OR "tinnitus") AND ("temporal resolution" OR "gap detection" OR "gap in noise" OR "gap" OR "intermittent" OR "GIN" OR "silent interval") AND ((MH "Evoked Potentials, Auditory, Brainstem") OR (MM "Evoked Potentials, Auditory") OR (MH "Brain Stem") OR (MH "Auditory Steady-State Response") OR (MM "Evoked Potentials") OR "ERP" or "encephalo" or "N1" or "P1" or "N2" or "P2" or "P3a" or "P3b" or "P300" or "ERP" or "ABR" or "evoked brain stem auditory response" or "brain stem response" or "evoked brain stem response" OR (MH "Electroencephalography"))	Any Field: Tinnitus OR Any Field: tinn* OR Any Field: ear* OR Any Field: buzz* OR Any Field: ring* OR Any Field: roar* OR Any Field: pulsat* OR Any Field: pulse* AND Any Field: temporal resolution OR Any Field: gap detection OR Any Field: gap in noise* OR Any Field: gap* OR Any Field: intermitt* OR Any Field: GIN OR Any Field: silent interval* AND (Any Field: Evoked Potentials, Auditory, Brainstem OR Any Field: Evoked Potentials, Auditory OR Any Field: Brain Stem OR Any Field: Auditory Steady-State Response* OR Any Field: Evoked Potential* OR Any Field: EEG* OR Any Field: encephalo* OR Any Field: N1 OR Any Field: P1 OR Any Field: N2 OR Any Field: P2 OR Any Field: P3a OR Any Field: P300 OR Any Field: P3b OR Any Field: EEG OR Any Field: ABR OR Any Field: evoked brain stem auditory response OR Any Field: brain stem response OR Any Field: evoked brain stem response OR Any Field: Electroencephalography)

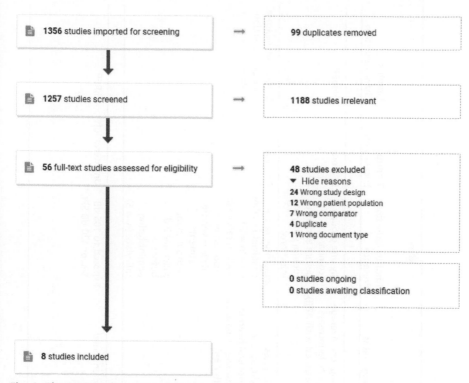

Fig. 1. The PRISMA flowchart of study selection.

age of the human tinnitus groups was between 35 and 53 years old and the control group mean age was between 35 and 55 years old. The standard deviation of age was as high as 20 years in one study.[29] For the animal studies, the mean age was reported as 2 to 4 months old in Lowe and Walton[24]; however, it was not reported in either article by Berger and colleagues.[23,25] The matching procedures varied between the studies, that is, if they were mentioned at all. In 3 of the human studies, the subjects were matched by sex, age, and/or hearing status. In 2 animal studies, the animals were their own controls and tested before and after tinnitus induction. Matching procedures were not reported in 3 articles.

Hearing status was reported in 7 of the 8 articles. Hearing was described as an average threshold increase measured using the auditory brainstem response in 2 of the 3 animal studies. Berger and colleagues[23] did not mention hearing status. Among the human studies, hearing was evaluated by determining the pure tone threshold of detection. Normal hearing was defined in relation to frequency. For Mahmoudian and colleagues[26,27] and Mohebbi and colleagues,[30] normal hearing was characterized as equal to or less than 20 dBHL from 250 to 2000 Hz and less than 40 dBHL at 4000 and 8000 Hz. Ku and colleagues[28] allowed thresholds to be less than 20 dBHL at 600 and 1000 Hz and less than 40 dBHL at 8000 Hz. Morse and Vander Werff[29] permitted less than 20 dBHL for the pure tone average at 500, 1000, and 2000 Hz. Generally, the accepted hearing threshold was higher for the higher frequencies of 4000 or 8000 Hz (n = 3) or not reported (n = 1), compared with the frequencies less than 2000 Hz, which were all below 20 dBHL. No human studies reported hearing thresholds higher than 8 kHz.

Table 2
Population demographics of the yielded studies (n = 8)

Study	Species	Groups	Mean Age	Hearing Status	Tinnitus Induction/ Presence	Tinnitus Localization	Tinnitus Characterization
Sodium salicylate etiology							
Lowe and Walton,[24] 2015	CBA/CaJ mice	Tinnitus (n = 12) Control (n = 12) Each animal is its own control	2–4 months old	Hearing loss: Average threshold increase (measured with ABR)	Only one group (comparison before and after sodium salicylate injections)	Bilateral	Gap-PPI
Berger et al,[25] 2017	Tricolor guinea pigs	Tinnitus (n = 8) Control (n = 5)	Not mentioned	Hearing loss: Reductions in peripheral hearing sensitivity (measured with ABR)	Sodium salicylate dissolved in saline only (n = 3); Sodium salicylate dissolved in saline + vehicle treatment without saline salicylate 2 d before administering salicylate (n = 5)	Bilateral	Behavioral measure of gap detection ability
Noise-induced etiology							
Berger et al,[23] 2018	Guinea pigs	Tinnitus (n = 9 ears) Control (n = 9 ears) Each animal is its own control	Not mentioned	Not mentioned	Exposed to 105 dB SPL or 120 dB SPL	Unilateral left	GiREP

Idiopathic etiology

Study	Subject	Groups	Age	Hearing	Condition	Laterality	Measures
Mahmoudian et al,[26] 2013	Humans	Tinnitus (n = 28) Control (n = 33) Age and sex matched	Tinnitus = 35.3 y (SD 7.0) Control = 35.2 y (SD 6.9)	Normal hearing: ≤20 dB HL in octave frequencies of 250–2000 Hz and no more than 40 dB HL in frequencies of 4000 and 8000 Hz	Tinnitus or no tinnitus	Left (n = 7) Right (n = 4) Head (n = 17)	TQ-P and THI-P questionnaires, minimal masking level, residual inhibition, pitch, and loudness matching
Mahmoudian et al,[27] 2015	Humans	Residual inhibition (n = 13) No residual inhibition (n = 15)	35.3 y (22–45 years old) (SD 7.0)	Normal hearing: <20 dB HL in octave frequencies of 250–2000 Hz, and <40 dB HL in frequencies of 4000 and 8000 Hz	Tinnitus with residual inhibition or no residual inhibition treated with auditory electrical stimulation or placebo electrical stimulation	Left (n = 6) Right (n = 7) Bilateral (n = 15)	TQ-P,THI-P, VAS, and pitch and loudness matching of tinnitus, minimal masking level, residual inhibition
Ku et al,[28] 2017	Humans	Tinnitus (n = 16) Control (n = 18) Age and hearing loss matched	Tinnitus = 59.2 y (SD = 8) Control = 59.2 y (SD = 6)	Normal hearing: 8 kHz = 39.1 (tinnitus) and 34.4 (control). 600 Hz = 13.1 (tinnitus) and 16.1 (control). 1 kHz = 17.4 (tinnitus) and 17.2 (control)	Tinnitus or no tinnitus	Bilateral (n = 9) or unilateral (n = 7)	Tinnitus pitch and loudness matching test

(continued on next page)

Table 2 (continued)							
Study	Species	Groups	Mean Age	Hearing Status	Tinnitus Induction/ Presence	Tinnitus Localization	Tinnitus Characterization
Mohebbi et al,[30] 2019	Humans	Compensated tinnitus (n = 20) Decompensated tinnitus (n = 20) Control (n = 20)	Compensated tinnitus = 44.4 y (SD = 11.5) Decompensated tinnitus = 42.4 (SD = 11.3) Control = 40.1 (SD = 11.6)	Normal hearing: ≤20 dBHL in octave frequencies of 250–2000 Hz, and <40 dB HL in frequencies of 4000 and 8000 Hz in both ears	Compensated or decompensated tinnitus or no tinnitus	Left (n = 15) Right (n = 11) Bilateral (n = 14)	VAS, THI, and TQ questionnaires + Loudness and pitch matching of tinnitus, minimal masking level, residual inhibition
Morse and Vander Werff,[29] 2019	Humans	Tinnitus (n = 13) Control (n = 13) Age, sex, and hearing loss matched	Tinnitus = 52.9 y (SD = 19.3) Control = 54.5 y (SD = 18.0)	Normal hearing: Pure tone average = 18.9 (SD 11.0) (tinnitus) and 20.2 (SD 15.4) (control)	Chronic tinnitus or no tinnitus	Bilateral or unilateral	THI questionnaire + tinnitus pitch- and loudness matching

Abbreviations: ABR, auditory brainstem response; dB, decibel; Gap-PPI, Gap-prepulse inhibition; GIREP, gap-induced reduction in evoked potentials; HL, hearing loss; SD, standard deviation; THI(-P), (Persian) tinnitus handicap inventory; TQ(-P), (Persian) tinnitus questionnaire; VAS, visual analog scale.

Tinnitus was identified in the human populations using tinnitus pitch and loudness matching procedures (n = 4) and tinnitus questionnaires: Tinnitus Questionnaire (n = 3), Tinnitus Handicap Inventory (n = 4), or a Visual Analog Scale (n = 2). In the animal population, tinnitus was induced using salicylate (n = 2) or noise exposure (n = 1) and the presence of tinnitus was determined using the gap-induced reduction paradigm with evoked potentials (n = 1), behavioral measures of gap detection (n = 1), or the gap-prepulse inhibition test (n = 1). Residual inhibition was measured in one study.[27] The main difference between groups was the presence or absence of tinnitus (n = 4), although one study separated the groups by treatment using electrical stimulation. This study also was the only one that did not present a control group.[27] Of the 3 animal studies, groups were separated based on levels of noise exposure (n = 1) or based on the moment of tinnitus induction, for example, before and after salicylate injection (n = 2). Tinnitus localization in the human studies included both bilateral and unilateral tinnitus (n = 5) but was either exclusively bilateral (n = 2) or unilateral (n = 1) in the animal studies.

Methods

The characteristics of the EEG recording technique can be found in **Table 3**. The animal studies investigated either the auditory brainstem response to gaps (n = 1) or the amplitude ratios of the electrocorticography (EcoG; n = 2). For these studies, between 3 and 8 electrodes were used. Two animal studies used system 3 interface by Tucker Davis Technologies (TDT;[24,25]) and Berger and colleagues[23] did not report their recording system. All 3 animal studies and one study on humans[30] presented the stimuli through speakers. All studies using human participants reported long latency potentials (n = 5). Of these studies, 3 (of the same laboratory) reported values of the Mismatch Negativity response, 2 reported the N1 and P2, and one study reported the P1. These evoked potentials were recorded with a minimum of 4 to 5 electrodes (n = 2) and 32 to 64 electrodes (n = 3) at the maximum. All the studies investigating the MMN used the Brain Quick system (Micromed, Treviso, Italy) and the 2 studies on the N1, P2, and/or P1 used either the SynAmpsRT system by Neuroscan (Charlotte, NC)[29] or an analog-digital converter.[28] The stimuli were presented either under earphones, ER-3A (n = 3) or ER-2 (n = 1), or through free-field speakers.

Stimuli used are summarized in **Table 4**. Most of the studies used narrowband noises with various center frequencies in which gaps were inserted (n = 7). These frequencies ranged from 500 to 24,000 Hz, although human data was only reported up to 8500 Hz. The remaining studies used broadband noises (n = 3; note that Berger and colleagues[23,25] used both NBN and BBN). Stimulus presentation levels were typically at 55 to 85 dB SPL (n = 3) except for 2 studies that presented levels relative to audiometric thresholds at 20 dB SL (n = 1) or 50 dB SL (n = 1). Within these stimuli, gaps of various lengths were inserted. The length of the gaps were either subthreshold at 0 to 2 ms (n = 3), at the threshold of detection that was determined behaviorally (n = 1), or at suprathreshold values of 4 to 16 ms (n = 4), 20 to 25 (n = 3), 50 ms (n = 3) or 100 ms (n = 1).

Outcomes

The paradigms, outcomes, and results for each study are found in **Table 4**. Three main paradigms were investigated: the GIN test (n = 2), the GPIAS reflex (n = 3), and the multideviant paradigm (MMN; n = 3). In the GIN tests, the response was recorded for the offset of the gap (ie, the onset of the stimulus following the gap). The GPIAS reflex was recorded as the response to the onset of the loud startling stimulus of 65 dB SL[28] or of 95, 100, or 105 dB SPL[23] following the gap. The multideviant

Table 3
Methodologies and equipment used in the yielded studies (n = 8)

Study	Recording System	Transducer	Recording Filters (Hz)	Sampling Rate	Electrodes (n)	AEP Studied	Type and Localization of Electrodes
Mice							
Lowe and Walton,[24] 2015	System III hardware (TDT) data-acquisition system and averaged with BioSig software	Multi-field (MF1) magnetic speaker	300 Hz–3 kHz	Not reported	3	ABR	Active (noninverting) electrode at the vertex, the reference (inverting) below the RE, and the ground below the LE
Guinea pigs							
Berger et al,[25] 2017	TDT Medusa headstage amplifier connected to a TDT System 3 interface and BrainWare software	Free-field via a single ³/₄-inch tweeter (Tymphany XT19TD00)	Filtered online between 0.5–300 Hz	Not reported	8	EcoG	Implanted silver-ball electrodes positioned over left and right rostral AC, caudal AC and cerebellum + reference and ground
Berger et al,[23] 2018	TDT Medusa headstage amplifier connected to a TDT System 3 interface and BrainWare software	Free-field via a single ³/₄-inch tweeter (Tymphany XT19TD00)	Filtered online between 60 and 300 Hz	Not reported	8 ? (not explicitly reported)	EcoG	Implanted silver-ball electrodes positioned over left and right rostral AC, caudal AC and cerebellum + reference and ground
Humans							
Mahmoudian et al,[26] 2013	BRAIN QUICK LTM	ER-3A	Online bandpass filtered 0.00–100 Hz	1024 Hz	64	MMN	64-channel Ag/AgCl electrodes, the ground was on Fz and the reference on the nose
Mahmoudian et al,[27] 2015	Micromed BRAIN QUICK system	ER-3A	Online bandpass filtered 0.00–100 Hz	1024 Hz	32	MMN	32-channel Ag/AgCl electrodes, ground on the forehead and reference on the nose

Ku et al,[28] 2017	Analog-digital conversion (ADC)	ER-2	Bandpass filter of 1–100 Hz	1000 Hz	4	P1-N1-P2	10-mm gold disc electrode (F-E5GH) on the vertex (Cz) for the active electrode; disposable and adhesive silver-silver chloride electrodes on the ipsilateral mastoid = reference (A1 or A2) and ground = Fpz
Morse and Vander Werff,[29] 2019	Compumedics Neuroscan Stim; Neuroscan Synamps RT system	ER-3A	Online bandpass filtered from 0.1 to 100 Hz	1000 Hz	5	P1-N1-P2	Three-channel recording montage with midline noninverting electrodes (Pz, Cz, Fz, a forehead ground, mastoids reference)
Mohebbi et al,[30] 2019	BRAIN QUICK LTM	2 Speakers with 45° angle and 1.5 m distance facing the subjects	Online bandpass filtered 0.4–200 Hz and 50 Hz notch filter (power line interference)	1024 Hz	64	MMN	64-channel Ag/AgCl electrodes, the ground was on Fz and the reference on the nose

Abbreviations: AC, auditory cortex; AEP, auditory evoked potential; EcoG, electrocorticography; LE, left ear; MMN, mismatch negativity; RE, right ear; TDT, Tucker Davis Technologies.

Table 4
Stimuli, outcomes and results in the yielded studies (n = 8)

Study	Paradigm Used	Stimuli	Gap Duration	Outcomes Considered	Tinnitus Frequency	Major Findings
Mice						
Lowe and Walton,[24] 2015	Modified GIN test	150-m 70 dB NBN centered at 6, 12, 16, 20, 24 or 36 kHz presented with or without a silent gap	2, 4, 8, 12, 16, 25, and 50 ms	Neural gap detection threshold: maximum gap length where a postgap onset (ie, gap offset) ABR P1 or P4 amplitude is significantly smaller than the pregap onset response	GPIAS deficit for 12 and 16 kHz	Neural gap detection threshold **increase** after SS at 16 kHz only for P1 (mean: **8–25 ms**) and at 12, 16, and 20 kHz for P4. The behavioral PPI was similar with significant difference after SS at 12 and 16 kHz
Guinea pigs						
Berger et al,[25] 2017	GPIAS & Modified GIN test	MGDT: 200 ms BBN followed by various length gaps and a 50 ms postgap BBN burst all at 70 dB SPL. GIREP: Background BBN noise or NBN at 5, 9, 13, or 17 kHz presented at 50, 60 or 70 dB SPL; followed by 50 ms gap and a startling BBN at 95, 100 or 105 dB SPL.	1, 2, 4, 8, 10, 20, 50, and 75 ms	Neural gap detection threshold (MGDT) minimum gap length where a significant amplitude increase of the postgap EcoG response to the burst relative to baseline Neural GPI (or GIREP) ratio (gap/no gap) using the amplitudes P1-N1 in response to onset of startling sound following gap	GPIAS deficit for BBN	Neural gap detection threshold **increase** with BBN after SS greater in the rostral than the caudal AC (median: **8–15 ms**) Neural GPI ratio **increase for 50 ms gap** in rostral AC for the BBN and 4–6 kHz after SS similar to the behavioral GPI which also increased for BBN

Berger et al,[23] 2018	GPIAS	GIREP: Background BBN or NBN at 5, 9, 13, or 17 kHz presented at 55, 60, or 70 dB SPL; followed by 50 ms gap and a startling BBN at 95, 100, or 105 dB SPL	50 ms	Neural GPI (or GIREP) ratio (gap/no gap) using the amplitudes P1-N1 in response to onset of startling sound following gap	Not assessed	Neural GPI ratio **increase** for **50 ms gap** after 120 dB noise exposure, in right rostral, caudal for 8–10 kHz and Left rostral and caudal AC for BBN
Humans						
Mahmoudian et al,[26] 2013	Multiple deviant paradigm	Standard stimuli were 75 ms pure tones of 500 Hz, 1 kHz, and 1.5 kHz at 65 dB SPL with multiple deviants in frequency, intensity, duration, location, and silent gap duration	7 ms	Standard-deviant difference wave where the MMN occurs 100–250 ms following the offset of the gap	Not reported	MMN amplitude and AUC **reduced** for gap duration deviant in Tinnitus compared with NH Controls
Mahmoudian et al,[27] 2015	Multiple deviant paradigm	Standard stimuli were 75 ms pure tones of 500 Hz, 1 kHz, and 1.5 kHz at 65 dB SPL with multiple deviants in frequency, intensity, duration, location, and silent gap duration	7 ms	Standard-deviant difference wave where the MMN occurs 100–250 ms following the offset of the gap	Not reported	AES treatment recovered the MMN amplitude and AUC for other deviants but **not gap**
Mohebbi et al,[30] 2019	Multiple deviant paradigm	Standard stimuli were 75 ms pure tones of 500 Hz, 1 kHz, and 1.5 kHz at 65 dB SPL with multiple deviants in frequency, intensity, duration, location, and silent gap duration	7 ms	Standard-deviant difference wave in which the MMN occurs 100–250 ms following the offset of the gap	7.50 ± 1.6 kHz[a] for compensated and 7.60 ± 1.42 kHz for decompensated Tinnitus group (2 AFC pitch matching method)	MMN amplitude and AUC **reduced** for the gap duration deviant in decompensated Tinnitus group compared with Controls and compensated Tinnitus

(continued on next page)

Table 4
(continued)

Study	Paradigm Used	Stimuli	Gap Duration	Outcomes Considered	Tinnitus Frequency	Major Findings
Morse and Vander Werff,[29] 2019	Modified GIN Test	3-s white noise stimuli at 50 dB SL in which a gap is inserted	2 ms, individual threshold + 2 ms, 20 ms	Gap-evoked P1-N1-P2 amplitude, latency, and area	Not reported	Neural gap detection threshold: No significant differences by Tinnitus group for any of the peak amplitudes, latencies or AUC below, at or above gap threshold. P1 latency **decreased** for **threshold** and **20 ms gap** in BBN for Tinnitus group
Ku et al,[28] 2017	Similar to GPIAS	20 dB SL background pure tones of 600 Hz & 8 kHz with a startling 1-kHz tone burst of 20-ms duration at 65-dB SL	20 ms, 50 ms, and 100 ms	Neural GPI ratio (gap/no gap) using the N1-P2 amplitude to the intense sound stimulus following the gap or no gap. Lower ratio indicates greater inhibition because the N1-P2 amplitude of gap would be smaller	Pure tone 8 kHz (2 AFC pitch matching method)	Neural GPI ratio **increase** at 8 kHz for **20 ms gap** durations but not 50 or 100 ms which indicates less inhibition by gap than Controls. No group separation at 600 Hz as both groups showed an increased GPI ratio

Abbreviations: 2 AFC, 2 alternative forced choice method; AC, auditory cortex; AES, auditory electrical stimulation; AUC, area under the curve; BBN, broadband noise; GIN, gap in noise; GIN, gaps in noise; GIREP, gap-induced reductions in evoked potentials; GPI, gap-prepulse inhibition; GPIAS, gap-prepulse inhibition of the acoustic startle; MGDT, minimum gap detection threshold; MMN, mismatch negativity; NBN, narrowband noise; NH, normal hearing; PPI, prepulse inhibition; SL, sensation level; SPL, sound pressure level; SS, salicylate.

[a] Unit not reported but presumably kHz. The EEG components examined by each study in underlined, and the corresponding main results are in Bold.

paradigm measured the change in response to a gapped stimulus that was played in alternation with a control stimulus (ie, the standard) and a series of other deviant stimuli.

Of the 2 studies using the GIN test, one was on mice and the other was on humans. The Lowe and Walton[24] study showed, in mice, a decrease of salience to the gap at the frequency of the tinnitus, which was measured using the amplitude of the first positivity of the auditory brainstem response (<1 ms from the onset of the postgap stimulus). The human data[29] measured the amplitude of the cortical response, the P1 (<100 ms from the onset of the postgap stimulus) and found a decrease in latency for threshold and suprathreshold gaps in the tinnitus group using a white noise stimulus. Three studies investigated the GPIAS reflex, of which 2 were studies on guinea pigs and one was on humans. The guinea pig studies found a gap-prepulse inhibition ratio increase (ie, larger peak-to-peak P1-N1 differences) after tinnitus was induced either by noise exposure or salicylate. An increase was also seen as an N1-P2 peak-to-peak difference in humans with tinnitus for 20-m gaps but not for 50-m or 100-m gaps. Three studies investigated the amplitude of the MMN to the gap duration deviant using the multiple deviant paradigm. These studies found the MMN amplitude and the area under the curve in tinnitus participants to be reduced compared with the normal hearing controls using a 7-m gap. These studies also showed no change in MMN amplitude in those with compensated tinnitus[30] and residual inhibition (**Fig. 2**).[27]

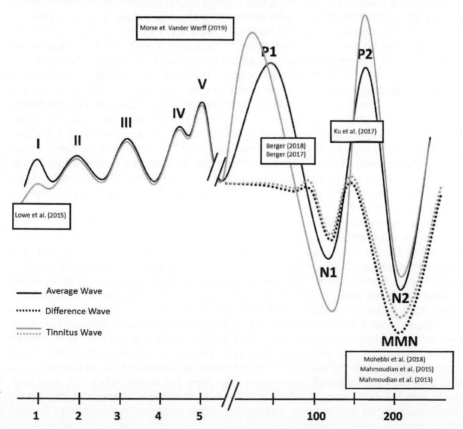

Fig. 2. Summary schema of the findings in the reviewed studies.

DISCUSSION

The behavioral GPIAS has already been identified as a method for determining the presence of tinnitus in animals.[2] However, this paradigm has not been successfully replicated in humans.[13] For this reason, an electrophysiological method that investigates the neural response to gaps is of interest. A search of the literature to determine if the gap-elicited EEG has the potential to detect auditory changes related to tinnitus yielded 8 articles. Three studies involved mice and guinea pigs and 5 studies involved humans. Three approaches to gap-elicited evoked potentials have been identified: (1) the GIN paradigm to measure the neural gap detection threshold, (2) the GPIAS paradigm to measure the neural gap-prepulse inhibition, and (3) the MMN multideviant paradigm to measure gap-elicited responses.

Given the literature reviewed here, does tinnitus alter the activation of the EEG elicited by gaps? Using the neural gap detection threshold in which the minimum gap length that could elicit a significantly different EEG amplitude at the offset of the gap (ie, the onset of the stimulus following of the gap), studies showed an increase of the neural gap detection threshold in those with salicylate-induced tinnitus.[24] This procedure is essentially a modification of the psychoacoustic GIN test in which the threshold is defined as the minimum gap length that can be correctly identified with approximately 50% accuracy. In the human data there was no significant change between groups when using the P1-N1-P2 response to a gap length below, at, and above threshold.[29] This suggests that the neural gap detection threshold may not be different between those with and without tinnitus. Indeed, human behavioral studies on gap detection showed no group separation for stimuli matched or unmatched to the frequency of the tinnitus.[31–32] However, the Morse and Vander Werff study[29] did not use the same method as the studies by Berger and colleagues[23],[25] or Lowe and Walton.[24] In the latter studies, a minimum gap duration that elicited a significant postgap change in the neural response was used to determine the gap duration. Thus, the EEG was used as an indicator of the gap detection threshold. In contrast, the Morse and Vander Werff[29] study used behavioral gap detection threshold to define the 3 conditions. A future study on humans using a method similar to the studies by Berger and colleagues[23,25] or Lowe and Walton[24] would be relevant to determine the neural gap threshold. As such, the pregap and postgap P1-N1-P2 response to gap durations of 1 or 2 ms up to above 20 ms could be used to determine the gap threshold. The resulting neural gap thresholds could then be compared between the human and animal studies.

Using a neural gap-prepulse inhibition as an indicator for separating the tinnitus group from the controls (a modification of the gap-prepulse inhibition of the acoustic startle), Berger and colleagues[23] showed that the neural GPI increased (eg, gap detection decreased) for broadband noise in guinea pigs with salicylate-induced and noise-induced tinnitus. GPI also increased using narrowband noise centered around 4 to 6 kHz and 8 to 10 kHz for salicylate and noise-induced tinnitus, respectively. This pattern was also found in Ku and colleagues,[28] showing a neural GPI ratio increase at 8 kHz in humans with a putative 8 kHz tonal tinnitus. However, this group separation occurred for only the 20-m gaps and not for the 50-m and 100-m gaps, and was absent at the lower-frequency condition (600 Hz). These results suggest that the neural GPI might reveal an effect of tinnitus frequency on gap inhibition that was not seen previously using the startle reflex.[13] It also suggests that the 50-m gap duration, which elicits significant changes in the animal literature, may be too long to induce the same changes in the human tinnitus population.

Finally, using the MMN amplitude to determine the neural activation of the gap, studies showed that there was a significant increase in the amplitude and the area under the curve for participants with reported tinnitus and in those with decompensated tinnitus.[30] Unlike the studies on the neural GPI, this effect does not appear to be frequency-specific, as the participants were not separated based on tinnitus frequency and the stimulus was not matched. It is unclear if the same effect would be seen for gap durations higher or lower than 7 ms because only one gap duration was used. Therefore, future studies to be conducted on the MMN should use a range of gap durations and test the MMN response to stimuli that are matched and unmatched to the frequency of the tinnitus.

Is the EEG-gap activated differently for short-latency versus long-latency potentials? The only short-latency EEG that was recorded was the ABR study by Lowe and Walton,[24] which showed a change in the neural gap detection threshold in mice with salicylate tinnitus. This effect has not yet been replicated in humans with tinnitus. A future study on the neural gap detection threshold using the ABR in humans with tinnitus would be valuable. All of the remaining studies investigated the cortical response to the gap. They indicate that the response to a startling stimulus following a gap of 50 or 20 ms may be reduced in populations with tinnitus. Further studies are necessary to examine if this effect can be measured for gap durations shorter than 20 ms.

Possible limitations must be considered when interpreting the results, which relate to the effects of attention, methodology, hearing loss, and tinnitus frequency. Briefly, the effect of attentional bias on EEG responses is well known, especially the N1-gap responses, which can be modified by actively attending to the stimulus[33–35] Another potential limitation when comparing between the animal and human data are not only the differences between populations, but also the electrode setup. The electrodes in humans are always surface adhesives or cap-electrodes that capture responses at the level of the scalp. For animals, the electrodes are subcutaneous or even directly positioned over the cortex and, therefore, much closer to the source of the response. For this reason, the level of noise is lower and thus a better signal-to-noise ratio can be achieved. It is therefore possible that differences obtained in animals may be masked by higher skin impedances in humans. In addition, population differences occur at the level of tinnitus etiology. The animal data have known tinnitus origins, because they are artificially produced within the laboratory. This is unlike patients with tinnitus who have a variety of tinnitus origins, many of which are idiopathic. To illustrate the effect of tinnitus origin on the data, the 2 studies by Berger and colleagues[23,25] induced tinnitus using either salicylate or noise, and although they used the same EEG methods, the frequencies that showed significant effect differed between the 2 methods of induction. It is conceivable that given the heterogeneity of tinnitus origins in humans, frequency-specific effects may be masked depending on the subtypes of tinnitus within the study sample and by the presence of (at least some degree of) hearing loss. The effects of hearing loss and tinnitus frequency are other possible confounds in some of the present findings. Only 3 studies reviewed here assessed or reported tinnitus frequency in relation to their findings,[24,25,28] among which only one was a human study.[28] Yet the method used for tinnitus pitch matching, the 2 alternative forced choice method (2-AFC), is known to have reliability issues.[1] These issues mostly have to do with tinnitus encompassing a range of frequencies rather than a single frequency (eg, Refs.[36,37]) and that these frequencies typically lie within the hearing loss bandwidth. Hearing loss in itself represents a challenge to tinnitus research and has been controlled for in all studies except for one.[23]

SUMMARY

In summary, this review demonstrates that although the need for an objective measure of tinnitus is warranted, very few studies exist on the gap-elicited EEG, and even fewer have considered gap detection at the tinnitus frequency. Therefore, given the current available evidence, the answer to the question as to whether the gap response is affected or not by tinnitus is equivocal. Although some studies reported that gap detection was impaired in tinnitus, others reported findings difficult to interpret. Given the small number of studies yielded from this review, there were many different methodologies used making it insufficient for conducting a meta-analysis of the data. Each study needed to be considered separately from the others because of variability among stimuli used, paradigms, populations, outcomes, and methods. Future research that expand the methodologies described in the literature is necessary to better understand the effect of tinnitus on the auditory processing of various gap durations. It is also important to have more peripheral data on the gap-elicited EEG to make comparisons on the signal processing of temporal information in a tinnitus population compared with a normal-hearing group. The mismatch negativity appears to show tinnitus population separation; however, this is based on the results of only a single laboratory using a single paradigm. Replication of these findings in other laboratories is necessary to confirm the reported effects.

ACKNOWLEDGMENTS

This study was supported by a research grant from the Natural Sciences and Engineering Research Council of Canada.

DISCLOSURE

The authors have nothing to disclose.

REFERENCES

1. Hébert S. Individual reliability of the standard clinical method vs patient-centered tinnitus likeness rating for assessment of tinnitus pitch and loudness matching. JAMA Otolaryngol Head Neck Surg 2018;144(12):1136–44.
2. Turner JG, Brozoski TJ, Bauer CA, et al. Gap detection deficits in rats with tinnitus: a potential novel screening tool. Behav Neurosci 2006;120(1):188–95.
3. Yang G, Lobarinas E, Zhang L, et al. Salicylate induced tinnitus: behavioral measures and neural activity in auditory cortex of awake rats. Hear Res 2007; 226(1–2):244–53.
4. Turner JG, Parrish J. Gap detection methods for assessing salicylate-induced tinnitus and hyperacusis in rats. Am J Audiol 2008;17(2):S185–92.
5. Wang H, Brozoski TJ, Turner JG, et al. Plasticity at glycinergic synapses in dorsal cochlear nucleus of rats with behavioral evidence of tinnitus. Neuroscience 2009; 164(2):747–59.
6. Holt AG, Bissig D, Mirza N, et al. Evidence of key tinnitus-related brain regions documented by a unique combination of manganese-enhanced MRI and acoustic startle reflex testing. PLoS One 2010;5(12):e14260.
7. Ralli M, Lobarinas E, Fetoni AR, et al. Comparison of salicylate- and quinine-induced tinnitus in rats: development, time course, and evaluation of audiologic correlates. Otol Neurotol 2010;31(5):823–31.
8. Longenecker RJ, Galazyuk AV. Development of tinnitus in CBA/CaJ mice following sound exposure. J Assoc Res Otolaryngol 2011;12(5):647–58.

9. Engineer ND, Riley JR, Seale JD, et al. Reversing pathological neural activity using targeted plasticity. Nature 2011;470(7332):101–4.

10. Mao JC, Pace E, Pierozynski P, et al. Blast-induced tinnitus and hearing loss in rats: behavioral and imaging assays. J Neurotrauma 2012;29(2):430–44.

11. Zhang J, Zhang Y, Zhang X. Auditory cortex electrical stimulation suppresses tinnitus in rats. J Assoc Res Otolaryngol 2011;12(2):185–201.

12. Middleton JW, Tzounopoulos T. Imaging the neural correlates of tinnitus: a comparison between animal models and human studies. Front Syst Neurosci 2012; 6:35.

13. Fournier P, Hebert S. Gap detection deficits in humans with tinnitus as assessed with the acoustic startle paradigm: does tinnitus fill in the gap? Hear Res 2013; 295:16–23.

14. Campbell J, LaBrec A, Bean C, et al. Auditory gating and extended high-frequency thresholds in normal-hearing adults with minimal tinnitus. Am J Audiol 2019;28(1S):209–24.

15. Andersson G, McKenna L. The role of cognition in tinnitus. Acta Otolaryngol Suppl 2006;(556):39–43.

16. Duda-Milloy V, Tavakoli P, Campbell K, et al. A time-efficient multi-deviant paradigm to determine the effects of gap duration on the mismatch negativity. Hear Res 2019;377:34–43.

17. Naatanen R, Jiang D, Lavikainen J, et al. Event-related potentials reveal a memory trace for temporal features. Neuroreport 1993;5(3):310–2.

18. Muller-Gass A, Stelmack RM, Campbell KB. The effect of visual task difficulty and attentional direction on the detection of acoustic change as indexed by the Mismatch Negativity. Brain Res 2006;1078(1):112–30.

19. Sussman ES, Horvath J, Winkler I, et al. The role of attention in the formation of auditory streams. Percept Psychophys 2007;69(1):136–52.

20. Milloy V, Fournier P, Benoit D, et al. Auditory brainstem responses in tinnitus: a review of who, how, and what? Front Aging Neurosci 2017;9:237.

21. Arksey H, O'Malley L. Scoping studies: Towards a methodological framework. Int J Soc Res Methodol 2005;8:19–32.

22. Levac D, Colquhoun H, O'Brien KK. Scoping studies: advancing the methodology. Implement Sci 2010;5:69.

23. Berger JI, Owen W, Wilson CA, et al. Gap-induced reductions of evoked potentials in the auditory cortex: a possible objective marker for the presence of tinnitus in animals. Brain Res 2018;1679:101–8.

24. Lowe AS, Walton JP. Alterations in peripheral and central components of the auditory brainstem response: a neural assay of tinnitus. PLoS One 2015;10(2): e0117228.

25. Berger JI, Coomber B, Wallace MN, et al. Reductions in cortical alpha activity, enhancements in neural responses and impaired gap detection caused by sodium salicylate in awake guinea pigs. Eur J Neurosci 2017;45(3):398–409.

26. Mahmoudian S, Farhadi M, Najafi-Koopaie M, et al. Central auditory processing during chronic tinnitus as indexed by topographical maps of the mismatch negativity obtained with the multi-feature paradigm. Brain Res 2013;1527:161–73.

27. Mahmoudian S, Farhadi M, Mohebbi M, et al. Alterations in auditory change detection associated with tinnitus residual inhibition induced by auditory electrical stimulation. J Am Acad Audiol 2015;26(4):408–22.

28. Ku Y, Ahn JW, Kwon C, et al. The gap-prepulse inhibition deficit of the cortical N1-P2 complex in patients with tinnitus: the effect of gap duration. Hear Res 2017; 348:120–8.

29. Morse K, Vander Werff KR. Comparison of silent gap in noise cortical auditory evoked potentials in matched tinnitus and no-tinnitus control subjects. Am J Audiol 2019;28(2):260–73.
30. Mohebbi M, Daneshi A, Asadpour A, et al. The potential role of auditory prediction error in decompensated tinnitus: an auditory mismatch negativity study. Brain Behav 2019;9(4):e01242.
31. Boyen K, Baskent D, van Dijk P. The gap detection test: can it be used to diagnose tinnitus? Ear Hear 2015;36(4):e138–45.
32. Campolo J, Lobarinas E, Salvi R. Does tinnitus "fill in" the silent gaps? Noise Health 2013;15(67):398–405.
33. Campbell K, Macdonald M. The effects of attention and conscious state on the detection of gaps in long duration auditory stimuli. Clin Neurophysiol 2011; 122(4):738–47.
34. Harris KC, Wilson S, Eckert MA, et al. Human evoked cortical activity to silent gaps in noise: effects of age, attention, and cortical processing speed. Ear Hear 2012;33(3):330–9.
35. Alain C, McDonald KL, Ostroff JM, et al. Aging: a switch from automatic to controlled processing of sounds? Psychol Aging 2004;19(1):125–33.
36. Basile CE, Fournier P, Hutchins S, et al. Psychoacoustic assessment to improve tinnitus diagnosis. PLoS One 2013;8(12):e82995.
37. Roberts L, Moffat G, Baumann M, et al. Residual inhibition functions overlap tinnitus spectra and the region of auditory threshold shift. J Assoc Res Otolaryngol 2008;9(4):417–35.

Tinnitus Neuroimaging

Meredith E. Adams, MD, MS[a],*, Tina C. Huang, MD[a],
Srikantan Nagarajan, PhD[b,c], Steven W. Cheung, MD[c]

KEYWORDS

- Tinnitus • Neuroimaging • Functional connectivity • Striatal gating

KEY POINTS

- Human neuroimaging provides insights into the neurophysiologic and neuroanatomic bases of tinnitus in both clinical and investigational realms.
- Chronic subjective tinnitus is associated with heterogeneous changes in auditory and nonauditory central nervous system networks and structures.
- Functional neuroimaging aims to identify treatment-responsive biomarkers that inform clinical decision making and novel treatment targets that motivate development of pharmacologic, behavioral, and neuromodulatory approaches for mitigation of bothersome tinnitus.

INTRODUCTION

Tinnitus is a disorder of auditory perception in the absence of physical sound stimuli. Individuals with tinnitus may describe auditory phantoms as ringing, buzzing, roaring, or other sounds in the ear(s) or head that cannot be observed by an examiner. Many people with tinnitus adapt well, but sufferers may find that auditory phantoms intrude on activities of daily living, exacerbate behavioral and emotional distress, impair mental concentration, and disrupt sleep.[1] As such, tinnitus is characterized not only by its perceptual features (eg, loudness, pitch, duration, and laterality) but also by reactions[2] and distress.[3,4]

The pathophysiology of the genesis and persistence of tinnitus is not fully understood. Furthermore, tinnitus perception and severity-related reactions have additional complexity due to variations in the weighing of critical factors among individuals. For many, tinnitus may be initiated by hearing loss with concomitant loss of sensory input from the cochlea to the central auditory pathways (ie, peripheral deafferentation).[1,5]

[a] Department of Otolaryngology–Head and Neck Surgery, University of Minnesota, 420 Delaware Street Southeast, MMC 395, Minneapolis, MN 55455, USA; [b] Department of Radiology and Biomedical Imaging, University of California San Francisco, 513 Parnassus Avenue S362, San Francisco, CA 94143-0628, USA; [c] Department of Otolaryngology–Head and Neck Surgery, University of California San Francisco, 2233 Post Street Suite 341, San Francisco, CA 94115-1225, USA
* Corresponding author.
E-mail address: meadams@umn.edu

Otolaryngol Clin N Am 53 (2020) 583–603
https://doi.org/10.1016/j.otc.2020.04.002
0030-6665/20/© 2020 Elsevier Inc. All rights reserved.

Accordingly, this article provides guidance on the clinical use of imaging to identify relevant auditory lesions when evaluating tinnitus patients. Furthermore, an expanding body of evidence points to tinnitus as having strong neural correlates in the human central nervous system (CNS).[6] After introducing the anatomy and imaging modalities most pertinent to tinnitus neuroscience, this article reviews tinnitus-associated alterations in key auditory and nonauditory CNS networks. Emphasis is placed on how these findings support proposed models of tinnitus and how this line of investigation is relevant to practicing clinicians.

IMAGING FOR TINNITUS IN THE CLINICAL SETTING

In the clinical setting, imaging is indicated for the subset of tinnitus patients who display features suggestive of concerning underlying medical conditions. The evaluation of tinnitus begins with the clinical history, physical examination, and audiometric testing. Tinnitus should be characterized as subjective or objective and as pulsatile or nonpulsatile. Subjective tinnitus implies that only the patient is able to hear the auditory phantom. In contrast, objective tinnitus may be perceived by an external observer and often has an identifiable anatomic source. Pulsatile tinnitus, whether objective or subjective, may be a symptom of various vascular lesions that are best evaluated with neuroimaging, as reviewed by Eisenman and colleagues[7] and Hertzano and colleagues.[8] This review is focused on subjective tinnitus. Subjective tinnitus may be idiopathic, secondary to sensorineural hearing loss, or attributable to another specific underlying cause that may or may not require imaging to identify.[9] Etiologies range from cerumen impaction, middle ear disease, and cochlear and labyrinthine disorders to retrocochlear lesions, such as vestibular schwannoma.

According to clinical practice guidelines[9] and published appropriateness criteria,[10] imaging is not routinely indicated for the evaluation of symmetric or bilateral subjective, nonpulsatile tinnitus in the absence of other symptoms, because the yield is likely to be low. Evaluation for retrocochlear lesions using magnetic resonance imaging (MRI) with gadolinium is warranted for patients with subjective nonpulsatile tinnitus who have 1 or more of the following: (1) unilateral tinnitus, (2) asymmetric or unilateral sensorineural hearing loss, and (3) focal neurologic symptoms.[9,10] Asymmetric hearing loss is best defined as asymmetry of greater than or equal to 20 decibels Hearing Level (dB HL) at 2 contiguous frequencies or greater than or equal to 15 dB HL at any 2 frequencies between 2000 Hz and 8000 Hz,[11,12] or a significant difference in word recognition based on an established binomial model.[13] Fewer than 5% of patients with tinnitus and asymmetric hearing loss are found to have a vestibular schwannoma,[14,15] but early tumor identification may prevent further morbidity. If the accompanying hearing loss is conductive, temporal bone computed tomography may assist in lesion characterization and treatment selection, such as in cases of otosclerosis or superior semicircular canal dehiscence.[16]

WHY ARE OBJECTIVE NEUROIMAGING MEASURES OF SUBJECTIVE TINNITUS NEEDED?

The use of neuroimaging to identify the neuroanatomic and physiologic correlates of tinnitus has high diagnostic and therapeutic relevance. At present, tinnitus diagnosis and measures of severity are largely dependent on subjective self-reported surveys and corroborative examination findings. This can be frustrating for patients trying to comprehend the biological basis of their condition and for clinicians who seek an objective test to confirm and characterize the diagnosis. Because tinnitus perceptions and reactions are highly heterogeneous, neuroimaging may provide the power to delineate tinnitus subtypes. Knowledge of biologic mechanisms of tinnitus also is crucial for designing interventions to alleviate tinnitus perception (awareness) and distress (severity). Ideally, effective interventions demonstrate improvement not only in patient-reported outcomes but also in affected CNS regions. Thus, objective neuroimaging measures are critical for assessments of treatment efficacy.

NEUROIMAGING MODALITIES USED IN TINNITUS RESEARCH
Functional Imaging Methods

Functional neuroimaging methods are used to characterize the location, extent, and magnitude of neural activity and connections within the CNS.[17] Different brain regions are considered functionally connected when their neural activity is temporally correlated or coherent. Distinct regions with highly correlated/coherent activity are identified as neural networks.[18] Functional imaging modalities employed in tinnitus research include functional MRI (fMRI), PET, electroencephalography (EEG), and magnetoencephalographic imaging (MEGI).

Both fMRI and PET exploit the fact that changes in neural activity alter local cerebral perfusion and metabolism.[17] As oxygen levels increase in active brain regions, fMRI indirectly detects changes in neural activity via blood oxygen level–dependent (BOLD) responses that manifest as changes in the T2* signal of echo planar MR images.[19] T2* relaxation reflects the decay of transverse magnetization from spin-spin interactions (T2) and inhomogeneities in the magnetic field. Task-based fMRI studies compare BOLD levels during an experimental task to a baseline state.[19] In contrast, resting state fMRI (RS-fMRI) detects temporal correlations in spontaneous low-frequency (<0.1 Hz) fluctuations in BOLD signals across brain regions while participants are in a state of wakeful rest, unengaged by stimuli or tasks.[18] Functional connectivity of brain regions is inferred by synchronous BOLD signal fluctuation.[20] Tinnitus likely alters resting state activity given that awareness and distress persist when individuals are ostensibly at rest, unengaged in attentional tasks.[18] Although fMRI has high spatial resolution, disadvantages for tinnitus research include scanner noise interference with auditory processing and resting state achievement and longer temporal resolution (seconds) compared with EEG and MEGI.[21] **Figs. 1** and **2** provide examples of fMRI functional connectivity analysis, described later.

PET spatially maps regions of brain activity by measuring regional cerebral blood flow elevation in response to rising oxygen and glucose demands. After administration, radiolabeled tracers, such as fluorodeoxyglucose (FDG), accumulate in active brain regions and then decay, evidenced by PET-detectable photon emission.[17] PET has advantages of being silent and compatible with ferromagnetic implants (eg, cochlear implants), but its spatial and temporal resolution are inferior to fMRI. **Fig. 3** shows an application of PET to the study of neurobiological heterogeneity in tinnitus subgroups.[22] In this instance, investigators sought evidence of sex-related differences in resting state brain activity. Note that PET color maps often are superimposed on an average of the structural MRIs for study participants for anatomic reference, and the color scale indicates activity levels, with red/orange indicating highest activity and blue/violet representing lowest activity.

EEG and MEGI are electrophysiologic methods of recording electric potentials (EEG) and magnetic fields (MEGI) generated by spontaneous (resting state) or evoked brain activity. Neural activity produces time-varying electrical currents that create local voltage differences (EEG) or magnetic fields (MEGI), measured using

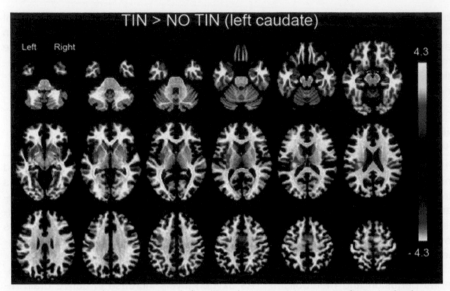

Fig. 1. Increased left corticostriatal functional connectivity on RS-fMRI in bothersome tinnitus with single-sided deafness. Cohort comparisons between subjects with tinnitus (TIN, N = 15) and without (NO TIN, N = 15) show significant differences (*P*<.05 false discovery rate cluster-mass corrected). The color bar represents the *t* statistic of differences in functional connectivity between cohorts. Positive values (*red colors*) indicate increased connectivity and negative values (*blue colors*) indicate decreased connectivity. Deaf ear distribution in TIN cohort: 7 left and 8 right.

sensitive arrays placed on the scalp surface. The detection of these signals requires a sufficient mass of active neurons to be coordinated in space and time.[23] Synchronous fluctuations in the activity of coordinated groups of neurons produce oscillations, or rhythms, in a range of frequencies (eg, delta, theta, alpha, beta, and gamma). Rather than being epiphenomena, these oscillations may reflect the mechanism by which neurons are brought together into assemblies to integrate signals into perceptions.[24] The profile of oscillations in neural activity can be used to describe altered neural activity in resting state networks. EEG and MEGI have excellent temporal resolution (milliseconds) and improved spatial resolution arising from novel source reconstruction algorithms.[25–28] **Fig. 3** provides an example of RS-MEGI, described later.

Structural Imaging Methods

Functional changes in the CNS of individuals with tinnitus may be accompanied by changes in the neuroanatomic structures or neural circuits that mediate function.[29] Neuroanatomic structure may be altered by changes in cell size, number of neurons, or synapses[30] that can accompany neurologic disorders. Structural imaging methods used most commonly in tinnitus research are voxel-based morphometry (VBM) and diffusion tensor imaging (DTI). VBM quantifies regional gray-matter volume using high-resolution structural MRI. Voxels are the 3-dimensional analog of pixels that form images. To detect changes, VBM statistically compares gray-matter volumes voxel by voxel between individuals either on a whole-brain or region-of-interest basis.[29] Surface-based morphometry (SBM) yields analogous measures regarding the thickness, surface area, and curvature of surface gray

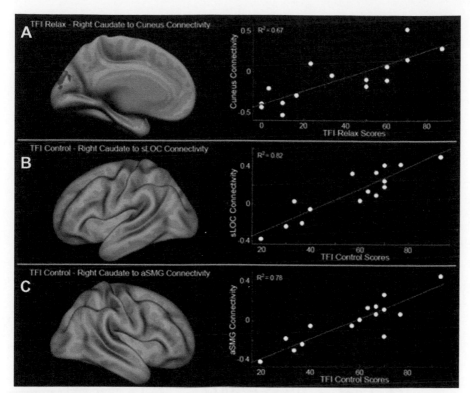

Fig. 2. Strength of connectivity on RS-fMRI between caudate nucleus and nonauditory structures is correlated with TFI subscales in bothersome tinnitus with single-sided deafness. (A) Connectivity between caudate nucleus and cuneus is correlated with difficulty to relax attributed to tinnitus. (B) Connectivity between caudate nucleus and superior lateral occipital cortex (sLOC) and (C) between caudate nucleus and anterior supramarginal gyrus (aSMG) is correlated with lower control over the tinnitus percept. Yellow indicates significant increased connectivity (P<.05 false discovery rate cluster-mass corrected).

matter.[29] **Fig. 4** demonstrates use of VBM analysis to examine the effect of mild tinnitus of greater than 1-year duration on gray-matter volume of a limbic system structure, the anterior cingulate cortex.[31] The statistical maps show voxels that differ between groups, with the t statistic indicated by the color scale. Note that volumetric analyses provide statistical cohort–level inferences only and are not yet adequately sensitive for providing individual subject-level information. Clinicians do not routinely detect volume changes on individual images, but this is an exciting area for patient centric research.

Another MRI modality, DTI, characterizes anatomic changes in white mater connecting brain regions. DTI assesses the strength and directionality of the diffusion of water molecules within white-matter structures in order to infer white-matter density or integrity and to reconstruct white-matter tracts.[32] **Fig. 5** is an example of use of DTI to compare white-matter tract orientation between individuals with hearing loss and tinnitus, hearing loss and no tinnitus, and normal hearing controls without tinnitus. Fractional anisotropy is a measure of directionality.[33] There were no differences between the group with tinnitus and those without.

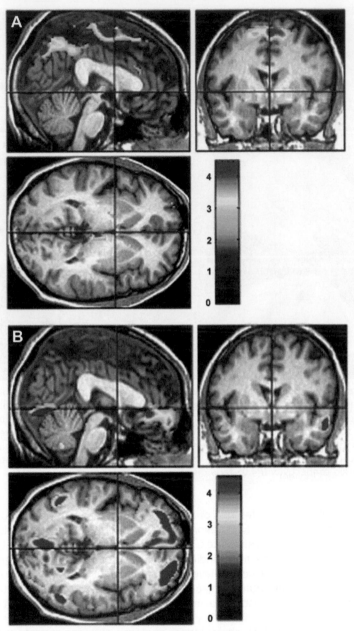

Fig. 3. PET imaging, showing (A) increased metabolic activity preferentially in temporal and parietal brain regions in female tinnitus patients compared with male tinnitus patients and (B) increased metabolic activity in frontal and occipital regions in male tinnitus patients compared with female tinnitus patients.[22] (Reprinted from Progress in Brain Research, P. Eichhammer, G. Hajak, T. Kleinjung, M. Landgrebe, B. Langguth, Functional imaging of chronic tinnitus: the use of positron emission tomography, Page 86, Copyright (2007), with permission from Elsevier.)

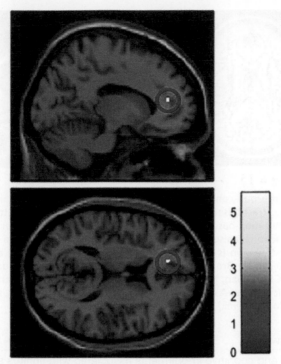

Fig. 4. Cluster showing a significant effect of tinnitus on gray-matter volume of the left anterior cingulate (MLTIN_1> NH). Cluster showing a significant effect (P<.05 family-wise error corrected) of tinnitus in the left anterior cingulate in the whole-brain VBM analysis. Highlighted area corresponds to a positive effect (increase in volume for the tinnitus group vs the normal hearing control group). MLTIN_1, mild, long-term tinnitus patients; NH, normal hearing controls.[31] (Reprinted from Brain Research, Vol. 1697, SA Schmidt, B Zimmerman, RO Bido Medina, JR Carpenter-Thompson, FT Husain. Changes in gray and white matter in subgroups within the tinnitus population, Pages 64-74, Copyright (2017), with permission from Elsevier.)

TINNITUS-RELEVANT NEUROANATOMY
Central Auditory System

The pathway transducing sound to the CNS begins as cochlear hair cells transmit signals via the auditory nerve to the ipsilateral cochlear nucleus in the pons. From there, most fibers of the tonotopically arranged lemniscal (or classical auditory) pathway cross midline to synapse in the superior olivary complex. Neurons then ascend via the lateral lemniscus to synapse in the inferior colliculus (IC) in the midbrain. The IC relays signals to the medial geniculate body (MGB) of the thalamus, from which neurons project to the primary auditory cortex (AC) in Heschl gyrus of the temporal lobe. In the nontonotopic, extralemniscal (or nonclassical auditory) pathway, neurons project from the peripheral shell of the IC to intermix with inputs from other sensory modalities (eg, vision and somatosensation) in the brainstem reticular formation on the way to thalamic nuclei, which then send information to association cortices.[5,34] The thalamus is of particular interest in tinnitus pathophysiology because it regulates the flow of sensory information to and from the AC via connections with both auditory and nonauditory networks, including the limbic system.[1,34]

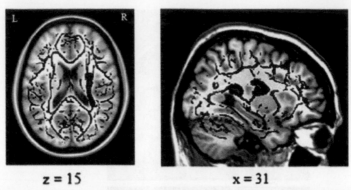

Fig. 5. Whole-brain group comparisons (Hearing loss (HL) < Normal hearing (NH)) of DTI data obtained using tract-based spatial statistics of FSL (corrected for multiple comparisons at P<.1 using permutation-based tests). The statistically significant clusters are depicted in red color over a fractional anisotropy skeleton map in blue color. Only the HL < NH comparison was significant. Shown is an axial slice at (*left*) z = 15 and (*right*) a sagittal slice at x = 31.[33] (Reprinted from Brain Research, Vol 1369, FT Husain, RE Medina, CW Davis, Y Szymko-Bennett, K Simonyan, NM Pajor, B Horwitz, Neuroanatomical changes due to hearing loss and chronic tinnitus: A combined VBM and DTI study, Pages 74-88, Copyright (2011), with permission from Elsevier.)

Nonauditory Networks

As the emotional and cognitive impairments associated with tinnitus suggest, nonauditory networks and structures factor prominently in tinnitus neuroscience, including the limbic system, striatum, attention networks, and the default mode network. The limbic system is a group of interconnected CNS structures engaged in processing emotion, affect, moods, and certain forms of memory.[29,35] Limbic system and related structures include the hippocampus, amygdala, anterior cingulate cortex, and posterior cingulate cortex, adjacent prefrontal cortex, insula, and interconnections with the hypothalamus, thalamus, and ventral striatum (nucleus accumbens [NAc]) of the basal ganglia. The caudate nucleus, a portion of the dorsal striatum, also is implicated in tinnitus.[36] Attentional networks, also known as global awareness networks, involve frontal and parietal cortical areas.[18] Unlike the other networks, discussed previously, the default mode network is most active during wakeful rest and less active with task engagement. Comprised of nodes from the ventromedial prefrontal cortex (vmPFC), posterior cingulate cortex, precuneus, and superior frontal gyrus, the default mode network likely is active in self-referential processing and episodic memory.[37]

NEUROIMAGING CORRELATES OF TINNITUS IN THE CENTRAL AUDITORY SYSTEM

Given that tinnitus is an auditory phantom, it is logical to seek its neural substrate in the auditory system. Hearing loss from cochlear or other peripheral auditory injury is a leading risk factor for tinnitus but is insufficient for its maintenance, particularly because tinnitus persists after auditory nerve transection[38] and in individuals without hearing loss (although hearing loss may go undetected by standard audiometry).[39] Thus, although peripheral deafferentation may initiate tinnitus, central neuroplastic responses maintain the perception.[40,41] Animal models of tinnitus, induced by peripheral deafferentation, demonstrate central auditory system (CAS) changes that may lead to tinnitus perception, including tonotopic map reorganization, neural hyperactivity, and increased neural synchrony.[42–44] If analogous CAS changes are responsible for human tinnitus perception, effects should be observable on neuroimaging. Selected studies addressing these models and CAS structural changes are reviewed.

Tonotopic map reorganization in the AC was observed in animals deafferented by noise trauma, such that neurons in regions corresponding to hearing loss shift their tuning to respond preferentially to frequencies at the edge of the loss instead.[42] The overrepresentation of edge frequencies by cortical neurons could increase neural synchrony and spontaneous activity, generating the tinnitus percept. Some EEG and MEGI studies support the general presence of map reorganization.[45,46] In comparing frequency maps between tinnitus patients and controls using MEGI and fMRI of field strengths up to 7T, however, tinnitus patients do not appear to have gross changes in tonotopic mapping at hearing loss or edge frequencies.[47–50] Although changes could occur at levels below MEGI and fMRI resolution, gross map reorganization is not essential for tinnitus perception.

Increased spontaneous firing rates in cortical neurons have also been sought among individuals with tinnitus. The firing rate of auditory neurons increases when an external sound source is present. It is hypothesized that pathologically increased spontaneous firing rates could lead to auditory phantom perception.[17] Investigations using resting state FDG-PET to compare the relative amount of metabolic activity in left and right primary ACs observed significantly more asymmetry in tinnitus patients than controls, with left AC having greater resting activity than right AC.[51–53] A subsequent comparison of FDG-PET, however, in 20 tinnitus patients to 19 controls found no tinnitus-associated hyperactivity. Rather, in both groups, primary AC activity was greater on the left than the right,[54] suggesting hemispheric asymmetries in metabolic activity may be a normal brain characteristic.

Tinnitus-associated neural hyperactivity has been investigated further through neuroimaging observations of central auditory responses after sound stimulation. Broadband sound-evoked fMRI activation of the subcortical IC was compared between tinnitus and nontinnitus subjects in 2 studies.[55,56] Both found greater sound-evoked activation of IC in the tinnitus group, suggesting abnormal gain within the auditory pathway. This finding held for groups matched for hearing, age, and emotional status[55] but not for hyperacusis. When normal hearing participants with and without tinnitus were assessed for sound level tolerance before sound-evoked fMRI, those with hyperacusis had elevated activation of IC, thalamus, and primary AC. Increased activation of the primary AC (and not IC or thalamus), however, was related to tinnitus alone, suggesting the disproportionate response to sound by IC neurons was related to hyperacusis rather than tinnitus.[57] AC hyperactivity to sound was observed in other studies. In 2 separate cohorts, in response to narrow-band sounds matched to tinnitus frequency, participants with tinnitus showed greater BOLD responses than matched controls in the primary AC.[58,59] Although these findings suggest tinnitus-associated AC hyperactivity, another study, comparing participants with tinnitus and hearing loss and hearing-matched controls, found no differences in sound-evoked fMRI AC activation.[60] Whether AC hyperactivity is the cause or a consequence of tinnitus perception remains to be determined.

Changes in neural synchrony associated with tinnitus have been examined using EEG and MEGI. These modalities examine oscillations from synchronous activity of neuronal populations, rather than the synchronous activity between neuron pairs reported in animal tinnitus models.[61,62] EEG and MEGI have been used to test if tinnitus arises from thalamocortical dysrhythmia.[63,64] Auditory stimuli increase thalamocortical rhythms from baseline alpha to gamma.[65] The thalamocortical dysrhythmia model predicts that, as peripheral deafferentation reduces excitatory thalamic inputs, thalamocortical oscillations decrease to low-frequency delta and theta rhythms, reducing the lateral inhibition in the AC that alpha rhythms usually sustain. Consequently, gamma oscillations increase at AC edge frequencies, which lead to the tinnitus percept. RS-MEGI and EEG measurements from AC of individuals with tinnitus compared with controls demonstrated findings consistent with this model, including reductions in alpha rhythm[66,67] and increases in slow-wave delta[67] and gamma rhythms.[67,68] Other investigators, however, have not observed these effects[69,70] or observed an inverse of alpha and gamma activity in both tinnitus and control groups,[71] suggesting this pattern is not essential for tinnitus perception. In another study using RS-MEGI before and after tinnitus masking, gamma activity was not correlated with tinnitus or hearing loss, but effective tinnitus masking was associated with decreased delta activity, suggesting delta rhythm as a correlate of tinnitus perception.[72] Rather than underlying the tinnitus percept, gamma rhythms may be responsible for tinnitus loudness, because positive correlations between gamma activity in contralateral AC and reported tinnitus intensity were observed.[73]

Morphologic changes in the CAS of tinnitus patients have been observed with structural imaging, although findings have been inconsistent. A significant challenge with these data, as in many tinnitus neuroimaging studies, is difficulty in separating tinnitus effects from those of comorbid hearing loss.[74] Studies using structural MRI with VBM or SBM to compare tinnitus to nontinnitus control groups reported gray-matter reductions in AC[75,76] and IC,[77] interpreted by some as evidence of tinnitus-associated increased nerve-firing, excitotoxicity, and cell death.[78] Others, including studies controlling for hearing loss and a structural meta-analysis, observed gray-matter increases in primary or secondary AC volume.[33,79,80] Additional findings are emerging, suggesting that AC gray-matter volumes differ based on tinnitus duration[31] and, possibly, based on emotional reactions to tinnitus. In a well-powered study that examined the association between tinnitus distress and gray-matter volume, distress was negatively correlated with AC volume,[81] but a positive correlation was reported by others using a different distress questionnaire.[80]

NEUROIMAGING CORRELATES OF TINNITUS INVOLVING NONAUDITORY NETWORKS AND STRUCTURES
Networks

Resting state functional connectivity measurements have demonstrated that tinnitus is associated with changes in widely distributed nonauditory brain areas as well as the CAS. Thus, the various facets of tinnitus awareness and distress may be driven by altered connections between multiple overlapping brain networks, including those responsible for emotional processing, attention, and memory.[82] Variations between individuals in the involvement of specific networks may be responsible for clinically observed tinnitus heterogeneity.[82] Several themes have emerged, including alterations of attention-related networks,[83–85] decreased coherency in default mode connectivity,[84,86–88] auditory-limbic interactions,[84,89] and auditory-visual interactions.[83] For excellent reviews of specific RS-functional connectivity changes in tinnitus, see Husain and Schmidt[90] and Shahsavarani and colleagues.[18]

As an example, a recent MEGI-RS functional connectivity study using a whole-brain approach identified brain regions altered in chronic tinnitus and, importantly, that their connectivity strength was correlated with tinnitus severity.[91] Specifically, RS-MEGI examination of neural synchrony at oscillatory frequencies associated with local computation (gamma) and inter-regional coordination (theta, alpha, and beta) revealed that global functional connectivity was correlated with tinnitus severity, as measured with the Tinnitus Functional Index (TFI).[4] (**Fig. 6**). In the theta band, global functional

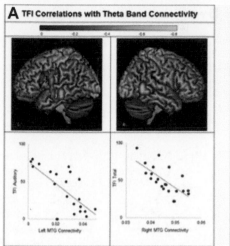
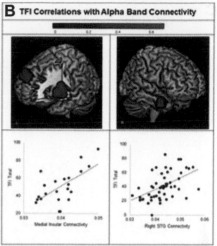

Fig. 6. RS-MEGI functional connectivity using a whole-brain approach shows that specific brain regions have alterations in chronic tinnitus and connectivity strength is correlated with tinnitus severity. Positive correlations are shown in a pink color scale and negative correlations in a cyan color scale. In the theta band, global functional connectivity of the left MTG and right MTG is negatively correlated with the TFI auditory subscale (A). In the alpha band, global functional connectivity of the left medial insula and right middle temporal regions is correlated positively with TFI total scores (B). In the beta band, global functional connectivity of the left MTG and right middle occipital gyrus is correlated inversely with the TFI auditory subscale (C). Finally, in the low gamma band, global functional connectivity in left precentral and prefrontal brain regions is correlated negatively with the TFI auditory subscale (D).

connectivity of the left middle temporal gyrus (MTG) and MTG was negatively correlated with the TFI auditory subscale, which estimates auditory difficulties attributed to tinnitus (see **Fig. 6**A). In the alpha band, global functional connectivity of the left medial insula and right middle temporal regions was correlated positively with total TFI scores (see **Fig. 6**B). In the beta band, global functional connectivity of the left MTG and right middle occipital gyrus (MOG) was inversely correlated with the TFI auditory subscale (see **Fig. 6**C). Finally, in the low gamma band, global functional connectivity in left precentral and prefrontal brain regions is negatively correlated with the TFI auditory subscale (see **Fig. 6**D).

In keeping with this, a recent meta-analysis of 9 whole-brain resting state studies of brain abnormalities in chronic subjective tinnitus[54,86,89,92–97] identified consistent regions of increased resting state activity in tinnitus patients compared with controls, including MTG, frontal cortex (inferior frontal and superior frontal gyri), limbic structures (parahippocampus and insula), cuneus, and cerebellum.[98] A subsequent meta-analysis of 8 VBM data sets[31,74,77,80,99–102] showed complementary structural changes, with tinnitus patients having increased gray-matter volume in MTG, superior temporal gyrus, angular gyrus, and decreased gray-matter volume in caudate nucleus, superior frontal gyrus, and the supplementary motor area.[79]

Caudate Nucleus in Tinnitus

There is growing evidence from human neurostimulation[36,103,104] and RS-fMRI[105–107] neuroimaging studies that another portion of the striatum, the caudate nucleus, plays

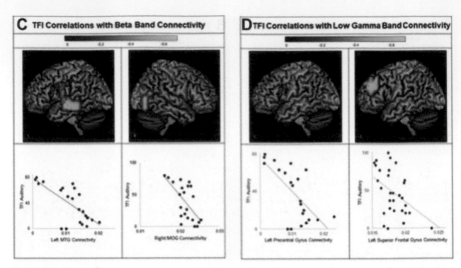

Fig. 6. (continued)

an important role in the perception of tinnitus, with diagnostic and therapeutic implications. In a phase I clinical trial on 5 subjects evaluating deep-brain stimulation of
the caudate nucleus to mitigate moderately severe or more serious treatment-
resistant tinnitus, the clinically significant treatment response rate was 60% to
80%.[103] Consistent with this human clinical trial data, a complementary RS-fMRI
study that compared chronic tinnitus patients adjusted for hearing loss level against
matched controls with normal hearing revealed increased caudate nucleus to AC
functional connectivity in the tinnitus cohort.[106]

MODELS OF TINNITUS

Recently 3 tinnitus models have emerged. One model suggests that tinnitus arises
from an expectation mismatch within the auditory system.[108,109] Specifically, this
model posits a disparity between what the brain predicts it should be hearing (predic-
tions based on aberrant neural activity occurring in cortical frequency regions affected
by hearing loss and underlying the tinnitus percept) and the acoustic information that
is delivered to the brain by a damaged cochlea. In this framework, a disparity between
the predicted and delivered signals causes auditory attention facilitated by subcortical
neuromodulatory systems that is manifested as tinnitus awareness.[109]

A second model suggests that tinnitus is driven by auditory-limbic interactions[58,59,110] The model posits a key role for a limbic-corticostriatal-thalamic network
in governing awareness of auditory phantoms. The model presumes that hearing loss
leads to neural hyperactivity. Although the circuit mechanisms that lead to global hyperactivity are unclear, it can be speculated that the loss of inhibitory GABAergic input
is involved. The signal ascends via the lemniscal pathway to AC and via the extralemniscal pathway that connects with limbic and striatal structures, including amygdala,
ventral striatum (NAc), and vmPFC. It is believed that limbic and auditory brain areas
interact at the thalamic level for noise cancellation of tinnitus percepts and this process is abnormal in persistent tinnitus. In support of this model, VBM studies demonstrated reductions in gray-matter volume in the NAc[99] and vmPFC[58,99] of individuals
with tinnitus compared with controls matched for hearing[111]; increased vmPFC

responses to sound matched to tinnitus frequency on fMRI[59]; and a negative correlation between white-matter integrity in the vmPFC and tinnitus loudness on DTI.[112]

A third model suggests that tinnitus arises from abnormal corticostriatal gating mechanisms (**Fig. 7**)[104] that was inspired by related work on basal ganglia circuitry and function,[113,114] with the following key assumptions: (1) instruction on details of phantom percepts are represented in the central auditory system,[17,115–117] (2) permission to gate candidate phantom percepts for conscious awareness is controlled by the dorsal striatum,[118–120] and (3) tinnitus severity is modulated by a limbic and paralimbic system-NAc-ventral striatum loop.[121,122] This model aims to account for clinical modulators of tinnitus perception and to motivate studies to identify candidate brain targets for treatment-responsive biomarker development and tinnitus mitigation by device-based (eg, deep-brain stimulation) and device-free (eg, magnetic resonance–guided ultrasound) neuromodulation approaches.

It is posited that corticostriatal connectivity between sensory cortex and the dorsal caudate nucleus (dorsal striatum) is a key pathway to convey transformed auditory phantom representations to the basal ganglia for action.[123–125] Striatal gate control normally is restrictive but can become pathologically permissive to allow awareness of phantom percepts in response to alterations of phantom representations in central nervous structures and behavioral and mood circuits in limbic cortex. Tinnitus perception also may be modulated by external auditory stimuli[126–128] and, because the basal ganglia are central to sensorimotor integration, somatosensory stimuli,[129–131] sensorimotor jaw protrusion[132,133] and neck contracture[134,135] movements, and motor gaze-evoked events.[136–138] Moreover, limbic cortex, paralimbic structures, NAc, and the ventral striatum constitute an ensemble of networks that may be critical to the genesis and maintenance of behavioral and emotional distress associated with tinnitus. Those circuits may change striatal gate permissiveness of the dorsal striatum through intrastriatal and nigrotegmental pathways that connect the dorsal and ventral striatum.[139] Alteration in the balance of excitation and inhibition either within the caudate nucleus or its projections to sensory cortex[140,141] may modulate dorsal striatal gate permissiveness.

In additional support of this model, RS-fMRI functional connectivity using a caudate nucleus seeded approach differentiated those with chronic tinnitus from those without tinnitus in cohorts matched for hearing loss.[105] In a comparison study on single-sided

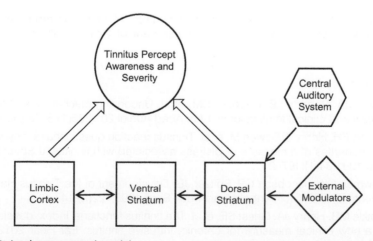

Fig. 7. Striatal gate control model.

deafness, the cohort with chronic tinnitus exhibited increased auditory corticostriatal functional connectivity localized to the left caudate nucleus (see **Fig. 1**). Furthermore, voxel-wise connectivity strength was correlated with subscales of a standardized measure of tinnitus disability, the TFI, for the single-sided deafness tinnitus cohort. **Fig. 2** shows increased connectivity between the right caudate and cuneus for the TFI relaxation subscale, where increased connectivity is correlated with higher interference with the ability to relax. There also was increased connectivity between the right caudate and superior lateral occipital cortex and the right caudate and anterior supramarginal gyrus for the control subscale, where increased connectivity was correlated with the sense of reduced control over the tinnitus percept.

Additional models of tinnitus have arisen from observations in animal models and humans. One such model suggests a role in tinnitus generation or modulation for the cerebellum,[142,143] which receives ascending and descending inputs from auditory pathways.[144] In a rat model of acoustic trauma–induced tinnitus, inactivation or ablation of the paraflocculus of the cerebellum eliminated preexisting tinnitus.[142] Consistent with this observation, human neuroimaging has revealed that the cerebellum in tinnitus sufferers has increased perfusion on nuclear medicine scans (including PET),[145–147] increased activity on RS-fMRI,[98] and increased functional connectivity with other CNS regions that correlates with tinnitus handicap scores.[148] Further tests of this model (and others) may be performed in humans in future studies using the methodologies introduced in this article.

SUMMARY AND FUTURE DIRECTIONS

Human neuroimaging continues to provide insights into the neurophysiologic and neuroanatomic bases of subjective chronic tinnitus in clinical and investigational realms. Intriguingly, one of the most prevalent themes in human tinnitus neuroimaging is heterogeneity among studies. As functional neuroimaging gains traction in clinical medicine, there is optimism that multimodal fMRI and MEGI treatment-responsive biomarkers will be developed to inform clinical decision making and that novel treatment targets will be identified that are suitable for innovative pharmacologic, behavioral, and neuromodulatory approaches for mitigation of bothersome tinnitus.

DISCLOSURE

The authors have no commercial or financial conflicts of interest to report. A portion of the work presented was funded by Department of Defense W81XWH1810741 (SWC, SN).

REFERENCES

1. Henry JA, Roberts LE, Caspary DM, et al. Underlying mechanisms of tinnitus: review and clinical implications. J Am Acad Audiol 2014;25(1):5–22 [quiz: 126].

2. Wilson PH, Henry J, Bowen M, et al. Tinnitus reaction questionnaire: psychometric properties of a measure of distress associated with tinnitus. J Speech Hear Res 1991;34(1):197–201.

3. Newman CW, Jacobson GP, Spitzer JB. Development of the Tinnitus Handicap Inventory. Arch Otolaryngol Head Neck Surg 1996;122(2):143–8.

4. Meikle MB, Henry JA, Griest SE, et al. The tinnitus functional index: development of a new clinical measure for chronic, intrusive tinnitus. Ear Hear 2012;33(2): 153–76.

5. Elgoyhen AB, Langguth B, De Ridder D, et al. Tinnitus: perspectives from human neuroimaging. Nat Rev Neurosci 2015;16(10):632–42.
6. Piccirillo JF, Rodebaugh TL, Lenze EJ. Tinnitus. JAMA 2020. https://doi.org/10.1001/jama.2020.0697.
7. Eisenman DJ, Raghavan P, Hertzano R, et al. Evaluation and treatment of pulsatile tinnitus associated with sigmoid sinus wall anomalies. Laryngoscope 2018;128(Suppl 2):S1–13.
8. Hertzano R, Teplitzky TB, Eisenman DJ. Clinical Evaluation of Tinnitus. Neuroimaging Clin N Am 2016;26(2):197–205.
9. Tunkel DE, Bauer CA, Sun GH, et al. Clinical practice guideline: tinnitus. Otolaryngol Head Neck Surg 2014;151(2 Suppl):S1–40.
10. Kessler MM, Moussa M, Bykowski J, et al. ACR Appropriateness Criteria(®) Tinnitus. J Am Coll Radiol 2017;14(11s):S584–91.
11. Durakovic N, Valente M, Goebel JA, et al. What defines asymmetric sensorineural hearing loss? Laryngoscope 2019;129(5):1023–4.
12. Margolis RH, Saly GL. Asymmetric hearing loss: definition, validation, and prevalence. Otol Neurotol 2008;29(4):422–31.
13. Carney E, Schlauch RS. Critical difference table for word recognition testing derived using computer simulation. J Speech Lang Hear Res 2007;50(5):1203–9.
14. Ahsan SF, Standring R, Osborn DA, et al. Clinical predictors of abnormal magnetic resonance imaging findings in patients with asymmetric sensorineural hearing loss. JAMA Otolaryngol Head Neck Surg 2015;141(5):451–6.
15. Choi KJ, Sajisevi MB, Kahmke RR, et al. Incidence of retrocochlear pathology found on MRI in patients with non-pulsatile tinnitus. Otol Neurotol 2015;36(10):1730–4.
16. Cunnane MB. Imaging of Tinnitus. Neuroimaging Clin N Am 2019;29(1):49–56.
17. Lanting CP, de Kleine E, van Dijk P. Neural activity underlying tinnitus generation: results from PET and fMRI. Hear Res 2009;255(1–2):1–13.
18. Shahsavarani S, Khan RA, Husain FT. Tinnitus and the brain: a review of functional and anatomical magnetic resonance imaging studies. Perspect ASHA Spec Interest Groups 2019;4:896–909.
19. Husain FT. Neural networks of tinnitus in humans: Elucidating severity and habituation. Hear Res 2016;334:37–48.
20. Beckmann CF, DeLuca M, Devlin JT, et al. Investigations into resting-state connectivity using independent component analysis. Philos Trans R Soc Lond B Biol Sci 2005;360(1457):1001–13.
21. Perrachione TK, Ghosh SS. Optimized design and analysis of sparse-sampling FMRI experiments. Front Neurosci 2013;7:55.
22. Eichhammer P, Hajak G, Kleinjung T, et al. Functional imaging of chronic tinnitus: the use of positron emission tomography. Prog Brain Res 2007;166:83–8.
23. Adjamian P. The application of electro- and magneto-encephalography in tinnitus research - methods and interpretations. Front Neurol 2014;5:228.
24. Weisz N, Obleser J. Synchronisation signatures in the listening brain: a perspective from non-invasive neuroelectrophysiology. Hear Res 2014;307:16–28.
25. Cai C, Diwakar M, Chen D, et al. Robust Empirical Bayesian Reconstruction of Distributed Sources for Electromagnetic Brain Imaging. IEEE Trans Med Imaging 2020;39(3):567–77.
26. Owen JP, Wipf DP, Attias HT, et al. Performance evaluation of the Champagne source reconstruction algorithm on simulated and real M/EEG data. Neuroimage 2012;60(1):305–23.

27. Wipf D, Nagarajan S. A unified Bayesian framework for MEG/EEG source imaging. Neuroimage 2009;44(3):947–66.
28. Wipf DP, Owen JP, Attias HT, et al. Robust Bayesian estimation of the location, orientation, and time course of multiple correlated neural sources using MEG. Neuroimage 2010;49(1):641–55.
29. Adjamian P, Hall DA, Palmer AR, et al. Neuroanatomical abnormalities in chronic tinnitus in the human brain. Neurosci Biobehav Rev 2014;45(100):119–33.
30. May A, Gaser C. Magnetic resonance-based morphometry: a window into structural plasticity of the brain. Curr Opin Neurol 2006;19(4):407–11.
31. Schmidt SA, Zimmerman B, Bido Medina RO, et al. Changes in gray and white matter in subgroups within the tinnitus population. Brain Res 2018;1679:64–74.
32. Le Bihan D. Looking into the functional architecture of the brain with diffusion MRI. Nat Rev Neurosci 2003;4(6):469–80.
33. Husain FT, Medina RE, Davis CW, et al. Neuroanatomical changes due to hearing loss and chronic tinnitus: a combined VBM and DTI study. Brain Res 2011; 1369:74–88.
34. Ryan D, Bauer CA. Neuroscience of Tinnitus. Neuroimaging Clin N Am 2016; 26(2):187–96.
35. Mayberg HS. Limbic-cortical dysregulation: a proposed model of depression. J Neuropsychiatry Clin Neurosci 1997;9(3):471–81.
36. Cheung SW, Larson PS. Tinnitus modulation by deep brain stimulation in locus of caudate neurons (area LC). Neuroscience 2010;169(4):1768–78.
37. Raichle ME. The brain's default mode network. Annu Rev Neurosci 2015;38: 433–47.
38. House JW, Brackmann DE. Tinnitus: surgical treatment. Ciba Found Symp 1981; 85:204–16.
39. Liberman MC, Kujawa SG. Cochlear synaptopathy in acquired sensorineural hearing loss: Manifestations and mechanisms. Hear Res 2017;349:138–47.
40. Roberts LE, Eggermont JJ, Caspary DM, et al. Ringing ears: the neuroscience of tinnitus. J Neurosci 2010;30(45):14972–9.
41. Baguley D, McFerran D, Hall D. Tinnitus. Lancet 2013;382(9904):1600–7.
42. Rajan R, Irvine DR. Neuronal responses across cortical field A1 in plasticity induced by peripheral auditory organ damage. Audiol Neurootol 1998;3(2–3): 123–44.
43. Noreña AJ, Tomita M, Eggermont JJ. Neural changes in cat auditory cortex after a transient pure-tone trauma. J Neurophysiol 2003;90(4):2387–401.
44. Seki S, Eggermont JJ. Changes in spontaneous firing rate and neural synchrony in cat primary auditory cortex after localized tone-induced hearing loss. Hear Res 2003;180(1–2):28–38.
45. Weisz N, Wienbruch C, Dohrmann K, et al. Neuromagnetic indicators of auditory cortical reorganization of tinnitus. Brain 2005;128(11):2722–31.
46. Wienbruch C, Paul I, Weisz N, et al. Frequency organization of the 40-Hz auditory steady-state response in normal hearing and in tinnitus. Neuroimage 2006; 33(1):180–94.
47. Sereda M, Adjamian P, Edmondson-Jones M, et al. Auditory evoked magnetic fields in individuals with tinnitus. Hear Res 2013;302:50–9.
48. Ghazaleh N, Zwaag WV, Clarke S, et al. High-resolution fmri of auditory cortical map changes in unilateral hearing loss and tinnitus. Brain Topogr 2017;30(5): 685–97.
49. van Dijk P, Langers DR. Mapping tonotopy in human auditory cortex. Adv Exp Med Biol 2013;787:419–25.

50. Langers DR, de Kleine E, van Dijk P. Tinnitus does not require macroscopic to-notopic map reorganization. Front Syst Neurosci 2012;6:2.
51. Arnold W, Bartenstein P, Oestreicher E, et al. Focal metabolic activation in the predominant left auditory cortex in patients suffering from tinnitus: a PET study with [18F]deoxyglucose. ORL J Otorhinolaryngol Relat Spec 1996;58(4):195–9.
52. Wang H, Tian J, Yin D, et al. Regional glucose metabolic increases in left auditory cortex in tinnitus patients: a preliminary study with positron emission tomography. Chin Med J (Engl) 2001;114(8):848–51.
53. Schecklmann M, Landgrebe M, Poeppl TB, et al. Neural correlates of tinnitus duration and distress: a positron emission tomography study. Hum Brain Mapp 2013;34(1):233–40.
54. Geven LI, de Kleine E, Willemsen AT, et al. Asymmetry in primary auditory cortex activity in tinnitus patients and controls. Neuroscience 2014;256:117–25.
55. Melcher JR, Levine RA, Bergevin C, et al. The auditory midbrain of people with tinnitus: abnormal sound-evoked activity revisited. Hear Res 2009;257(1–2): 63–74.
56. Lanting CP, De Kleine E, Bartels H, et al. Functional imaging of unilateral tinnitus using fMRI. Acta Otolaryngol 2008;128(4):415–21.
57. Gu JW, Halpin CF, Nam EC, et al. Tinnitus, diminished sound-level tolerance, and elevated auditory activity in humans with clinically normal hearing sensitivity. J Neurophysiol 2010;104(6):3361–70.
58. Leaver AM, Renier L, Chevillet MA, et al. Dysregulation of limbic and auditory networks in tinnitus. Neuron 2011;69(1):33–43.
59. Seydell-Greenwald A, Leaver AM, Turesky TK, et al. Functional MRI evidence for a role of ventral prefrontal cortex in tinnitus. Brain Res 2012;1485:22–39.
60. Boyen K, de Kleine E, van Dijk P, et al. Tinnitus-related dissociation between cortical and subcortical neural activity in humans with mild to moderate sensorineural hearing loss. Hear Res 2014;312:48–59.
61. Ochi K, Eggermont JJ. Effects of salicylate on neural activity in cat primary auditory cortex. Hear Res 1996;95(1–2):63–76.
62. Adjamian P, Sereda M, Hall DA. The mechanisms of tinnitus: perspectives from human functional neuroimaging. Hear Res 2009;253(1–2):15–31.
63. Llinás RR, Ribary U, Jeanmonod D, et al. Thalamocortical dysrhythmia: A neurological and neuropsychiatric syndrome characterized by magnetoencephalography. Proc Natl Acad Sci U S A 1999;96(26):15222–7.
64. Llinás RR, Steriade M. Bursting of thalamic neurons and states of vigilance. J Neurophysiol 2006;95(6):3297–308.
65. Kaiser J, Lutzenberger W. Cortical oscillatory activity and the dynamics of auditory memory processing. Rev Neurosci 2005;16(3):239–54.
66. Schlee W, Schecklmann M, Lehner A, et al. Reduced variability of auditory alpha activity in chronic tinnitus. Neural Plast 2014;2014:436146.
67. Weisz N, Muller S, Schlee W, et al. The neural code of auditory phantom perception. J Neurosci 2007;27(6):1479–84.
68. Vanneste S, Heyning PV, Ridder DD. Contralateral parahippocampal gamma-band activity determines noise-like tinnitus laterality: a region of interest analysis. Neuroscience 2011;199:481–90.
69. Zobay O, Palmer AR, Hall DA, et al. Source space estimation of oscillatory power and brain connectivity in tinnitus. PLoS One 2015;10(3):e0120123.
70. Zobay O, Adjamian P. Source-space cross-frequency amplitude-amplitude coupling in tinnitus. Biomed Res Int 2015;2015:489619.

71. Lorenz I, Müller N, Schlee W, et al. Loss of alpha power is related to increased gamma synchronization-A marker of reduced inhibition in tinnitus? Neurosci Lett 2009;453(3):225–8.
72. Adjamian P, Sereda M, Zobay O, et al. Neuromagnetic indicators of tinnitus and tinnitus masking in patients with and without hearing loss. J Assoc Res Otolaryngol 2012;13(5):715–31.
73. van der Loo E, Gais S, Congedo M, et al. Tinnitus intensity dependent gamma oscillations of the contralateral auditory cortex. PLoS One 2009;4(10):e7396.
74. Melcher JR, Knudson IM, Levine RA. Subcallosal brain structure: correlation with hearing threshold at supra-clinical frequencies (>8 kHz), but not with tinnitus. Hear Res 2013;295:79–86.
75. Schneider P, Andermann M, Wengenroth M, et al. Reduced volume of Heschl's gyrus in tinnitus. Neuroimage 2009;45(3):927–39.
76. Aldhafeeri FM, Mackenzie I, Kay T, et al. Neuroanatomical correlates of tinnitus revealed by cortical thickness analysis and diffusion tensor imaging. Neuroradiology 2012;54(8):883–92.
77. Landgrebe M, Langguth B, Rosengarth K, et al. Structural brain changes in tinnitus: grey matter decrease in auditory and non-auditory brain areas. Neuroimage 2009;46(1):213–8.
78. Leaver AM, Seydell-Greenwald A, Rauschecker JP. Auditory-limbic interactions in chronic tinnitus: Challenges for neuroimaging research. Hear Res 2016;334:49–57.
79. Cheng S, Xu G, Zhou J, et al. A Multimodal Meta-Analysis of Structural and Functional Changes in the Brain of Tinnitus. Front Hum Neurosci 2020;14:28.
80. Boyen K, Langers DR, de Kleine E, et al. Gray matter in the brain: differences associated with tinnitus and hearing loss. Hear Res 2013;295:67–78.
81. Schecklmann M, Lehner A, Poeppl TB, et al. Auditory cortex is implicated in tinnitus distress: a voxel-based morphometry study. Brain Struct Funct 2013;218(4):1061–70.
82. De Ridder D, Vanneste S, Weisz N, et al. An integrative model of auditory phantom perception: tinnitus as a unified percept of interacting separable subnetworks. Neurosci Biobehav Rev 2014;44:16–32.
83. Burton H, Wineland A, Bhattacharya M, et al. Altered networks in bothersome tinnitus: a functional connectivity study. BMC Neurosci 2012;13:3.
84. Schmidt SA, Akrofi K, Carpenter-Thompson JR, et al. Default mode, dorsal attention and auditory resting state networks exhibit differential functional connectivity in tinnitus and hearing loss. PLoS One 2013;8(10):e76488.
85. Schmidt SA, Carpenter-Thompson J, Husain FT. Connectivity of precuneus to the default mode and dorsal attention networks: A possible invariant marker of long-term tinnitus. Neuroimage Clin 2017;16:196–204.
86. Leaver AM, Turesky TK, Seydell-Greenwald A, et al. Intrinsic network activity in tinnitus investigated using functional MRI. Hum Brain Mapp 2016;37(8):2717–35.
87. Carpenter-Thompson JR, Schmidt SA, Husain FT. Neural Plasticity of Mild Tinnitus: An fMRI Investigation comparing those recently diagnosed with tinnitus to those that had tinnitus for a long period of time. Neural Plast 2015;2015:161478.
88. Lanting C, WoźAniak A, van Dijk P, et al. Tinnitus- and task-related differences in resting-state networks. Adv Exp Med Biol 2016;894:175–87.
89. Maudoux A, Lefebvre P, Cabay JE, et al. Auditory resting-state network connectivity in tinnitus: a functional MRI study. PLoS One 2012;7(5):e36222.

90. Husain FT, Schmidt SA. Using resting state functional connectivity to unravel networks of tinnitus. Hear Res 2014;307:153–62.
91. Demopoulos C, Duong X, Hinkley LB, et al. Global resting state functional connectivity of neural oscillations in tinnitus with and without hearing loss. Human brain mapping, 2020. [epub ahead of print].
92. Laureano MR, Onishi ET, Bressan RA, et al. Memory networks in tinnitus: a functional brain image study. PLoS One 2014;9(2):e87839.
93. Chen YC, Zhang J, Li XW, et al. Aberrant spontaneous brain activity in chronic tinnitus patients revealed by resting-state functional MRI. Neuroimage Clin 2014;6:222–8.
94. Ueyama T, Donishi T, Ukai S, et al. Alterations of Regional Cerebral Blood Flow in Tinnitus Patients as Assessed Using Single-Photon Emission Computed Tomography. PLoS One 2015;10(9):e0137291.
95. Chen YC, Xia W, Feng Y, et al. Altered interhemispheric functional coordination in chronic tinnitus patients. Biomed Res Int 2015;2015:345647.
96. Yang H, Zheng Y, Ou Y, et al. Regional homogeneity on resting state fMRI in patients with tinnitus. J Otol 2014;9(4):173–8.
97. Chen YC, Feng Y, Xu JJ, et al. Disrupted brain functional network architecture in chronic tinnitus patients. Front Aging Neurosci 2016;8:174.
98. Chen YC, Wang F, Wang J, et al. Resting-state brain abnormalities in chronic subjective tinnitus: a meta-analysis. Front Hum Neurosci 2017;11:22.
99. Mühlau M, Rauschecker JP, Oestreicher E, et al. Structural brain changes in tinnitus. Cereb Cortex 2006;16(9):1283–8.
100. Allan TW, Besle J, Langers DR, et al. Neuroanatomical alterations in tinnitus assessed with magnetic resonance imaging. Front Aging Neurosci 2016;8:221.
101. Han Q, Feng Y, Liu D, et al. MRI analysis of regional homogeneity and gray matter structure in chronic subjective tinnitus. Chinese Journal of Medical Imaging Technology 2018;34:30–4.
102. Krick CM, Grapp M, Daneshvar-Talebi J, et al. Cortical reorganization in recent-onset tinnitus patients by the Heidelberg Model of Music Therapy. Front Neurosci 2015;9:49.
103. Cheung SW, Racine CA, Henderson-Sabes J, et al. Phase I trial of caudate deep brain stimulation for treatment-resistant tinnitus. J Neurosurg 2019;1–10. https://doi.org/10.3171/2019.4.JNS19347.
104. Larson PS, Cheung SW. Deep brain stimulation in area LC controllably triggers auditory phantom percepts. Neurosurgery 2012;70(2):398–405 [discussion: 405–6].
105. Henderson-Sabes J, Shang Y, Perez PL, et al. Corticostriatal functional connectivity of bothersome tinnitus in single-sided deafness. Sci Rep 2019;9(1):19552.
106. Hinkley LB, Mizuiri D, Hong O, et al. Increased striatal functional connectivity with auditory cortex in tinnitus. Front Hum Neurosci 2015;9:568.
107. Perez PL, Wang SS, Heath S, et al. Human caudate nucleus subdivisions in tinnitus modulation. J Neurosurg 2019;1–7. https://doi.org/10.3171/2018.10.JNS181659.
108. Eggermont JJ, Roberts LE. The neuroscience of tinnitus. Trends Neurosci 2004;27(11):676–82.
109. Roberts LE, Husain FT, Eggermont JJ. Role of attention in the generation and modulation of tinnitus. Neurosci Biobehav Rev 2013;37(8):1754–73.
110. Rauschecker JP, Leaver AM, Mühlau M. Tuning out the noise: limbic-auditory interactions in tinnitus. Neuron 2010;66(6):819–26.

111. Leaver AM, Seydell-Greenwald A, Turesky TK, et al. Cortico-limbic morphology separates tinnitus from tinnitus distress. Front Syst Neurosci 2012;6:21.
112. Seydell-Greenwald A, Raven EP, Leaver AM, et al. Diffusion imaging of auditory and auditory-limbic connectivity in tinnitus: preliminary evidence and methodological challenges. Neural Plast 2014;2014:145943.
113. Graybiel AM. Habits, rituals, and the evaluative brain. Annu Rev Neurosci 2008; 31:359–87.
114. Joel D, Niv Y, Ruppin E. Actor-critic models of the basal ganglia: new anatomical and computational perspectives. Neural Netw 2002;15(4–6):535–47.
115. De Ridder D, De Mulder G, Verstraeten E, et al. Primary and secondary auditory cortex stimulation for intractable tinnitus. ORL J Otorhinolaryngol Relat Spec 2006;68(1):48–54 [discussion: 54–5].
116. Eggermont JJ. Role of auditory cortex in noise- and drug-induced tinnitus. Am J Audiol 2008;17(2):S162–9.
117. Kaltenbach JA. Summary of evidence pointing to a role of the dorsal cochlear nucleus in the etiology of tinnitus. Acta Otolaryngol 2006;(556):20–6.
118. Pomata PE, Belluscio MA, Riquelme LA, et al. NMDA receptor gating of information flow through the striatum in vivo. J Neurosci 2008;28(50):13384–9.
119. Schneider JS. Basal ganglia role in behavior: importance of sensory gating and its relevance to psychiatry. Biol Psychiatry 1984;19(12):1693–710.
120. Villablanca JR. Why do we have a caudate nucleus? Acta Neurobiol Exp (Wars) 2010;70(1):95–105.
121. Jastreboff PJ. Tinnitus retraining therapy. Prog Brain Res 2007;166:415–23.
122. LeDoux JE. Emotion circuits in the brain. Annu Rev Neurosci 2000;23:155–84.
123. Reale RA, Imig TJ. Auditory cortical field projections to the basal ganglia of the cat. Neuroscience 1983;8(1):67–86.
124. Selemon LD, Goldman-Rakic PS. Longitudinal topography and interdigitation of corticostriatal projections in the rhesus monkey. J Neurosci 1985;5(3):776–94.
125. Yeterian EH, Pandya DN. Corticostriatal connections of the superior temporal region in rhesus monkeys. J Comp Neurol 1998;399(3):384–402.
126. Stouffer JL, Tyler RS. Characterization of tinnitus by tinnitus patients. J Speech Hear Disord 1990;55(3):439–53.
127. Tyler R, Coelho C, Tao P, et al. Identifying tinnitus subgroups with cluster analysis. Am J Audiol 2008;17(2):S176–84.
128. Tyler RS, Baker LJ. Difficulties experienced by tinnitus sufferers. J Speech Hear Disord 1983;48(2):150–4.
129. Bernstein JM. Cutaneous-evoked tinnitus: first reported case without preceding posterior fossa surgery. Int Tinnitus J 2007;13(2):159–60.
130. Cacace AT, Cousins JP, Parnes SM, et al. Cutaneous-evoked tinnitus. II. Review Of neuroanatomical, physiological and functional imaging studies. Audiol Neurootol 1999;4(5):258–68.
131. Moller AR, Moller MB, Yokota M. Some forms of tinnitus may involve the extra-lemniscal auditory pathway. Laryngoscope 1992;102(10):1165–71.
132. Pinchoff RJ, Burkard RF, Salvi RJ, et al. Modulation of tinnitus by voluntary jaw movements. Am J Otol 1998;19(6):785–9.
133. Rubinstein B, Axelsson A, Carlsson GE. Prevalence of signs and symptoms of craniomandibular disorders in tinnitus patients. J Craniomandib Disord 1990; 4(3):186–92.
134. Abel MD, Levine RA. Muscle contractions and auditory perception in tinnitus patients and nonclinical subjects. Cranio 2004;22(3):181–91.

135. Levine RA, Abel M, Cheng H. CNS somatosensory-auditory interactions elicit or modulate tinnitus. Exp Brain Res 2003;153(4):643–8.
136. Biggs ND, Ramsden RT. Gaze-evoked tinnitus following acoustic neuroma resection: a de-afferentation plasticity phenomenon? Clin Otolaryngol Allied Sci 2002;27(5):338–43.
137. Coad ML, Lockwood A, Salvi R, et al. Characteristics of patients with gaze-evoked tinnitus. Otol Neurotol 2001;22(5):650–4.
138. Lockwood AH, Wack DS, Burkard RF, et al. The functional anatomy of gaze-evoked tinnitus and sustained lateral gaze. Neurology 2001;56(4):472–80.
139. Pennartz CM, Berke JD, Graybiel AM, et al. Corticostriatal Interactions during Learning, Memory Processing, and Decision Making. J Neurosci 2009;29(41): 12831–8.
140. Calabresi P, Centonze D, Gubellini P, et al. Synaptic transmission in the striatum: from plasticity to neurodegeneration. Prog Neurobiol 2000;61(3):231–65.
141. Goubard V, Fino E, Venance L. Contribution of astrocytic glutamate and GABA uptake to corticostriatal information processing. J Physiol 2011;589(Pt 9): 2301–19.
142. Bauer CA, Kurt W, Sybert LT, et al. The cerebellum as a novel tinnitus generator. Hear Res 2013;295:130–9.
143. Brozoski TJ, Ciobanu L, Bauer CA. Central neural activity in rats with tinnitus evaluated with manganese-enhanced magnetic resonance imaging (MEMRI). Hear Res 2007;228(1–2):168–79.
144. Azizi SA, Burne RA, Woodward DJ. The auditory corticopontocerebellar projection in the rat: inputs to the paraflocculus and midvermis. An anatomical and physiological study. Exp Brain Res 1985;59(1):36–49.
145. Mirz F, Pedersen B, Ishizu K, et al. Positron emission tomography of cortical centers of tinnitus. Hear Res 1999;134(1–2):133–44.
146. Shulman A, Strashun A. Descending auditory system/cerebellum/tinnitus. Int Tinnitus J 1999;5(2):92–106.
147. Osaki Y, Nishimura H, Takasawa M, et al. Neural mechanism of residual inhibition of tinnitus in cochlear implant users. Neuroreport 2005;16(15):1625–8.
148. Feng Y, Chen YC, Lv H, et al. Increased Resting-State Cerebellar-Cerebral Functional Connectivity Underlying Chronic Tinnitus. Front Aging Neurosci 2018;10:59.

Current Validated Medical Treatments for Tinnitus
Cognitive Behavioral Therapy

Laurence McKenna, PhD, MClinPsychol[a,b,]*, Florian Vogt, PhD, ClinPsyD[c], Elizabeth Marks, ClinPsyD[a]

KEYWORDS

- Tinnitus • Cognitive behavioral therapy • Mindfulness • MBCT • Acceptance
- Insomnia

KEY POINTS

- Cognitive behavioral therapy (CBT) is an effective treatment for tinnitus distress and endorsed by governing bodies.
- CBT is not widely available to people suffering from tinnitus despite a variety of modalities having been shown to be beneficial; service provision should change to reflect the evidence base.
- New acceptance-based treatments grounded in cognitive and behavioral processes are promising to be additional treatments.

INTRODUCTION

The overall experience of distressing tinnitus represents a weave among physical, cognitive, attentional, and emotional threads. The interconnected nature of these threads means that a reduction in one element might be expected to reduce the overall suffering. Interestingly, however, observations show that the physical/acoustic characteristics of tinnitus do not predict tinnitus-related disability, nor do the acoustic characteristics tend to change following successful therapy.[1] This lends support to the suggestion that psychological therapies focusing on cognitive, behavioral, and emotional aspects of tinnitus will be valuable in the care of people with distressing tinnitus.

[a] Department Clinical Psychology, Royal National Ear Nose Throat and Eastman Dental Hospital, University College Hospital London, 6th Floor West, Ground Floor North, 250 Euston Road, London WN1 2PG, UK; [b] UK & Ear Institute, University College London, 332 Grays Inn Rd, London WC1X 8EE, UK; [c] Department of Psychology, University of Bath, Claverton Down, Bath BA2 7AY, UK
* Corresponding author.
E-mail address: Laurence.mckenna@nhs.net

Otolaryngol Clin N Am 53 (2020) 605–615
https://doi.org/10.1016/j.otc.2020.03.007
0030-6665/20/© 2020 Elsevier Inc. All rights reserved.

The best evidence for psychological approaches to tinnitus exists for cognitive behavioral therapies (CBT). CBT developed from 2 main schools of psychological thinking: behavioral therapy and psychoanalysis. Behavioral therapy grew from the learning theories of Pavlov and Skinner, and used techniques for changing behavioral responses to situations (eg, desensitization and counterconditioning) as a way of changing emotional responses.[2,3] Later, Ellis[4] and Beck[5] expanded on this understanding of psychology to recognize the role of cognition, based on the fundamental premise that individuals are affected not only by external events but also by the way they perceive and interpret such events. Thus, an individual's response to any situation depends more on how they think about that situation than on the situation itself.

THE COGNITIVE BEHAVIORAL THERAPY MODEL

A simple way to understand this is the "ABC model." An Activating Event (A) leads to Beliefs (cognitions and interpretations) about the event (B) that in turn result in emotional, behavioral, physical, and attentional Consequences (C). Examples of how this might relate to tinnitus are shown in **Table 1**.

Interpretations of tinnitus that are more negative and threatening will lead to greater levels of distress compared with more neutral interpretations. The Consequences themselves will feed back into the tinnitus and beliefs. The individual who becomes increasingly anxious and focused on tinnitus, and who adopts behavioral excesses or limitations to fit around tinnitus, will become increasingly distressed by tinnitus. This leads to further negative beliefs and the individual is caught in a vicious cycle that perpetuates distress.[6] An example of this formulation of tinnitus is shown in **Fig. 1**.

INFORMATION PROCESSING BIASES AND THINKING STYLES

We are all prone to information processing biases that tend to intensify in a context of threat and loss. Thoughts arise in our mind automatically and quickly and are often taken to reflect a "truth" of a situation to which we then react. Such automatic thinking can allow us to navigate the world intuitively with little effort and using judgments based on heuristics.[7] This "quick thinking" approach becomes unhelpful when it involves particular thinking styles. For example, a focus on threat will lead to more anxiety-filled thoughts; a focus on loss or negative self-evaluation will lead to more

Table 1 Different cognitive responses to tinnitus lead to different emotional, attentional, physical, and behavioral consequences		
A **Activating Event**	**B** **Belief (Thoughts)**	**C** **Consequences**
Tinnitus enters awareness	This noise means there's something wrong with my body. It will get worse and I won't be able to concentrate. I'll have to stop work.	Emotional: Anxiety. Physical: Bodily tension, increase in tinnitus. Attentional: Focus more on tinnitus. Behavioral: Take time off work.
Tinnitus enters awareness	This noise is a bit annoying, but I know it's just tinnitus and is not dangerous. I have work stress at the moment, and I know tinnitus gets worse when I'm stressed.	Minimal emotional, physical or attentional changes. Behavioral: Take action to reduce stress levels.

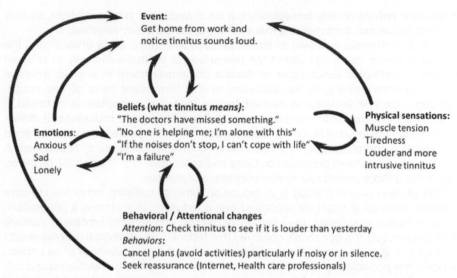

Fig. 1. Cognitive behavioral formulation of persistent tinnitus distress (a "vicious flower").

negative and depressive thoughts. Thus, the biases in information processing intrinsic to our brains often result in interpretations that do not match the available evidence.[7]

Thinking styles affect how we perceive physical sensations. Although most people would prefer not to have tinnitus, profound distress emerges only in approximately 10% of people with tinnitus. A CBT approach postulates that suffering is worsened through information processing biases that lead to *overly* negative interpretations of tinnitus.

CBT was originally developed to treat psychiatric disorders.[8,9] It is also effective at alleviating distress and improving quality of life across a range of other distressing long-term physical health conditions, such as chronic pain,[10] somatic complaints,[11] insomnia,[12] and tinnitus.[13]

THE COGNITIVE BEHAVIORAL TREATMENT MODEL AND ITS RATIONALE IN TINNITUS CARE

The use of CBT in a tinnitus context has been proposed by several investigators.[14–18] This was underpinned by the suggestion that the natural history of tinnitus is characterized by the process of habituation[19] and that successful management of tinnitus will support habituation and remove factors that impede it. Thus treatment should reduce physiologic arousal, encourage exposure, and reduce the negative emotional significance of the tinnitus. This inspired the use of CBT in the management of tinnitus before the development of a fully coherent conceptual CBT model of tinnitus distress.

In 2014, McKenna and colleagues[20] posited the cognitive behavioral model of tinnitus whereby an overly negative interpretation of tinnitus leads to increased sympathetic autonomic arousal, selective attention, and monitoring of tinnitus. This results in greater detection of tinnitus and becomes an iterative process. When overly negative thinking and stress arousal are sustained, they may cause increased levels of anxiety or low mood that, in turn, worsen the negative cognition. To try to cope with the impact of tinnitus, the individual engages in behaviors that attempt to keep them safe, and usually involve avoidance, suppression, and escape. These "safety-seeking behaviors" reduce anxiety immediately but are maladaptive in the long-term, as they prevent the person from realizing that their thoughts are *overly* negative.

Selective attention is known to distort perception in other areas of life,[21] and the model suggests that it can distort the perception of tinnitus sufficiently to account for the catastrophic descriptions of tinnitus commonly heard in a clinic. There is good evidence pointing to the existence of the component parts of this model, although stronger evidence is needed for the idea that perception is distorted.[20] The model involves both psychosomatic and somatopsychic processes. It differs slightly from the focus of Hallam and colleagues[19] in that a greater emphasis is placed on vigilance and orientation to tinnitus rather than simply a failure of habituation. A similar model has been proposed by Cima and colleagues.[22,23] This model, however, attributes a more central role to fear-avoidance processes.

The ultimate goal of therapy is to reduce or eliminate suffering rather than to cure tinnitus. Although it might be supposed that a reduction in tinnitus is a prerequisite for a reduction in suffering, the interplay of psychic and somatic processes indicate that this is not so. It is commonly observed that reducing psychological distress results in a reduction in the intrusiveness of tinnitus and in the pervasiveness of its impact. Indeed, one possible implication of the model of tinnitus suffering of McKenna and colleagues[20] is that removal of tinnitus *per se* might not even be sufficient to remove suffering if the iterative processes have become chronic and patients begin worrying about tinnitus returning.

A change in cognition is key to reducing tinnitus suffering.[24] A standard CBT package has been described,[25] but there is no precise prescription about how cognitive change should be achieved. Indeed, Cima and colleagues[23] emphasize the diversity of techniques used in CBT. Nonetheless, cognitive restructuring, behavioral experiments, and relaxation exercises are well recognized and commonly used components of CBT. Some of these elements are also found in other approaches.[23] The directive counseling element of Tinnitus Retraining Therapy (TRT) could be said to be a cognitive manipulation, albeit a "one-size-fits-all" manipulation. With this in mind, CBT should work carefully alongside other interventions, such as sound therapy. For some, sound therapy may offer a "stepping stone" that at first reduces distress. It can, however, become an unhelpful behavior if the patient believes that he or she will be unable to cope without constant use of a sound device. This represents a form of avoidance maintaining overly negative thoughts. The cognitive context is key, as the same behavior might serve different functions.

THIRD-WAVE COGNITIVE BEHAVIORAL THERAPY: MINDFULNESS AND ACCEPTANCE

In recent decades, "acceptance-based" approaches developed and extended existing CBT while continuing to recognize that distress is maintained by cognitive behavioral factors. This has been referred to as a "Third Wave" of CBT. The emphasis is on changing the *relationship* with difficult or uncomfortable thoughts and feelings, and learning to *accept* these rather than seeking to modify them. Suffering is regarded as a normal part of life, and the philosophy suggests that attempts to resist or change suffering often lead to its perpetuation or exacerbation.[26] The ephemeral nature of thoughts and experiences is stressed. So, patients do not change *what* they think about tinnitus, but rather recognize thoughts, emotions, and sensations simply as part of their moment-by-moment experience that will arise, linger, and then change.

Behavioral change encourages patients to allow all experiences to be present, without attempting to escape or avoid them. There are 2 overlapping strands: acceptance and commitment therapy (ACT) and mindfulness-based therapies, such as mindfulness-based cognitive therapy (MBCT). Both schools make use of mindfulness meditations (MMs), and it is possible that the practice of MMs, sitting in stillness while allowing tinnitus to be present in awareness involves, at least in part, behavioral exposure. Another possibility is that MMs enhance meta-cognitive awareness and skills that reduce the engagement in repetitive negative thinking. The frequent paradoxic impact of avoidance behavior is highlighted, for example, the attempt to "not think of tinnitus" often results in greater awareness of it. ACT also encourages the patient to invest his or her energy in the pursuit of meaningful values rather than in unsuccessful efforts to remove the aversive experience.

Acceptance-based therapies have been found to be beneficial in the treatment of emotional disorders and long-term physical conditions.[27–30]

SLEEP MANAGEMENT

Sleep disturbance is a major factor in tinnitus.[31] Still, little research has been done on the subject. Sleep disturbance has only occasionally been measured in outcome studies and been a target for therapy in even fewer.[32] There is, however, good evidence that CBT is an effective approach to managing primary insomnia and insomnia secondary to other health problems.[33] A consensus statement by the British Association for Psychopharmacology recommends that CBT should be the first line of treatment for insomnia.[34] In chronic pain states, it has been suggested that treating insomnia as the primary therapeutic target, rather than the pain, leads to better outcomes for both insomnia and pain. There is some evidence that using CBT to manage insomnia in patients with tinnitus is successful in improving sleep and reducing tinnitus distress.[35] This has provided a basis for a randomized controlled trial (RCT) into CBT management of tinnitus-related insomnia.[36] The process of CBT for insomnia shares the same features as set out previously, although there is a considerable emphasis on monitoring actual sleep patterns and aligning the behavior of being in bed to these and to the circadian rhythm.

EVIDENCE FOR COGNITIVE BEHAVIORAL THERAPY

Meta-analyses have indicated the beneficial effects of CBT on tinnitus-related distress.[1,13] Across 24 studies (n = 700), CBT showed strong to moderate effect sizes on tinnitus annoyance posttreatment and at follow-up[1] and it (Cohen's d = 1.1) was more effective than other psychological treatments (Cohen's d = 0.30). Smaller effect sizes were obtained for measures of negative affect and sleep problems. Effects on tinnitus loudness were weaker and disappeared at follow-up. The largest meta-analysis to date of 15 RCTs (n = 1091) found CBT to have an impact on tinnitus-related distress (effect sizes ranging from 0.44 to 0.7) as well as a positive effect on mood. The benefits of CBT remained significant at follow-ups up to 18 months.[13] A recent Cochrane review of CBT for tinnitus[37] found CBT reduced the impact of tinnitus on quality of life when compared with no intervention/waiting list control, audiological care, TRT, and other active controls (standard mean differences range from −0.56 to −0.3).

RCTs also support "third-wave" CBT. For example, MBCT is an effective treatment for tinnitus, superior to applied relaxation in reducing tinnitus-related distress,[38,39] and ACT is effective for tinnitus-related distress, compared with TRT.[40]

A systematic review and meta-analysis of RCTs examining tinnitus management found the efficacy of most interventions for tinnitus (including hearing aids, maskers, and TRT) was not demonstrated conclusively.[41] Only studies examining CBT were numerous and similar enough to perform a meta-analysis and the efficacy of CBT (moderate effect size) appears to be reasonably established. A recent systematic review specifically of mindfulness-based therapies for tinnitus concluded that this approach is of benefit in tinnitus management but recognized that further studies are needed.[42] Another review of the literature examined 31 trials of CBT for tinnitus, including a number of acceptance-based therapy trials.[23] The investigators concluded that CBT "is the most evidence-based choice for effectively relieving tinnitus complaints so far"[23] (p. 38); there is evidence for long-term benefits of CBT-based treatments over periods of 15 years. In a large trial, CBT has been demonstrated to be effective as part of a stepped care intervention in which audiological diagnostics, treatment, and consultation, as well as CBT-treatment elements are combined.[43] Importantly, it also has been demonstrated to be a cost-effective intervention.[44]

A number of tinnitus management guidelines, based on systematic reviews, have either "recommended" or "strongly recommended" the use of CBT in tinnitus management,[45–47] while noting that the currently available evidence is not sufficient to support the recommendation of many other approaches (eg, acoustic therapeutic measures, transcranial magnetic or direct current stimulation, and specific forms of acoustic stimulation: noise/masker, retraining therapy, music). The latest Cochrane review of CBT for tinnitus concludes[37] that "...policy-makers and service providers should feel confident that CBT for tinnitus is beneficial for patients." Within the United Kingdom, the National Institute for Health and Care Excellence has produced tinnitus management guidelines. Based on the available evidence, the guidelines again point to the use of CBT (including acceptance-based therapies).[48]

Access to Cognitive Behavioral Therapy for Tinnitus

Accessing CBT for tinnitus can be difficult, as relatively few centers offer it. In spite of the evidence, a recent survey of UK tinnitus services revealed that only a minority of tinnitus services offered some form of CBT or of mindfulness.[49] Very few UK services involved psychologists, and this provision was only within England (not the other UK countries). In most cases, these CBT services were offered by audiologists. These services might be more properly described as a CBT-based approach rather than the provision of full CBT. There is as yet only one study of audiology-led CBT for tinnitus,[50] and the use of CBT in this context needs to be further investigated. In contrast, the survey revealed that most UK tinnitus services offered some form of sound therapy.[50] This is interesting because although there is some evidence of the benefits of sound-based therapy,[51–54] that evidence is less robust[55] than for CBT.

Interest has grown in alternative ways of accessing CBT, including self-help and Internet-based services. Self-help manuals can offer significant benefits, enhanced by minimal therapist support. Attrition rates are high,[56,57] however, and effect sizes are smaller than in regular CBT.[1,13,37] Internet-based CBT has the potential to increase access to evidence-based services that manage tinnitus. Self-help is delivered via computer, with therapist support provided by email. Outcomes are superior to self-help manuals in relieving tinnitus distress and depression, with studies reporting benefits equivalent to regular CBT.[58–60] Importantly, a recent study has demonstrated that guided Internet-based CBT, delivered by an appropriately trained audiologist, led to benefits in reducing tinnitus distress,[50] including at follow-up 12 months after treatment.[61] The same study group also noted that the Internet-based CBT was as effective as standard face-to-face care for tinnitus.[62] High attrition rates may be problematic in Internet therapy.[63] Currently, improved access to CBT for tinnitus via the Internet remains a future prospect; the present reality is that it is not routinely available through most tinnitus centers.

A basic rule of economics is that supply and demand move to meet one another, and it is, therefore, possible that there is an interplay between these 2 forces that limit the provision of CBT as a form of tinnitus care. The issue is one of demand as well as supply. More than 25 years ago, a leading UK otologist noted that only 2% of consultants dealing with tinnitus regularly referred patients for psychological assessment or therapy.[64] It is likely that today the current limited supply of CBT reflects a similar hesitation in requesting the service. Clinical practice guidelines for diagnosis and treatment of tinnitus in Japan acknowledged that despite the possible benefits, it is seen as difficult to perform psychotherapy alongside otorhinolaryngology.[65] The investigators opined that sound therapy is more likely to be carried out. It is just as likely that this reflects a medical, or care, culture as a national culture. For CBT to be acceptable in a tinnitus context, a biopsychosocial model of health and illness is needed. This is certainly not a new concept, but it must be asked how pervasively it is embraced within otolaryngology and audiology. It is likely that a cultural change is required among clinical gatekeepers for services. It is also likely that a change is needed among health insurance companies who are often unwilling to fund nonmedical therapies for patients with tinnitus and so effectively deny their clients access to meaningful evidence-based support. A cultural change is also needed among patients. It has been noted that people with distressing tinnitus want a pharmacologic solution rather than a management strategy.[66] If this perspective is to change (while a cure is awaited) then better marketing of CBT is needed.

SUMMARY

CBT for tinnitus involves identifying and modifying maladaptive behaviors, thoughts, and feelings by means of practical hands-on work and homework assignments. CBT has been practised for many years but is still not widely used in tinnitus management. This is unfortunate, as evidence suggests that this approach benefits many patients when tinnitus is a significant source of distress in the patient's life. It is desirable, however, to continue to develop and implement CBT treatments. An argument can be made that tinnitus services should redeploy some resources to follow the evidence and have substantive provision of CBT rather than continuing to invest in less-evidenced strategies. The financial implications of this are likely to be small but it will require a cultural change. Such a change will be needed among patients as well as clinicians and funders. It is appropriate that clinicians take a lead in this by being mindful of the evidence and moving away from the rhetoric of "no cure; you must learn to live with it" and espousing the benefits of CBT, a therapeutic approach that reduces tinnitus suffering. Such a change may influence the choices patients and funders make.

DISCLOSURE

The authors have nothing to disclose.

REFERENCES

1. Andersson G, Lyttkens L. A meta-analytic review of psychological treatments for tinnitus. Br J Audiol 1999;33(4):201–10.
2. Pavlov IP. Lectures on conditioned reflexes: twenty-five years of objective study of the higher nervous activity (behaviour) of animals. New York: Liverwright Publishing Corporation; 1928. https://doi.org/10.1037/11081-000.
3. Skinner BF. Operant behavior. Am Psychol 1963;18(8):503–15.

4. Ellis A. Rational psychotherapy and individual psychology. J Individ Psychol 1957;13:38–44.
5. Beck AT. Depression: causes and treatment. Philadelphia: University of Pennsylvania Press; 1967.
6. Salkovskis PM, Warwick HM, Deale AC. Cognitive-behavioral treatment for severe and persistent health anxiety (hypochondriasis). Brief Treat Crisis Interv 2003; 3(3):353–67.
7. Kahneman D. Thinking, fast and slow. Penguin, UK: Farrar, Straus and Giroux; 2011.
8. Persons J, Davidson J, Tompkins M. Essential components of cognitive-behavior therapy for depression. Washington, DC: American Psychological Association; 2001.
9. Butler AC, Chapman JE, Forman EM, et al. The empirical status of cognitive-behavioral therapy: a review of meta-analyses. Clin Psychol Rev 2006;26(1): 17–31.
10. Morley S, Eccleston C, Williams A. Systematic review and meta-analysis of randomized controlled trials of cognitive behaviour therapy and behaviour therapy for chronic pain in adults, excluding headache. Pain 1999;80(1–2):1–13.
11. Kroenke K. Efficacy of treatment for somatoform disorders: a review of randomized controlled trials. Psychosom Med 2007;69(9):881–8.
12. Morin CM, Culbert JP, Schwartz SM. Nonpharmacological interventions for insomnia: a meta-analysis of treatment efficacy. Am J Psychiatry 1994;151(8): 1172–80.
13. Hesser H, Weise C, Westin VZ, et al. A systematic review and meta-analysis of randomized controlled trials of cognitive-behavioral therapy for tinnitus distress. Clin Psychol Rev 2011;31(4):545–53.
14. Scott B, Lindberg P, Lyttkens L, et al. Psychological treatment of tinnitus. An experimental group study. Scand Audiol 1985;14(4):223–30.
15. Sweetow RW. Cognitive aspects of tinnitus patient management. Ear Hear 1986; 7(6):390–6.
16. Henry JL, Wilson PH. Tinnitus: a self-management guide for the ringing in your ears. 1st edition. Boston: Allyn & Bacon; 2001.
17. Andersson G. Psychological aspects of tinnitus and the application of cognitive-behavioral therapy. Clin Psychol Rev 2002;22(7):977–90.
18. Kröner-Herwig B, Frenzel A, Fritsche G, et al. The management of chronic tinnitus: comparison of an outpatient cognitive-behavioral group training to minimal-contact interventions. J Psychosom Res 2003;54(4):381–9.
19. Hallam R, Rachman S, Hinchcliffe R. Psychological aspects of tinnitus. In: Rachman S, editor. Contributions to medical psychology. 1984. p. 31–53. Oxford (England). Available at: https://scholar.google.com/scholar_lookup? title=Psychological+aspects+of+tinnitus&author=RS+Hallam&author=S+ Rachman&author=R+Hinchcliffe&publication_year=1984&hl=en. Accessed November 29, 2019..
20. McKenna L, Handscomb L, Hoare DJ, et al. A scientific cognitive-behavioral model of tinnitus: novel conceptualizations of tinnitus distress. Front Neurol 2014;5:196.
21. Tuschen-Caffier B, Bender C, Caffier D, et al. Selective visual attention during mirror exposure in anorexia and bulimia nervosa. PLoS One 2015;10(12): e0145886.
22. Cima RFF, Crombez G, Vlaeyen JWS. Catastrophizing and fear of tinnitus predict quality of life in patients with chronic tinnitus. Ear Hear 2011;32(5):634–41.

23. Cima RFF, Andersson G, Schmidt CJ, et al. Cognitive-behavioral treatments for tinnitus: a review of the literature. J Am Acad Audiol 2014;25(1):29–61.
24. Langguth B, Landgrebe M, Kleinjung T, et al. Tinnitus and depression. World J Biol Psychiatry 2011;12(7):489–500.
25. Baguley D, Andersson G, McFerran D, et al. Tinnitus: a multidisciplinary approach. 2nd edition. West Sussex, UK: Wiley-Blackwell; 2013. https://doi.org/10.1002/9781118783009.
26. Hayes SC. Acceptance and commitment therapy, relational frame theory, and the third wave of behavioral and cognitive therapies. Behav Ther 2004;35(4):639–65.
27. Crowe M, Jordan J, Burrell B, et al. Mindfulness-based stress reduction for long-term physical conditions: a systematic review. Aust N Z J Psychiatry 2016;50(1):21–32.
28. Khoury B, Lecomte T, Fortin G, et al. Mindfulness-based therapy: a comprehensive meta-analysis. Clin Psychol Rev 2013;33(6):763–71.
29. Veehof MM, Oskam M-J, Schreurs KMG, et al. Acceptance-based interventions for the treatment of chronic pain: a systematic review and meta-analysis. Pain 2011;152(3):533–42.
30. Ludwig DS, Kabat-Zinn J. Mindfulness in medicine. JAMA 2008;300(11):1350–2.
31. Sanchez L, Stephens D. A tinnitus problem questionnaire in a clinic population. Ear Hear 1997;18(3):210–7.
32. McKenna L, Daniel HC. The psychological management of tinnitus related insomnia. In: Tyler Richard, editor. Tinnitus treatments. New York: Thieme; 2005.
33. Morin CM, Bootzin RR, Buysse DJ, et al. Psychological and behavioral treatment of insomnia: update of the recent evidence (1998-2004). Sleep 2006;29(11):1398–414.
34. Wilson S, Anderson K, Baldwin D, et al. British Association for Psychopharmacology consensus statement on evidence-based treatment of insomnia, parasomnias and circadian rhythm disorders: an update. J Psychopharmacol 2019;33(8):923–47.
35. Marks E, McKenna L, Vogt F. Cognitive behavioural therapy for tinnitus-related insomnia: evaluating a new treatment approach. Int J Audiol 2019;58(5):311–6.
36. Marks E, McKenna L, Hallsworth C. Cognitive behavioural therapy for insomnia (CBTi) as a treatment for tinnitus-related insomnia: protocol for a randomised controlled trial. Trials 2019;20(1):667.
37. Fuller T, Cima R, Langguth B, et al. Cognitive behavioural therapy for tinnitus. Cochrane Database Syst Rev 2020;(1):CD012614.
38. McKenna L, Marks EM, Hallsworth CA, et al. Mindfulness-based cognitive therapy as a treatment for chronic tinnitus: a randomized controlled trial. Psychother Psychosom 2017;86(6):351–61.
39. Philippot P, Nef F, Clauw L, et al. A randomized controlled trial of mindfulness-based cognitive therapy for treating tinnitus. Clin Psychol Psychother 2012;19(5):411–9.
40. Westin VZ, Schulin M, Hesser H, et al. Acceptance and commitment therapy versus tinnitus retraining therapy in the treatment of tinnitus: a randomised controlled trial. Behav Res Ther 2011;49(11):737–47.
41. Hoare DJ, Kowalkowski VL, Kang S, et al. Systematic review and meta-analyses of randomized controlled trials examining tinnitus management. Laryngoscope 2011;121(7):1555–64.
42. Rademaker MM, Stegeman I, Ho-Kang-You KE, et al. The effect of mindfulness-based interventions on tinnitus distress. a systematic review. Front Neurol 2019;10. https://doi.org/10.3389/fneur.2019.01135.

43. Cima RFF, Maes IH, Joore MA, et al. Specialised treatment based on cognitive behaviour therapy versus usual care for tinnitus: a randomised controlled trial. Lancet 2012;379(9830):1951–9.
44. Maes IHL, Cima RFF, Anteunis LJC, et al. Cost-effectiveness of specialized treatment based on cognitive behavioral therapy versus usual care for tinnitus. Otol Neurotol 2014;35(5):787–95.
45. Tunkel DE, Bauer CA, Sun GH, et al. Clinical practice guideline: tinnitus. Otolaryngol Head Neck Surg 2014;151(2 Suppl):S1–40.
46. Zenner H-P, Delb W, Kröner-Herwig B, et al. A multidisciplinary systematic review of the treatment for chronic idiopathic tinnitus. Eur Arch Otorhinolaryngol 2017; 274(5):2079–91.
47. Cima RFF, Mazurek B, Haider H, et al. A multidisciplinary European guideline for tinnitus: diagnostics, assessment, and treatment. HNO 2019;67(Suppl 1):10–42.
48. Project information | Tinnitus: assessment and management | Guidance | NICE. Available at: https://www.nice.org.uk/guidance/ng155/chapter/Recommend ations. Accessed April 8, 2020.
49. Hoare DJ, Broomhead E, Stockdale D, et al. Equity and person-centeredness in provision of tinnitus services in UK National Health Service audiology departments. Eur J Pers Cent Healthc 2015;3(3):318–26.
50. Beukes EW, Baguley DM, Allen PM, et al. Audiologist-guided Internet-based cognitive behavior therapy for adults with tinnitus in the United Kingdom: a randomized controlled trial. Ear Hear 2018;39(3):423–33.
51. Searchfield GD, Kaur M, Martin WH. Hearing aids as an adjunct to counseling: tinnitus patients who choose amplification do better than those that don't. Int J Audiol 2010;49(8):574–9.
52. Trotter MI, Donaldson I. Hearing aids and tinnitus therapy: a 25-year experience. J Laryngol Otol 2008;122(10):1052–6.
53. dos Santos GM, Bento RF, de Medeiros IRT, et al. The influence of sound generator associated with conventional amplification for tinnitus control: randomized blind clinical trial. Trends Hear 2014;18. https://doi.org/10.1177/2331216514542657.
54. Bauer CA, Berry JL, Brozoski TJ. The effect of tinnitus retraining therapy on chronic tinnitus: a controlled trial. Laryngoscope Investig Otolaryngol 2017; 2(4):166–77.
55. Sereda M, Xia J, El Refaie A, et al. Sound therapy (using amplification devices and/or sound generators) for tinnitus. Cochrane Database Syst Rev 2018;(12). https://doi.org/10.1002/14651858.CD013094.pub2.
56. Kaldo V, Cars S, Rahnert M, et al. Use of a self-help book with weekly therapist contact to reduce tinnitus distress: a randomized controlled trial. J Psychosom Res 2007;63(2):195–202.
57. Malouff JM, Noble W, Schutte NS, et al. The effectiveness of bibliotherapy in alleviating tinnitus-related distress. J Psychosom Res 2010;68(3):245–51.
58. Kaldo-Sandström V, Larsen HC, Andersson G. Internet-based cognitive-behavioral self-help treatment of tinnitus: clinical effectiveness and predictors of outcome. Am J Audiol 2004;13(2):185–92.
59. Kaldo V, Levin S, Widarsson J, et al. Internet versus group cognitive-behavioral treatment of distress associated with tinnitus: a randomized controlled trial. Behav Ther 2008;39(4):348–59.
60. Andersson G, Strömgren T, Ström L, et al. Randomized controlled trial of internet-based cognitive behavior therapy for distress associated with tinnitus. Psychosom Med 2002;64(5):810–6.

61. Beukes EW, Allen PM, Baguley DM, et al. Long-term efficacy of audiologist-guided Internet-based cognitive behavior therapy for tinnitus. Am J Audiol 2018;27(3S):431–47.
62. Beukes EW, Andersson G, Allen PM, et al. Effectiveness of guided Internet-based cognitive behavioral therapy vs face-to-face clinical care for treatment of tinnitus: a randomized clinical trial. JAMA Otolaryngol Head Neck Surg 2018;144(12): 1126–33.
63. Abbott J-AM, Kaldo V, Klein B, et al. A cluster randomised trial of an Internet-based intervention program for tinnitus distress in an industrial setting. Cogn Behav Ther 2009;38(3):162–73.
64. Coles RR. A survey of tinnitus management in National Health Service hospitals. Clin Otolaryngol Allied Sci 1992;17(4):313–6.
65. Ogawa K, Sato H, Takahashi M, et al. Clinical practice guidelines for diagnosis and treatment of chronic tinnitus in Japan. Auris Nasus Larynx 2019. https://doi.org/10.1016/j.anl.2019.09.007.
66. McFerran DJ, Stockdale D, Holme R, et al. Why is there no cure for tinnitus? Front Neurosci 2019;13. https://doi.org/10.3389/fnins.2019.00802.

Current Validated Medical Treatments
Pharmacologic Interventions

Carol A. Bauer, MD

KEYWORDS

- Pharmacology • Tinnitus • Clinical trials • Psychoacoustic • Neurotransmitters
- Depression • Anxiety

KEY POINTS

- Drug therapies for tinnitus can be categorized into those directed at decreasing the sensation of tinnitus and those directed at decreasing the impact of tinnitus.
- All tinnitus intervention trials should clearly state their therapeutic objective or objectives, that is, treatment of sensation level or impact.
- There are no drug therapies universally effective in reducing the sensation of tinnitus, through either decreasing awareness or decreasing perceived loudness of the sensation.
- Categorizing tinnitus into subtypes has potential utility if drugs can be found to effectively treat individual subtypes.
- Clinical trials investigating drug efficacy must include appropriate controls that take into account the placebo response seen in all tinnitus treatments.

The search for an effective medication that will eliminate tinnitus has a very long history. Indeed, for as long as history has documented that humans have experienced, and been bothered by, tinnitus, there have been treatments in the form of drops, ointments, pills, and elixirs with claims of cures. Success has been elusive. Current pharmacologic interventions can be divided into those that attempt to eliminate the perception of tinnitus, and those that treat the negative comorbidities associated with tinnitus, thereby mitigating the negative impact of tinnitus on quality of life. One could also consider a third category of tinnitus drugs, which address a known pathologic condition that has tinnitus as an associated symptom (for example, Meniere's disease, otosclerosis, migraine-associated vertigo). This third category suffers from a paucity of research specifically directed at quantifying the modulation of tinnitus in these diseases and therefore is not addressed.

Department of Otolaryngology Head and Neck Surgery, Southern Illinois University School of Medicine, Springfield, IL 62794, USA
E-mail address: cbauer@siumed.edu

Otolaryngol Clin N Am 53 (2020) 617–626
https://doi.org/10.1016/j.otc.2020.03.009
0030-6665/20/© 2020 Elsevier Inc. All rights reserved.

The failure to find a drug that effectively cures tinnitus has multiple reasons. Treatments for any medical malady are most effectively developed when the underlying pathologic condition of the disease has been understood. Although there are multiple hypotheses regarding how and why tinnitus develops, there is no consensus at this time. Furthermore, it has not been clearly elucidated why there is a considerable range of reactions or levels of distress related to tinnitus. Factors that promote habituation to the tinnitus percept or that prevent habituation, thus resulting in bothersome intrusive tinnitus, have not been unequivocally established. Until such fundamental gaps in understanding the basic science of tinnitus have been addressed, the search for effective medications and/or the development of new pharmacologic interventions will be handicapped.

A second reason for failure to find an effective therapeutic is the wide range of methodologies used in tinnitus clinical trials. Optimized trial designs for testing treatment efficacy have been proposed but are infrequently followed.[1,2] There are many validated questionnaires and assessment tools available, but there is no consensus on the best measurements and metrics that should be used in tinnitus trials. Comparison of drug trials using different measurements can be challenging. Finally, the important issue of treatment significance, as opposed to statistical significance, should be considered when evaluating trial outcomes. A statistically significant change in severity score is not equivalent to a meaningful change for patient satisfaction and compliance.

Modern pharmacologic treatments of tinnitus rely primarily on adapting existing medications not developed for this indication and are therefore used "off-label." A common scenario for a specific drug or class of drugs used to treat tinnitus would unfold as follows. A medication is anecdotally reported to modulate tinnitus in one or several patients. Lidocaine, for example, was reported to decrease tinnitus loudness after topical application to the nose.[3] The first report of gabapentin reducing tinnitus loudness was in a patient taking the medication for chronic pain.[4] Tinnitus has features in common with neuropathic pain and has been associated with neural hyperactivity, potentially from loss of inhibitory tone in central auditory pathways. Drugs such as lidocaine and gabapentin therefore would seem to be worthy of further investigation (discussed later).

Uncontrolled trials or retrospective reports of clinical observations of a novel therapeutic often show promise.[5–7] Rarely, however, are such reports followed by basic experiments to confirm the therapeutic effect and reveal a mechanism of action. Gabapentin, for example, a congener of the inhibitory neurotransmitter gamma-aminobutyric acid (GABA) that does not directly act on GABA receptors, was found to effectively decrease psychophysical evidence of tinnitus in an animal model of noise-induced tinnitus.[8] However, subsequent blinded controlled clinical trials using standardized and validated measures did not yield consistent positive results.[9–12]

Why have drugs failed to consistently manage tinnitus? Several plausible reasons and knowledge gaps can be identified. First, what is the physiologic mechanism responsible for tinnitus, and is the mechanism universal? Is the perception of a phantom sound, regardless of its presumed clinical cause, the result of a set sequence of physiologic events? Is it reasonable to assume that the neural pathologic condition accompanying tinnitus associated with noise-induced hearing loss or sudden hearing loss is the same as that accompanying age-related hearing loss? The answers are not known and therefore identifying a drug with a mechanism that is universally effective may not be possible. Is there a different (or additional) mechanism involved in people who can somatically modulate the perceptual qualities of their tinnitus with neck or jaw or eye motion[13–16]? Is there an additional tinnitus-specific mechanism in play for people with tinnitus associated with severe distress, anxiety, and/or depression[17-19]? Is there an identifiable mechanism that can account for the bidirectional impact of sleep on tinnitus[20-22]? Finally, how do attentional mechanisms play into an individual's awareness and intrusiveness of their tinnitus[23-25]? The questions that arise from clinical observations all illuminate the complexity of the clinical problem and reinforce the challenges in finding an effective pharmacologic treatment that withstands repeated assessment in large-scale, blinded, placebo-controlled trials.

Several systematic reviews of pharmacologic treatments of tinnitus are available, and the reader interested in trial details and critiques is directed to these sources.[26-28] Among these, the review conducted by The Agency for Healthcare Research and Quality concluded that there is "low strength of evidence that all pharmacologic interventions include tinnitus specific quality of life; there is low strength of evidence that antidepressants improve anxiety and depression symptoms."[27] The American Academy of Otolaryngology Head and Neck Surgery Clinical Practice Guideline concluded that "[c]linicians should not routinely recommend antidepressants, anticonvulsants, anxiolytics, or intratympanic medications for a primary indication of treating persistent, bothersome tinnitus."[26] The most recent Cochrane Collaboration review of antidepressants and tinnitus reviewed 6 studies that evaluated 3 tricyclic antidepressants (amitriptyline, nortriptyline, trimipramine), 1 selective serotonin reuptake inhibitor (paroxetine), and 1 atypical antidepressant (trazodone) and concluded that there was insufficient evidence to prove efficacy in the management of tinnitus.[28]

ANTIDEPRESSANTS

The causal relationship between bothersome tinnitus and affective disorders, such as depression and anxiety, is still under debate. It is unclear if people with depression and/or anxiety are more prone to developing tinnitus; if tinnitus is a direct cause of depression and/or anxiety in some people; or if mood disorders simply exacerbate tinnitus severity independently from the pathologic mechanism or mechanisms responsible for tinnitus.[19,28] Several studies have demonstrated a higher prevalence of depression and anxiety in patients with bothersome tinnitus than in control sample populations.[29-31] It has been suggested that conclusions from small, potentially biased samples may not reflect the true prevalence of psychological disorders in people with tinnitus, and the reported prevalence may be subject to bias when data are drawn from population samples derived from psychiatry or mental-health clinics.[32] Notably, however, the 2007 National Health Interview Series, a household-based survey of adults older than 18 years of age conducted by trained interviewers, included for the first time a tinnitus module determining the prevalence and severity of tinnitus experienced over the past 12 months (defined as "no problem," "a small problem," "a moderate problem," "a big problem," "a very big problem"). Analysis of this general population sample showed a higher prevalence of depression (25.6%) and anxiety (26.1%) in adults reporting tinnitus than adults reporting no tinnitus (9.1% and 9.2%, respectively). However, the association between tinnitus and anxiety and depression was significant only for respondents endorsing tinnitus as "a big problem" or "a very big problem." In adults reporting tinnitus that categorically was less than "a big problem," the prevalence of anxiety and depression was similar to people without tinnitus.[19] Although the issue of causality has yet to be resolved, it is well recognized that concurrent mood disorders exert a negative impact on medical conditions, such as chronic pain and tinnitus severity.[33-35] Psychological distress and coping ability may be negatively correlated with bothersome tinnitus. If mood disorders exacerbate tinnitus, and this is mediated through innate or learned coping strategies, this suggests a possible avenue for treatment.[36] The question is: given the current state of information, should antidepressants and/or anxiolytics be used as primary treatments for tinnitus? Because depression can be a comorbid condition, and there is evidence of a negative interaction with tinnitus and because untreated depression can exacerbate coping ability, it is reasonable to conclude that clinicians should screen for depression in patients presenting with bothersome tinnitus and treat accordingly.

BENZODIAZEPINES

Benzodiazepines historically were commonly used medications for tinnitus. Specific drugs in the class include diazepam, clonazepam, and alprazolam. Purported benefits were related to treating the comorbidities of anxiety and insomnia that occur with chronic bothersome tinnitus. These compounds globally increase the levels of the inhibitory neurotransmitter GABA throughout the brain and therefore could directly modulate tinnitus, given that GABA downregulation has been identified as a potential tinnitus mechanism.[37–40] Significant concerns regarding abuse potential, and the interaction risk of overdose when GABA agonists are combined with opioids, have significantly reduced the use of these medications as a primary tinnitus therapeutic.

A recent review of the literature concluded there was low-quality evidence overall in controlled trials showing clinical efficacy for treating tinnitus with benzodiazepines.[41] Clonazepam was found to reduce tinnitus severity in 3 studies when compared with controls that included meclizine,[42] gabapentin,[43] and gingko biloba.[44] Tinnitus severity was assessed in these studies using a wide range of metrics, including visual analogue scale (VAS),[43,44] the Tinnitus Handicap Inventory (THI),[44] and assessment of tinnitus impact on sleep and activity.[42] These studies were limited, however, by inadequate blinding, lack of standardized assessments,[42] and potential cross-over effects from active comparator drugs. Alprazolam was first systematically studied by Johnson and colleagues[45] and was shown to reduce tinnitus loudness compared with saline placebo; however, there were no measures of changes in tinnitus severity reported in this trial. Conflicting results were found in a subsequent study comparing alprazolam with saline placebo.[46] In this study, which excluded subjects with clinical depression or anxiety, tinnitus loudness measured by psychophysical loudness matching procedure was unchanged with alprazolam. However, there was a significant reduction in tinnitus severity on a VAS with anchors of "no tinnitus" and "worst imaginable tinnitus," but there was no significant change in severity using a standardized questionnaire (THI).

ANTICONVULSANTS

The application of some classes of drugs to the treatment of tinnitus derived from analogies wherein tinnitus was viewed as an "auditory seizure" or an auditory manifestation of phantom pain.[47–49] Nonauditory sensory system deafferentation was known to result in pathologic neural hyperactivity and dysesthesia,[50,51] and a similar mechanism in the auditory system resulting in tinnitus was a reasonable conjecture. Early investigations of lidocaine and its oral congener tocainide were initially promising, but subsequent studies were less encouraging. The significant placebo effect and the variable response to lidocaine in a well-controlled trial dampened the initial enthusiasm for these medications.[52]

One of the most studied medications for tinnitus treatment in the past 2 decades is gabapentin. Originally developed as an antiepileptic drug for treating partial seizures, it eventually found wider use in treating diabetic neuropathic pain and postherpetic neuralgia. Gabapentin is presumed to enhance central inhibition by increasing

GABA synthesis through modulation of the GABA synthetic enzyme glutamic acid decarboxylase. Anecdotal reports of efficacy in reducing the loudness and salience of tinnitus aligned with the hypothetical mechanism of auditory deafferentation (hearing loss), leading to a pathologic loss of inhibitory neurotransmitter in central auditory pathways. The logic that enhanced neural inhibition would be effective in reducing neural hyperactivity and thus decrease the perception of tinnitus is reasonable. Research using an animal model of noise-induced hearing loss and tinnitus supported this reasoning as well.[8,53]

Four clinical trials have investigated gabapentin (Neurontin) for efficacy in treating tinnitus that is either acute onset (1 trial)[54] or chronic (3 trials).[9,10,55] Two additional placebo-controlled trials have been published but have methodologic limitations that constrain interpretation and generalization (for example, exclusion of subjects with bilateral tinnitus) and therefore will not be included in this summary.[11,12] Adults with acute tinnitus after noise trauma, present for less than 6 months, reported a significant decrease in tinnitus severity (rated with a multiquestion VAS) after 6 weeks' treatment with gabapentin 300 mg/d. The number of subjects achieving "success" criterion ($\geq$30% reduction in tinnitus severity VAS) was significantly greater in the gabapentin group (89%) compared with the patients receiving placebo (58%) ($P<.001$). Three randomized double-blinded placebo-controlled trials investigated chronic tinnitus. The definition of chronic varied from tinnitus present at least 3 months[9] to 12 months or more.[55] The studies varied also in drug protocol, severity, inclusion criteria, and secondary outcome measures (**Table 1**). Nevertheless, despite the different methodologies used in each study, efficacy was demonstrated in various metrics. Witsell and colleagues[9] showed that a significantly greater percentage of subjects reported global improvement in tinnitus after 2 weeks of gabapentin compared with placebo. Piccirillo and colleagues[10] showed a significantly greater decrease in THI score for subjects after 8 weeks of gabapentin (Δ 21.40) compared with placebo (Δ 1.75) among subjects with normal hearing ($P = .005$). The frequency composition for calculating threshold averages and categorizing as normal, mild, moderate, and severe was not reported, and therefore, the inclusion of subjects with evidence of noise-induced hearing loss at 4 kHz or greater in the normal hearing category is not known. Bauer and Brozoski[55] used a within-subject placebo-controlled study design and categorized subjects by tinnitus cause (noise-induced tinnitus vs presbycusis-induced tinnitus). Subjects with a history of noise-induced hearing loss and tinnitus showed a significant reduction in both annoyance and psychoacoustic measures of tinnitus loudness with daily gabapentin compared with measures and ratings while on placebo, an effect not seen in subjects with tinnitus related to presbycusis. An improvement in psychoacoustic tinnitus loudness match of 20 dB hearing level or greater was observed during gabapentin treatment relative to baseline in 30% of subjects categorized with noise-induced tinnitus experienced and 16% of subjects categorized with presbycusis-related tinnitus.

TINNITUS SUBTYPES AND TARGETED DRUG THERAPY

Identifying a drug that is universally and consistently effective for all people presumes that all tinnitus is alike. Current knowledge does not support the idea that a single pathologic mechanism is responsible for generating all types of tinnitus.[56] Drug development that acknowledges specific tinnitus modulators, such as stress, anxiety, depression, and sleep patterns, will be necessary if tinnitus can be treated as a problem of personalized medicine. Recent attempts at identifying circuit's responsible for the association between observed modulators and tinnitus is a promising area of

Table 1
Selected details of clinical trials investigating gabapentin for acute and chronic tinnitus

	Study Design Planned (Completed) Enrollment	Target Drug Dose and Schedule	Tinnitus Duration Highlighted Inclusion and Exclusion Criteria	Primary Outcome Measure (Secondary Outcome Measure)
Goljanian Tabrizi et al,[54] 2017	Randomized to drug or placebo Gabapentin 55 Placebo 48	600 mg/d × 6 wk	Tinnitus duration not specified Ages 18–50 y Tinnitus secondary to noise-trauma only Tinnitus severity not specified Depression not excluded	Tinnitus severity (VAS)
Witsell et al,[9] 2007	Randomized to drug or placebo Gabapentin 53 (49) Placebo 26 (16) Ten lost to follow-up	600 mg tid × 2 wk	≥3 mo Tinnitus severity not specified Depression not excluded	THI Profile of mood states Global tinnitus change (Likert scale)
Piccirillo et al,[10] 2007	Randomized to drug or placebo Gabapentin 70 (59) Placebo 65 (56)	3600 mg/d × 4 wk	≥6 mo THI ≥38 No depression	THI Global change (Likert scale) Global life disturbance
Bauer et al,[37] 2007	Repeated measures within-subject control Tinnitus categorized as secondary to noise-trauma or to presbycusis	Multiple doses and placebo assessed for each subject (900 mg/d, 1800 mg/d, 2400 mg/d)	≥12 mo THQ ≥30 No depression	Tinnitus Handicap Questionnaire Tinnitus experience questionnaire General health survey

Data from Refs.[9,10,37,54]

research.[57] Unfortunately, attempts at subtyping or categorizing tinnitus to facilitate individualized drug therapy plans are rare. Most clinical trials do not attempt to identify tinnitus subtypes and can miss what otherwise would be an effective drug in selected patients. Staccato or paroxysmal tinnitus may be a specific subtype that can be identified by clinical characteristics and is one example of this washout effect.[58–61] Although the evidence for efficacy is limited to small studies without placebo controls, the strength of the evidence is increased by the repeated positive results. Reviews that miss the exceptions can be misleading and result in missed opportunities for treatment successes.[62]

CHALLENGES OF ESTABLISHING TREATMENT EFFICACY

The search for a drug that can universally improve tinnitus loudness, intrusiveness, and impact on quality of life is ongoing. The history of tinnitus drug trials to date reveals important elements that can obscure drug identification and confound effective drug development if not addressed. It is clear that the strong placebo effect seen in clinical trials must be effectively controlled. Tinnitus impact and subjective distress can be challenging to assess. Stable baseline measures must be obtained to identify subjects who can provide high-fidelity data during exploratory drug investigations. Predefined criteria for clinically relevant improvement should be stated at the beginning of the trial, and these criteria should be clinically relevant and realistic. The enrolled subject groups must be clearly defined. It is important to determine if the drug is anticipated to have efficacy in treating new onset tinnitus or chronic persistent tinnitus. Significant improvement and spontaneous resolution occur in a not insignificant number of cases of acute tinnitus, and therefore, required diligence in establishing power estimates and control conditions.

DISCLOSURE

The author has no conflicts of interest to declare.

REFERENCES

1. Dobie RA. A review of randomized clinical trials in tinnitus. Laryngoscope 1999; 109(8):1202–11.
2. Landgrebe M, Azevedo A, Baguley D, et al. Methodological aspects of clinical trials in tinnitus: a proposal for an international standard. J Psychosom Res 2012;73(2):112–21.
3. Bárány R. Die Beeinflussing des Ohrensausens durch intravenous injizierte Lokalanasthetica. Acta Otolaryngol 1935;23:201–3.
4. Zapp JJ. Gabapentin for the treatment of tinnitus: a case report. Ear, nose, throat J 2001;80(2):114–6.
5. Melding PS, Goodey RJ, Thorne PR. The use of intravenous lignocaine in the diagnosis and treatment of tinnitus. J Laryngol Otol 1978;92(2):115–21.
6. Shea JJ, Harell M. Management of tinnitus aurium with lidocaine and carbamazepine. Laryngoscope 1978;88(9 Pt 1):1477–84.
7. Shulman A, Strashun AM, Goldstein BA. GABAA-benzodiazepine-chloride receptor-targeted therapy for tinnitus control: preliminary report. Int Tinnitus J 2002;8(1):30–6.
8. Bauer CA, Brozoski TJ. Assessing tinnitus and prospective tinnitus therapeutics using a psychophysical animal model. J Assoc Res Otolaryngol 2001;2(1):54–64.

9. Witsell DL, Hannley MT, Stinnet S, et al. Treatment of tinnitus with gabapentin: a pilot study. Otol Neurotol 2007;28(1):11–5.

10. Piccirillo JF, Finnell J, Vlahiotis A, et al. Relief of idiopathic subjective tinnitus: is gabapentin effective? Arch Otolaryngol Head Neck Surg 2007;133(4):390–7.

11. Bakhshaee M, Ghasemi M, Azarpazhooh M, et al. Gabapentin effectiveness on the sensation of subjective idiopathic tinnitus: a pilot study. Eur Arch Otorhinolaryngol 2008;265(5):525–30.

12. Dehkordi MA, Abolbashari S, Taheri R, et al. Efficacy of gabapentin on subjective idiopathic tinnitus: a randomized, double-blind, placebo-controlled trial. Ear Nose Throat J 2011;90(4):150–8.

13. Dehmel S, Cui YL, Shore SE. Cross-modal interactions of auditory and somatic inputs in the brainstem and midbrain and their imbalance in tinnitus and deafness. Am J Audiol 2008;17(2):S193–209.

14. Levine RA, Nam EC, Oron Y, et al. Evidence for a tinnitus subgroup responsive to somatosensory based treatment modalities. Prog Brain Res 2007;166:195–207.

15. Shore S, Zhou J, Koehler S. Neural mechanisms underlying somatic tinnitus. Prog Brain Res 2007;166:107–23.

16. Simmons R, Dambra C, Lobarinas E, et al. Head, neck, and eye movements that modulate tinnitus. Semin Hear 2008;29(4):361–70.

17. Halford JB, Anderson SD. Anxiety and depression in tinnitus sufferers. J Psychosom Res 1991;35(4–5):383–90.

18. Hebert S, Canlon B, Hasson D. Emotional exhaustion as a predictor of tinnitus. Psychother Psychosom 2012;81(5):324–6.

19. Bhatt JM, Bhattacharyya N, Lin HW. Relationships between tinnitus and the prevalence of anxiety and depression. Laryngoscope 2017;127(2):466–9.

20. Lazic K, Petrovic J, Ciric J, et al. REM sleep disorder following general anesthesia in rats. Physiol Behav 2017;168:41–54.

21. Folmer RL, Griest SE. Tinnitus and insomnia. Am J Otolaryngol 2000;21(5):287–93.

22. Hebert S, Carrier J. Sleep complaints in elderly tinnitus patients: a controlled study. Ear Hear 2007;28(5):649–55.

23. Dornhoffer J, Danner C, Mennemeier M, et al. Arousal and attention deficits in patients with tinnitus. Int Tinnitus J 2006;12(1):9–16.

24. Kaltenbach JA. The dorsal cochlear nucleus as a participant in the auditory, attentional and emotional components of tinnitus. Hear Res 2006;216-217:224–34.

25. Roberts LE, Husain FT, Eggermont JJ. Role of attention in the generation and modulation of tinnitus. Neurosci Biobehav Rev 2013;37(8):1754–73.

26. Tunkel DE, Bauer CA, Sun GH, et al. Clinical practice guideline: tinnitus. Otolaryngol Head Neck Surg 2014;151(2 Suppl):S1–40.

27. Pichora-Fuller MK, Santaguida P, Hammill A, et al. Evaluation and treatment of tinnitus: comparative effectiveness. Rockville (MD): Agency for Healthcare Research and Quality (U.S.); 2013.

28. Baldo P, Doree C, Molin P, et al. Antidepressants for patients with tinnitus. Cochrane Database Syst Rev 2012;(9):CD003853.

29. Sullivan MD, Katon W, Dobie R, et al. Disabling tinnitus. Association with affective disorder. Gen Hosp Psychiatry 1988;10(4):285–91.

30. Budd RJ, Pugh R. The relationship between locus of control, tinnitus severity, and emotional distress in a group of tinnitus sufferers. J Psychosom Res 1995;39(8):1015–8.

31. Harrop-Griffiths J, Katon W, Dobie R, et al. Chronic tinnitus: association with psychiatric diagnoses. J Psychosom Res 1987;31(5):613–21.
32. McFerran DJ, Baguley DM. Is psychology really the best treatment for tinnitus? Clin Otolaryngol 2009;34(2):99–101 [discussion: 02].
33. Folmer RL, Griest SE, Meikle MB, et al. Tinnitus severity, loudness, and depression. Otolaryngol Head Neck Surg 1999;121(1):48–51.
34. Ohayon MM, Schatzberg AF. Using chronic pain to predict depressive morbidity in the general population. Arch Gen Psychiatry 2003;60(1):39–47.
35. Fishbain DA, Cutler R, Rosomoff HL, et al. Chronic pain-associated depression: antecedent or consequence of chronic pain? A review. Clin J Pain 1997;13(2): 116–37.
36. Kirsch CA, Blanchard EB, Parnes SM. Psychological characteristics of individuals high and low in their ability to cope with tinnitus. Psychosom Med 1989; 51(2):209–17.
37. Bauer CA, Brozoski TJ. Gabapentin. In: Langguth B, Hajak G, Kleinjung T, et al, editors. Tinnitus: pathophysiology and treatment. New York: Elsevier; 2007. p. 287–301.
38. Brozoski T, Odintsov B, Bauer C. Gamma-aminobutyric acid and glutamic acid levels in the auditory pathway of rats with chronic tinnitus: a direct determination using high resolution point-resolved proton magnetic resonance spectroscopy (H-MRS). Front Syst Neurosci 2012;6:9.
39. Wang H, Brozoski TJ, Caspary DM. Inhibitory neurotransmission in animal models of tinnitus: maladaptive plasticity. Hear Res 2011;279(1–2):111–7.
40. Brozoski TJ, Caspary DM, Bauer CA, et al. The effect of supplemental dietary taurine on tinnitus and auditory discrimination in an animal model. Hear Res 2010;270(1–2):71–80.
41. Jufas NE, Wood R. The use of benzodiazepines for tinnitus: systematic review. J Laryngol Otol 2015;129(Suppl 3):S14–22.
42. Lechtenberg R, Shulman A. The neurologic implications of tinnitus. Arch Neurol 1984;41(7):718–21.
43. Bahmad FM Jr, Venosa AR, Oliveira CA. Benzodiazepines and GABAergics in treating severe disabling tinnitus of predominantly cochlear origin. Int Tinnitus J 2006;12(2):140–4.
44. Han SS, Nam EC, Won JY, et al. Clonazepam quiets tinnitus: a randomised crossover study with ginkgo biloba. J Neurol Neurosurg Psychiatry 2012;83(8):821–7.
45. Johnson RM, Brummett R, Schleuning A. Use of alprazolam for relief of tinnitus. A double-blind study. Arch Otolaryngol Head Neck Surg 1993;119(8):842–5.
46. Jalali MM, Kousha A, Naghavi SE, et al. The effects of alprazolam on tinnitus: a cross-over randomized clinical trial. Med Sci Monit 2009;15(11):PI55–60.
47. Melding PS, Goodey RJ. The treatment of tinnitus with oral anticonvulsants. J Laryngol Otol 1979;93(2):111–22.
48. Tonndorf J. The analogy between tinnitus and pain: a suggestion for a physiological basis of chronic tinnitus. Hear Res 1987;28(2–3):271–5.
49. Moller AR. Similarities between chronic pain and tinnitus. Am J Otol 1997;18(5): 577–85.
50. Loeser JD, Ward AA Jr, White LE Jr. Chronic deafferentation of human spinal cord neurons. J Neurosurg 1968;29(1):48–50.
51. Anderson LS, Black RG, Abraham J, et al. Neuronal hyperactivity in experimental trigeminal deafferentation. J Neurosurg 1971;35(4):444–52.
52. Duckert LG, Rees TS. Treatment of tinnitus with intravenous lidocaine: a double-blind randomized trial. Otolaryngol Head Neck Surg 1983;91(5):550–5.

53. Brozoski TJ, Bauer CA, Caspary DM. Elevated fusiform cell activity in the dorsal cochlear nucleus of chinchillas with psychophysical evidence of tinnitus. J Neurosci 2002;22(6):2383–90.
54. Goljanian Tabrizi A, Safavi Naini A, Baradaran N. Short-term effect of gabapentin on subjective tinnitus in acoustic trauma patients. Iran J Otorhinolaryngol 2017; 29(91):95–100.
55. Bauer CA, Brozoski TJ. Effect of gabapentin on the sensation and impact of tinnitus. Laryngoscope 2006;116(5):675–81.
56. Brozoski T, Odintsov B, Bauer C. Determination of GABA, glutamate and choline in the auditory pathway of animals with tinnitus, using high resolution proton magnetic resonance spectroscopy (1H-MRS). In: Atta-ur-Rahman, Choudhary MI, editors. Applications of NMR spectroscopy. Potomac (MD): Bentham Science Publishers, Bentham Ebook Series/NMR/EOI-03; 2016. p. 77–107.
57. Minen MT, Camprodon J, Nehme R, et al. The neuropsychiatry of tinnitus: a circuit-based approach to the causes and treatments available. J Neurol Neurosurg Psychiatry 2014;85(10):1138–44.
58. Mardini MK. Ear-clicking "tinnitus" responding to carbamazepine. N Engl J Med 1987;317(24):1542.
59. Levine RA. Typewriter tinnitus: a carbamazepine-responsive syndrome related to auditory nerve vascular compression. ORL J Otorhinolaryngol Relat Spec 2006; 68(1):43–6 [discussion: 46–7].
60. Brantberg K. Paroxysmal staccato tinnitus: a carbamazepine responsive hyperactivity dysfunction symptom of the eighth cranial nerve. J Neurol Neurosurg Psychiatry 2010;81(4):451–5.
61. Sunwoo W, Jeon YJ, Bae YJ, et al. Typewriter tinnitus revisited: the typical symptoms and the initial response to carbamazepine are the most reliable diagnostic clues. Sci Rep 2017;7(1):10615.
62. Hoekstra CE, Rynja SP, van Zanten GA, et al. Anticonvulsants for tinnitus. Cochrane Database Syst Rev 2011;(7):CD007960.

Current Device-based Clinical Treatments for Tinnitus

LaGuinn P. Sherlock, AuD[a,b,]*, David J. Eisenman, MD[c]

KEYWORDS

- Sound therapy • Hearing aids • Cochlear implants • Tinnitus treatment devices

KEY POINTS

- Current medical devices for tinnitus are intended to reduce the functional impact of bothersome tinnitus on sleep, concentration, mood, and hearing.
- Sound therapy devices and hearing aids serve to reduce the perceptual strength of the perceived tinnitus signal by offsetting the internal perception of sound with external sound and also reduce neural hyperactivity associated with tinnitus perception.
- Cochlear implants likely work in a manner similar to more conventional sound-based devices, by augmenting external sound perception and modulating neural activity.
- Devices other than hearing aids and cochlear implants are available and give patients more options to choose a device-based treatment compatible with personal preferences, lifestyle, and financial resources.

INTRODUCTION

Tinnitus is the perception of sound in the absence of an external sound source. An estimated 10% of the population has tinnitus, but only a subset of that population has tinnitus bothersome enough to disrupt or disturb sleep, concentration, and/or mood.[1,2] Tinnitus perception itself is not a problem; the problem is the reaction to tinnitus that is associated with these disruptions and disturbances. Reaction to tinnitus results in a cascade of events involving the limbic and autonomic nervous systems, such that the stress response is activated continuously, thereby affecting sleep, concentration, and mood. Many patients are told there is nothing that can be done. This

[a] Army Hearing Program, US Army Public Health Center, Aberdeen, MD, USA; [b] Audiology and Speech Pathology Center, Walter Reed National Military Medical Center, Bethesda, MD, USA; [c] Department of Otorhinolaryngology–Head and Neck Surgery, University of Maryland School of Medicine, 16 South Eutaw Street Suite 500, Baltimore, MD 21201, USA
* Corresponding author. National Military Audiology and Speech Pathology Center, Walter Reed National Military Medical Center, Building 19, Floor 5, 4954 North Palmer Road, Bethesda, MD 20889
E-mail address: laguinnsherlock@gmail.com

Otolaryngol Clin N Am 53 (2020) 627–636
https://doi.org/10.1016/j.otc.2020.03.010
0030-6665/20/© 2020 Elsevier Inc. All rights reserved.

negative counseling exacerbates the reaction and is counterproductive and incorrect. There are many options to reduce the negative reaction to tinnitus and facilitate habituation so that tinnitus no longer significantly affects quality of life.

Counseling therapies have the best evidence for reducing the impact of tinnitus on quality of life,[3] but there are medical devices available to facilitate a reduction in the perception of tinnitus and thus mitigate the reaction to tinnitus. Most patients with tinnitus also have hearing loss; some attribute problems caused by hearing loss to their tinnitus. These patients are particularly good candidates for hearing aids. Other patients have clinically normal hearing and may benefit from ear-level sound therapy. The use of external sound is an integral component of tinnitus management. Sound sources encompass nonmedical devices, such as sound apps on phones, to medical devices such as hearing aids and cochlear implants. The focus of this article is on medical devices that are now in use to help reduce the functional impact of tinnitus.

To date, there is no single therapeutic device that has been shown to universally reduce the perception of tinnitus. A multitude of factors play a role in the successful reduction of tinnitus perception and annoyance, including type of tinnitus (tonal vs noise), duration of tinnitus since onset, comorbidities (eg, anxiety, depression, other health issues), and patient willingness and ability to comply with a given treatment protocol.

CLINICAL PRACTICE GUIDELINE RECOMMENDATIONS FOR DEVICES FOR TINNITUS

The American Academy of Otolaryngology–Head and Neck Surgery published clinical practice guidelines for tinnitus in 2014.[3] Evidence for a series of 13 components of evaluation and management was examined to make evidence-based recommendations. The strength of each recommendation was categorically assigned 1 of 5 ratings (strong recommendation, recommendation, option, recommendation against, or no recommendation). With respect to medical devices available at the time the guidelines were developed, clinicians are advised to recommend a hearing aid evaluation for people with hearing loss and bothersome tinnitus. Clinicians may recommend sound therapy, but the evidence was judged to be insufficient to definitively recommend sound therapy. Cochlear implants and other medical devices were not evaluated as treatment options at the time the guidelines were developed.

INDICATIONS FOR SOUND THERAPY

Patients presenting with bothersome tinnitus may benefit from sound therapy to facilitate habituation. Broadly, sound therapy refers to enrichment of the sound environment. The intent of sound therapy is to reduce the perceptual contrast between the internal noise (tinnitus) and external noise (environmental sound). A candle in a dark room is a popular analogy to describe the role of sound therapy in reducing tinnitus intrusiveness. The lack of other visual stimuli makes the candle more prominent and therefore harder to ignore. When the lights are turned on, the candle is less noticeable and thus easier to ignore. Sound therapy can also be used to induce relaxation or to distract attention from the tinnitus, which helps to reduce the stress response that is activated by bothersome tinnitus. In addition to sound enrichment, avoidance of silence is recommended to facilitate habituation to tinnitus.

Sound enrichment can be accomplished with nonmedical and/or medical devices. Ear-level medical devices for sound enrichment include hearing aids, sound generators, and tinnitus treatment–specific devices. Cochlear implants also provide sound enrichment by directly stimulating auditory neurons to code sound in the brain.

There is a significant body of literature supporting the efficacy of sound enrichment when combined with counseling, but little evidence to support sound enrichment in isolation. Counseling is essential for reducing the negative emotional reactions to tinnitus. Sound enrichment is thought to facilitate a reduction in negative emotional reactions by interfering with the usual perception of tinnitus.

No study to date has compared the efficacy of tinnitus-specific counseling (eg, tinnitus retraining therapy) without device-based sound therapy (DBST) with standard-of-care counseling without DBST. It is therefore difficult to determine the relative influence of DBST on reductions in self-perceived tinnitus handicap. Evidence from a recent randomized double-blind clinical trial indicated that DBST did not result in significantly better outcomes than placebo DBST, but other evidence points to the synergistic benefit of sound therapy combined with counseling.[4,5]

NONMEDICAL DEVICES FOR MANAGEMENT OF TINNITUS

Sound has long been used to reduce the intrusiveness of tinnitus. Different types of sound can be used to achieve the patient's desired objective of distraction and/or relief, and these can be categorized as background, soothing, and interesting.[6] Background sound is any type of sound that is neutral and reduces the perceptual contrast between the internal sound of tinnitus and external environmental sound. Soothing sound is any type of sound that facilitates relaxation and is used to reduce the stress caused by tinnitus and provide relief. In addition, interesting sound is any type of sound that directs attention away from tinnitus by actively engaging attention. Although the objectives may differ, the different types of sounds may overlap in that an interesting sound may also be soothing, or a soothing sound may also be background sound.

Sources of background, soothing, and interesting sounds are environmental sounds, music, and speech. Examples of environmental sounds include fans, water fountains, and bedside sound generators (eg, https://marpac.com/collections/sound-machines). Soothing sounds include music and nonmusic sound apps, which are widely available for streaming through smart phones and external speakers, as well as sound spas. Music can also be used as an interesting sound when the person is actively listening. Interesting sound can be music or speech, such as a television show, a movie, or a podcast.

Sound therapy can be implemented without the use of medical devices and is therefore readily accessible to patients with bothersome tinnitus. Education about the purpose of sound enrichment is essential for successful outcomes and is available online (eg, https://www.ncrar.research.va.gov/Education/Documents/TinnitusDocuments/HowToManageYourTinnitus.pdf; https://medicine.uiowa.edu/oto/research/tinnitus-and-hyperacusis).

MEDICAL DEVICES FOR MANAGEMENT OF TINNITUS

The clinical concept of tinnitus masking using ear-level devices to reduce the intrusiveness of tinnitus has been around since the 1970s.[7] There has been considerable debate regarding the efficacy of total versus partial masking of the tinnitus perception; they have been established as equally effective for acute relief, but long-term efficacy seems to be better with partial masking.[8,9] The efficacy of sound therapy, as previously mentioned, has not been well established when studied at the population level.[4] Nonetheless, DBST is currently used and, anecdotally, patients report subjective benefit attributed to relief provided by an external sound that is less bothersome than the internal sound of tinnitus.

The plasticity of the central auditory system has been observed in both animals and humans and is the basis for using sound therapy.[10–12] The functional impact of reduced auditory input secondary to hearing loss is compensatory hyperactivity that may be perceived as tinnitus.[13] Animal models and functional imaging suggest that sound therapy reduces central auditory system hyperactivity to counteract the presumed maladaptive changes associated with the perception of tinnitus.[12,14–16]

Sound Generators

Ear-level sound generators, also referred to as tinnitus maskers, have been commercially available since 1976. The devices were initially referred to as tinnitus maskers because the original intent was to mask the tinnitus. They are more commonly referred to as sound generators now to achieve either total or partial masking of the tinnitus. Early versions produced broadband noise delivered to the ear via nonoccluding earmolds; manipulation of the broadband noise is available in current versions. Standalone ear-level sound generators are available (eg, https://generalhearing.com; https://solacefortinnitus.net/) at a lower cost than hearing aids. Recommended use time is at least 8 h/d but there are no studies of sound generator efficacy as a function of use time.

Devices combining amplification and sound generators were introduced to the market in the early 1990s and have grown in popularity since that time.

Hearing Aids

It has been well established that many patients with tinnitus attribute hearing difficulty to the presence of tinnitus, rather than the reverse.[17–19] Because most patients with tinnitus have some measurable degree of hearing loss, amplification is an appropriate intervention. Hearing aids providing prescribed amplification improve audibility, reducing the strain to hear. They amplify ambient sound, reducing exposure to excessively quiet environments (which tend to make tinnitus more audible) and provide natural sound therapy. Physiologically, compensation for peripheral loss of hearing may decrease the central gain associated with the tinnitus percept.[20]

Although the evidence overwhelmingly points to the efficacy and value of counseling in reducing the functional impact of tinnitus, hearing aid use has been validated as a contributing factor to reducing tinnitus distress,[21–25] and has been shown to reduce tinnitus annoyance without counseling.[26,27]

All of the major hearing aid manufacturers incorporate some form of sound therapy in their hearing aids, which can be used in isolation or combined with amplification. Sound options include broadband noise that can be customized by shaping the frequency response and modulation of the noise and fractal tones. Henry and colleagues[28] examined the validity of combination devices relative to amplification alone for reducing the functional impact of tinnitus as measured by the Tinnitus Functional Index and found that both resulted in a significant decline in subjective tinnitus handicap.

Notch Therapy

Notch therapy is based on the premise that decreasing external stimulation in the frequency region of the tinnitus may decrease hyperactivity in the corresponding regions of the central auditory system, thereby diminishing the perception of tinnitus. Tailor-made notched music training (TMNMT) has been shown to reduce tinnitus loudness[29] and is available online (https://www.audionotch.com/). TMNMT requires dedication to daily listening, which is disruptive to the normal daily routine for some patients.

An alternative to TMNMT is notched amplification, available from one of the hearing aid manufacturers (https://pro.signiausa.com). The advantage of notch therapy in hearing aids is the easy implementation of the therapy, combined with amplification to facilitate ease of listening. Study results provide evidence of greater subjective and objective improvements in tinnitus distress with notch therapy compared with traditional amplification.[30] Candidacy for this option is limited to patients with tonal tinnitus that is pitch-matched at less than 8000 Hz.

Other Medical Devices for Tinnitus Management

The use of music to reduce stress has been studied extensively, across medical and mental health care.[31] A novel device-based approach to tinnitus treatment using music was introduced in the United States in 2006 (http://neuromonics.com). Neuromonics Tinnitus Treatment (NTT) uses spectrally modified music customized to the patient's hearing loss to retrain the neural pathways. Recommended use time is 2 to 4 h/d for a minimum of 6 months. Nonrandomized, uncontrolled clinical trials have revealed significant declines in tinnitus intrusiveness.[32] The therapeutic sound is currently available for use through a patient's iPhone or iPad, under the direction of an audiologist. Recommended use time is substantially less than that for sound generators, but dedicated use time is required.

Newman and Sandridge[33] compared benefit and economic value between sound generators and NTT from a sample of clinical patients. Reductions in self-perceived tinnitus handicap were comparable. The sound generators were the more cost-effective alternative, but the investigators pointed out that patient preference variables (eg, lifestyle, acceptability of passive sound generator use vs active NTT use, and sound preference for broadband noise vs NTT music) are important considerations for individual management.

One medical device uses sound that mimics the patient's tinnitus to decrease tinnitus perception and is used while the patient is sleeping (https://otoharmonics.com). The device uses proprietary software, loaded onto an Apple iPad Air. A tinnitus sound print is created based on the patient's tinnitus pitch match. The sound print is loaded onto an Apple iPod touch and the patient is directed to use the device for 3 months, every night while sleeping. Sound is delivered to the ears via flexible ear buds and the patient adjusts the volume each night to match the volume of the tinnitus. The system incorporates the Tinnitus Functional Index to monitor the functional impact of tinnitus over time.

There is limited evidence to support the efficacy of this system, but a randomized controlled trial showed greater average reduction in the self-perceived functional impact of tinnitus as measured by the Tinnitus Functional Index and subjective tinnitus loudness for study participants using the device (sound print or broadband noise) compared with a bedside sound generator over a 3-month period.[34]

Cochlear Implants

Evidence from the earliest days of cochlear implantation has shown that most cochlear implant candidates have tinnitus, and, for many, tinnitus perception decreases following surgery and/or with use of their implants. Brackmann[35] reported that 80% (40 out of 50) of patients implanted with a House monopolar cochlear implant had varying degrees of preoperative tinnitus, and that, out of 29 of these 40 for whom data were available, 27% reported elimination and 52% reduction of tinnitus in the operated ear. A review of the literature from 1990 to 2006 revealed an incidence of tinnitus in cochlear implant candidates ranging from 65% to 100%, with a mean of 80%, although the percentage of those with bothersome tinnitus was unclear from the data.[36] Furthermore, most of the studies cited in the review showed a reduction in or elimination of tinnitus in the operated ear with monaural implantation. Another review showed many studies reporting contralateral tinnitus suppression as well.[37] A recent study, with newer generation devices, showed elimination of tinnitus and a decrease in tinnitus handicap in 28% of patients, with an estimated 75% of patients having some reduction in their symptoms.[38] Variables potentially affecting tinnitus outcomes are not known, and it is unclear what effect hearing preservation, electroacoustic stimulation, and bimodal stimulation would have on tinnitus. In addition, it has been shown that optimal stimulation parameters for hearing may not be the same as those for tinnitus suppression, and also that imperceptible electrical stimulation can suppress tinnitus. This finding implies that the benefit is not simply from enhanced sound perception but also from direct neuromodulation.[39,40] There have been analogous findings in hearing aid programming for tinnitus suppression.[41] For those patients in whom use of the cochlear implant itself does not provide sufficient tinnitus relief, sound therapy through a cochlear implant is potentially beneficial.[42]

Although these data are encouraging, cochlear implantation is still not indicated or considered the standard of care specifically for purposes of tinnitus treatment in patients who are not otherwise candidates for the procedure. However, where these data have become more relevant is in treatment of patients with single-sided deafness (SSD). Several studies over more than a decade have shown a significant decrease in tinnitus handicap in most patients with SSD undergoing cochlear implantation.[43–46] In this population, it is conceivable that implantation would be undertaken if not solely then at least more so, or even primarily, for purposes of tinnitus reduction in place of different hearing rehabilitation options such as Contralateral Routing of Signal (CROS), Bilateral Contralateral Routing of Signal (BiCROS), or implantable bone conduction devices.

Other, non–sound-based devices have been used or trialed for purposes of tinnitus reduction, but none has achieved universal recognition or become standard of care. These devices include repetitive transcranial magnetic stimulation,[47] direct auditory cortex stimulation,[48] and direct cochlear nerve stimulation.[49] None of these has been shown to be consistently beneficial over a sufficiently wide range of patients.

WILLINGNESS TO ACCEPT AND PAY

It is important for patients with bothersome tinnitus to have realistic expectations about tinnitus management using medical devices. Most, if not all, patients with tinnitus are seeking a solution that completely eliminates tinnitus perception. However, such a solution does not exist at this time for most patients with tinnitus.

A significant factor to consider regarding clinical device-based therapy is financial cost because the cost may present a potential barrier to willingness and/or ability to pursue a given device-based treatment option. Tinnitus-specific devices are generally not covered by insurance; out-of-pocket costs can reach more than $4000. Hearing aids with features such as notch therapy, sound therapy, and frequency lowering may be partially covered by insurance, but patients are likely to bear at least some of the cost, in the range of $2000 to $4000. Invasive devices such as cochlear implants are usually fully covered by insurance but involve surgical risk.

The individual's lifestyle and tinnitus symptoms are additional factors to consider. Commercially available medical devices for tinnitus management differ in the type and implementation of stimulation. Patient preference, psychosocial factors, tinnitus self-efficacy, and clinician expertise play a significant role in the successful management of tinnitus.[50] As such, a patient-centered approach that takes into consideration all of these factors has the greatest likelihood of resulting in a favorable outcome. In particular, tinnitus self-efficacy, which refers to the patients' confidence in their ability to perform specific skills (eg, use hearing aids or sound generators) to achieve a specific goal (ie, habituation to tinnitus), is central.[51]

Tyler[52] surveyed a large group of tinnitus self-help group attendees to determine what kinds of treatment and what costs people with tinnitus are willing to accept. The survey considered these 2 factors against 2 possible outcomes: reduction of tinnitus by half (eg, reducing perceived loudness and annoyance by half) and complete elimination of tinnitus. The survey revealed that noninvasive devices are more acceptable than invasive devices regardless of partial versus complete elimination. Most patients surveyed indicated willingness to spend $1000 to reduce tinnitus by half; most shifted to a willingness to spend $5000 to completely eliminate reduce tinnitus. Correlations between subjective ratings of loudness and annoyance were positive with the likelihood of using any type of treatment, but were not correlated with the amount participants were willing to pay. Individual financial circumstances and acceptance of risk influence willingness to pay for medical devices.

SUMMARY

In summary, current device-based clinical treatments for tinnitus encompass sound generators, hearing aids, cochlear implants, and tinnitus treatment devices. The primary indication for device use is tinnitus that is bothersome to the point of disrupting sleep and/or concentration, perceived as causing difficulty with hearing, and/or causing or increasing anxiety and/or depression. Devices vary in prescribed use time, application of sound, risk to patient, and cost. It is important to be aware that patients can experience significant reductions in self-perceived tinnitus handicap during and after DBST.

DISCLAIMER

The identification of specific products or scientific instrumentation is considered an integral part of the scientific endeavor and does not constitute endorsement, or implied endorsement, on the part of the author, Department of Defense, or any component agency. The views expressed in this article are those of the authors and do not reflect the official policy of the Department of Army/Navy/Air Force, Department of Defense, or US Government.

DISCLOSURE

The authors have nothing to disclose.

REFERENCES

1. Bhatt JM, Lin HW, Bhattacharyya N. Prevalence, severity, exposures, and treatment patterns of tinnitus in the United States. JAMA Otolaryngol Head Neck Surg 2016;142:959–65.
2. Shargorodsky J, Curhan GC, Farwell WR. Prevalence and characteristics of tinnitus among US adults. Am J Med 2010;123:711–8.
3. Tunkel DE, Bauer CA, Sun GH, et al. Clinical practice guidelines: tinnitus. Otolaryngol Head Neck Surg 2014;151:S1–40.
4. Tinnitus Retraining Therapy Trial Research Group, Scherer RW, Formby C. Effect of tinnitus retraining therapy vs. standard of care on tinnitus-related quality of life:

a randomized clinical trial. JAMA Otolaryngol Head Neck Surg 2019;145: 597–608.

5. Bauer CA, Brozoski TJ. Effect of tinnitus retraining therapy on the loudness and annoyance of tinnitus: a controlled trial. Ear Hear 2011;32:145–55.

6. Henry JA, Zaugg TL, Myers PJ, et al. Using therapeutic sound with progressive audiologic tinnitus management. Trends Amplif 2008;12:188–209.

7. Vernon J. The use of masking for relief of tinnitus. In: Silverstein H, Norrell H, editors. Neurological surgery of the ear volume II. Birmingham (England): Aesculapius Publishing; 1976. p. 104–18.

8. Henry JA, Schechter MA, Zaugg TL, et al. Clinical trial to compare tinnitus masking and tinnitus retraining therapy. Acta Otolaryngol Suppl 2006;556:649.

9. Tyler RS, Noble W, Coelho CB, et al. Tinnitus retraining therapy: mixing point and total masking are equally effective. Ear Hear 2012;33:588–94.

10. Engineer ND, Riley JR, Seale JD, et al. Reversing pathological neural activity using targeted plasticity. Nature 2011;470:101–4.

11. Yang S, Weiner BD, Zhang LS, et al. Homeostatic plasticity drives tinnitus perception in an animal model. Proc Natl Acad Sci U S A 2011;108:14974–9.

12. Shore SE, Roberts LE, Langguth B. Maladaptive plasticity in tinnitus – triggers, mechanisms and treatment. Nat Rev Neurol 2016;12:150–60.

13. Eggermont JJ. Neural substrates of tinnitus in animal and human cortex. HNO 2015;63:298–301.

14. Norena AJ, Eggermont JJ. Enriched acoustic environment after noise trauma abolishes neural signs of tinnitus. Neuroreport 2006;17:559–63.

15. Saunders JC. The role of central nervous system plasticity in tinnitus. J Commun Disord 2007;40:313–34.

16. Sedley W. Does gain explain? Neuroscience 2019;407:213–28.

17. Ratnayake SA, Jayarajan V, Bartlett J. Could an underlying hearing loss be a significant factor in the handicap caused by tinnitus? Noise Health 2009;111: 156–60.

18. Newman CW, Sandridge SA, Jacobson GP. Assessing outcomes of tinnitus intervention. J Am Acad Audiol 2014;25:76–105.

19. Henry JA, Griest S, Zaugg T, et al. Tinnitus and hearing survey: a screening tool to differentiate bothersome tinnitus from hearing difficulties. Am J Audiol 2015;24: 66–77.

20. Formby C, Gold S, Keaser M, et al. Secondary benefits from tinnitus retraining therapy: clinically significant increases in loudness discomfort level and expansion of the auditory dynamic range. Semin Hear 2007;28:227–60.

21. Henry JA, McMillan G, Dann S, et al. Tinnitus management: randomized controlled trial comparing extended-wear hearing aids, conventional hearing aids, and combination instruments. J Am Acad Audiol 2017;28:546–61.

22. Kochkin S, Tyler R. Tinnitus treatment and the effectiveness of hearing aids: hearing care professional perceptions. Hear Rev 2008;15:14–8.

23. Searchfield GD, Kaur M, Martin WH. Hearing aids as an adjunct to counseling: tinnitus patients who choose amplification do better than those that don't. Int J Audiol 2010;49:574–9.

24. Kochkin S, Tyler R, Born J. MarkeTrak VIII: the prevalence of tinnitus in the United States and the self-reported efficacy of various treatments. Hear Rev 2008;18: 10–27.

25. Shekhawat GS, Searchfield GD, Stinear CM. Role of hearing aids in tinnitus intervention: a scoping review. J Am Acad Audiol 2013;24:747–62.

26. Surr RK, Montgomery AA, Mueller HG. Effect of amplification on tinnitus among new hearing aid users. Ear Hear 1985;6:71–5.

27. Yakunina N, Lee WH, Ryu Y-J, et al. Tinnitus suppression effect of hearing aids in patients with high-frequency hearing loss: a randomized double-blind controlled trial. Otol Neurotol 2019;40:865–71.

28. Henry JA, Frederick M, Sell S, et al. Validation of a novel combination hearing aid and tinnitus therapy device. Ear Hear 2015;36:42–52.

29. Okamoto H, Stracke H, Stoll W, et al. Listening to tailor-made notched music reduces tinnitus loudness and tinnitus-related auditory cortex activity. Proc Natl Acad Sci U S A 2010;107:1207–10.

30. Haab L, Lehser C, Corona-Strauss FI, et al. Implementation and long-term evaluation of a hearing aid supported tinnitus treatment using notched environmental sounds. IEEE J Transl Eng Health Med 2019;7:1–9.

31. De Witte M, Spruit A, van Hooren S, et al. Effects of music interventions on stress-related outcomes: a systematic review and two meta-analyses. Health Psychol Rev 2019. https://doi.org/10.1080/17437199.2019.1627897.

32. Davis PB, Paki B, Hanley PJ. Neuromonics tinnitus treatment: third clinical trial. Ear Hear 2007;28:242–59.

33. Newman CW, Sandridge SA. A comparison of benefit and economic value between two sound therapy tinnitus management options. J Am Acad Audiol 2012;23:126–38.

34. Theodoroff SM, McMillan GP, Zaugg TL, et al. Randomized controlled trial of a novel device for tinnitus sound therapy during sleep. Am J Audiol 2007;26:543–54.

35. Brackmann DE. Reduction of tinnitus in cochlear-implant patients. J Laryngol Otol Suppl 1981;(4):163–5.

36. Baguley DM, Atlas MD. Cochlear implants and tinnitus. Prog Brain Res 2007;166:347–55.

37. Quaranta N, Wagstaff S, Baguley DM. Tinnitus and cochlear implantation. Int J Audiol 2004;43:245–51.

38. Kloostra FJJ, Verbist J, Hofman R, et al. A prospective study of the effect of cochlear implantation on tinnitus. Audiol Neurootol 2018;23(6):356–63.

39. McKerrow WS, Schreiner CE, Snyder RL, et al. Tinnitus suppression by cochlear implants. Ann Otol Rhinol Laryngol 1991;100:552–8.

40. Rubinstein JT, Tyler RS, Johnson A, et al. Electrical suppression of tinnitus with high-rate pulse trains. Otol Neurotol 2003;24:478–85.

41. Searchfield GD. Hearing aids and tinnitus. In: Tyler RS, editor. Tinnitus treatment: clinical protocols. New York: Thieme; 2005. p. 161–75.

42. Tyler RS, Owen RL, Bridges J, et al. Tinnitus suppression in cochlear implant patients using a sound therapy app. Am J Audiol 2018;27:316–23.

43. Häußler SM, Knopke S, Dudka S, et al. Improvement in tinnitus distress, health-related quality of life and psychological comorbidities by cochlear implantation in single-sided deaf patients. HNO 2019;67(11):863–73.

44. Holder JT, O'Connell B, Hedley-Williams A, et al. Cochlear implantation for single-sided deafness and tinnitus suppression. Am J Otolaryngol 2017;38:226–9.

45. Sladen DP, Frisch CD, Carlson ML, et al. Cochlear implantation for single-sided deafness: a multicenter study. Laryngoscope 2017;127:223–8.

46. Van de Heyning P, Vermeire K, Diebl M, et al. Incapacitating unilateral tinnitus in single-sided deafness treated by cochlear implantation. Ann Otol Rhinol Laryngol 2008;117:645–52.

47. Londero A, Bonfils P, Lefaucheur JP. Transcranial magnetic stimulation and subjective tinnitus. A review of the literature, 2014-2016. Eur Ann Otorhinolaryngol Head Neck Dis 2018;135:51–8.

48. Zhang J. Auditory cortex stimulation to suppress tinnitus: mechanisms and strategies. Hear Res 2013;295:38–57.

49. van den Berge MJ, van Dijk JM, Free RH, et al. Effect of direct stimulation of the cochleovestibular nerve on tinnitus: A long-term follow-up study. World Neurosurg 2017;98:571–7.

50. Searchfield GD, Durai M, Linford T. A state-of-the-art review: personalization of tinnitus sound therapy. Front Psychol 2017;8:1599.

51. Smith SL, Fagelson M. Development of the self-efficacy for tinnitus management questionnaire. J Am Acad Audiol 2011;22:424–40.

52. Tyler RS. Patient preferences and willingness to pay for tinnitus treatments. J Am Acad Audiol 2012;23:115–25.

Alternative Treatments of Tinnitus: Alternative Medicine

Friederike S. Luetzenberg, BS[f], Seilesh Babu, MD[g,h,i],
Michael D. Seidman, MD[a,b,c,d,e],*

KEYWORDS

- Tinnitus • Alternative medicine • Treatment

KEY POINTS

- Trials investigating acupuncture, herbs, vitamins, trace elements, melatonin, hypnosis, and others continue to present contradictory findings on the benefit in tinnitus treatment, yet many exhibit positive results.
- Because of the scarcity of well-designed studies and subsequent inconclusiveness of literature reviews, physicians remain skeptic of alternative treatment options that have been used in Eastern medicine for centuries.
- Based on study results, alternative treatments discussed should undergo trial periods for each tinnitus patient, as a treatment may not work for every patient alike.

INTRODUCTION

Tinnitus—the perception of sound in the ear or head in the absence of an external stimulus—is a symptom that approximately 10% to 15% of the world population suffer chronically and a burden to a patient's quality of life for which there is currently no universal cure.[1] Although alternative treatment options for tinnitus have not been recommended by the clinical practice guidelines published by the American Academy of Otolaryngology—Head and Neck Surgery,[2] many patients are dissatisfied with the results achieved by conventional medicine and open to a complementary-integrative

[a] Otologic/Neurotologic/Skull Base Surgery; [b] Wellness and Integrative Medicine; [c] Advent Health (Celebration and South Campuses); [d] Otolaryngology Head and Neck Surgery, University of Central Florida College of Medicine; [e] AdventHealth Medical Group- Otolaryngology-Head and Neck Surgery, 410Celebration Place Suite 305, Celebration, FL 34747, USA; [f] University of Central Florida College of Medicine, 6850 Lake Nona Boulevard, Orlando, FL 32827, USA; [g] Department of Otology, Neurotology, & Skull Base Surgery, Michigan Ear Institute, Farmington Hills, MI 48334, USA; [h] Ascension Macomb Otolaryngology Residency, 11800 East 12 Mile Road, Warren, MI 48093, USA; [i] Department of Otolaryngology, Wayne State University, Detroit, MI, USA
* Corresponding author. AdventHealth Medical Group- Otolaryngology-Head and Neck Surgery, 410 Celebration Place Suite 305, Celebration, FL34747.
E-mail address: Michael.seidman.md@adventhealth.com

Otolaryngol Clin N Am 53 (2020) 637–650
https://doi.org/10.1016/j.otc.2020.03.011
0030-6665/20/© 2020 Elsevier Inc. All rights reserved.

medical approach. In fact, some treatments such as acupuncture and herbal medicines have been used in Eastern cultures for centuries. Because of the lack of well-designed studies, however, Western physicians' skepticism persists. Yet it is important to acknowledge that no 2 patients are alike and what might benefit one person might not be of help for another. Instead of saying "you will have to live with it," we should listen to our patients and their preferences; we should consider all available options until we find a treatment that may be of benefit for that unique patient. In terms of alternative treatments, the following topics have yielded research, which, although not conclusive, can help provide viable treatment options that are noninvasive and generally speaking well tolerated.

ACUPUNCTURE

Acupuncture is a deeply seeded component of traditional Chinese medicine and has been used with the goal to rebalance action potentials of neurophysiological systems for centuries.[3,4] As such, acupuncture has been used in the treatment of tinnitus to influence the olivocochlear nucleus.[5] Although multiple studies have evaluated the effectiveness of acupuncture on tinnitus symptoms, the conclusions drawn by systematic reviews remain uncertain. Reviews cite the methodological flaws, sample size, and the bias of Chinese studies toward positive results as main critiques to decrease the studies'validity[3,4]; the differences concerning the number of treatment sessions and placement of acupoints and their effectiveness, unfortunately, were discussed to a lesser degree and deserve greater attention in future reviews. Studies conducting a single treatment session were less likely to report a statistically significant effect[6,7] than studies holding at least 10 acupuncture sessions.[8-10] This was confirmed by Lin and colleagues,[11] who analyzed various factors pertaining to patient demographics, tinnitus characteristics, and treatment and concluded that only the combination of acupoints and number of treatment sessions was statistically related to a better treatment outcome. Based on this review, a minimum of 17 to 24 acupuncture sessions should be the recommendation before determining if acupuncture is a valid treatment option for a particular patient. This being said, in the Center for Integrative Medicine started at Henry Ford Health System by MDS, they would provide 6 treatments over a 6-week time period and if the patient did not experience any improvement they were advised to discontinue. Specific acupoints seem to be an important component in improved tinnitus control. One of these points was shown to be along the vestibulocochlear line as laid out in Chinese scalp acupuncture (**Fig. 1**).[8] The study showed statistically significant improvements using validated tinnitus measures, such as visual analogue scale (VAS) and Tinnitus Handicap Inventory (THI) when compared with baseline and the control group.[8] Although the VAS assesses a patient's tinnitus severity based on pictures, the THI evaluates a patient's quality-of-life handicap through a series of questions regarding the patient's reactions to tinnitus in terms of emotional (eg, anger), functional (eg, difficulties concentrating), and catastrophic (eg,feelings of hopelessness) reactions.[12] No study reported any adverse effects of the treatment modality.

Furthermore, acupuncture has been evaluated for the possibility of affecting cochlear blood flow, which has been implicated as one of the etiologic contributors of tinnitus. Using infrared thermography, Cai and colleagues[7] suggested that a single acupuncture session could stabilize the capillary cochlear blood flow bilaterally, even if acupuncture was only applied on one side. Similarly, assessing cochlear neuronal activity using otoacoustic emissions (OAE) exhibited that acupuncture significantly increased the amplitude of OAE in both the needled and unneedled ears as compared

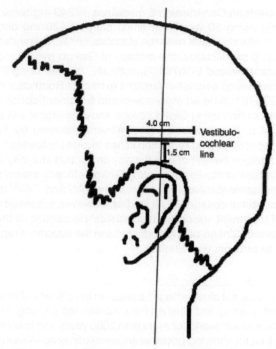

Fig. 1. Vestibulocochlear line according to Chinese scalp acupuncture. Effectiveness of acupuncture therapy as treatment of tinnitus: a randomized controlled trial. (*From* Doi MY, Tano SS, Schultz AR, Borges R, Marchiori LL. Effectiveness of acupuncture therapy as treatment for tinnitus: a randomized controlled trial. Braz J Otorhinolaryngol. 2016;82(4):458-465. https://doi.org/10.1016/j.bjorl.2016.04.002; with permission.)

with the control group, suggesting an effect of acupuncture on cochlear hair cells.[13] Unfortunately, most studies did not identify the form of tinnitus being treated, which may inadvertently affect the rate of success. Nonetheless, acupuncture seems to be a valid treatment option to offer patients suffering for tinnitus, given a sufficient number of treatment sessions.

HERBS
Ginkgo Biloba

The leaves of the ancient Chinese Ginkgo biloba tree have been used as health-enhancing remedies for thousands of years. Today, the herbal supplement is among the 5 most popular medications in the Western world and even licensed to treat cerebrovascular insufficiency in Germany.[14,15] Based on the German Commission E monograph, purified Ginkgo preparations, called EGb761, must contain certain percentages of flavonoids, proanthocyanidins, and terpenoids.[15] In the treatment of tinnitus, Ginkgo biloba has gained appreciable traction through a substantial number of studies assessing its efficacy and safety. Although many findings contradict each other, systematic reviews generally consider Ginkgo as a potential treatment option.[16,17]

Studies failing to detect superiority of Ginkgo biloba, as compared with a placebo group, may have used methodologically different protocols from studies concluding statistical significance. Considering that the recommended dosage of Ginkgo for tinnitus, based on German Commission E guidelines, is 240 mg twice daily,[18] it is not surprising that trials using 50 mg three times daily or 120 mg once daily do not conclude the herb's effectiveness over the placebo.[14,19] A review determined that in studies demonstrating significance, the efficacy of Ginkgo over placebo was related to the use of the standardized EGb761. Specifically, studies using EGb761 showed benefit versus studies using a nonstandardized extract.[20] Boetticher concluded standardized Ginkgo EGb761 to be an evidence-based treatment option for tinnitus.[20]

Another treatment option using Ginkgo biloba showing efficacy in the treatment of tinnitus consisted of a Ginkgo infusion pretreatment, followed by 12 weeks of oral Ginkgo.[21] This protocol displayed reduction in hearing loss following the infusion therapy, as well as an additive benefit of oral therapy on tinnitus intensity at the end of the trial.[21] One potential flaw of studies evaluating Ginkgo efficacy seems to be the lack of use of validated assessment measures, such as the VAS and THI,[22] and the only one that did, chose suboptimal dosages.[19] All studies, however, assessed the most important component of treatment success—the patients' perception of their own tinnitus. Based on this evidence, Ginkgo biloba ought to be in the treatment repertoire of a physician's approach to patients with tinnitus.

Other Herbs

Besides Ginkgo, more recent studies began assessing the efficacy of other herbal supplements, including red ginseng and Gushen Pian. Korean red ginseng, much like Ginkgo, has been used in the Eastern world for more than 2000 years and is known for antioxidative property as well as for showing potential antiapoptotic properties in an experimental model for cisplatinototoxicity.[23,24] Kim and colleagues[23] compared 3000 mg daily of red ginseng with 1500 mg of red ginseng with 80 mg twice daily of Ginkgo, assessing patients after 4 weeks of treatment using THI, VAS, and short-form 36 (SF-36). Ginkgo and low dose of red ginseng (1500 mg) did not demonstrate any improvement in THI, VAS, and SF-36 in this study. Patients given high-dose red ginseng had statistically significant improvement in their THI score compared with the Ginkgo group.

Gushen Pian, on the other hand, is a newly developed Chinese herbal medicine, which is being investigated for the treatment of sensorineural deafness and tinnitus.[25] Gushen Pian is a combination medicine consisting of Drynaria fortunei, Danshen, glycyrrhiza, and Calcined Ci Shi, which are said to "ventilate the ear"—or increase its blood circulation—increase overall circulation, balance herbal attributes, and decrease liver overactivity and strengthen bone, respectively.[25] Drynariafortunei by itself has also been shown to have protective properties against streptomycin-induced ototoxicity.[26] These herbs and the combination thereof are, according to traditional Chinese medicine, believed to alleviate tinnitus and sensorineural deafness by improving splenonephric perfusion, as it is believed that symptoms such as tinnitus are signals from the body indicating that the kidney's energy needs more support (the kidney is said to regulate the ear).[25,26] In its first trial, Gushen Pian displayed statistically significant therapeutic outcomes over placebo after 4 weeks of treatment in terms of tinnitus, dizziness, aural fullness, insomnia, and pure tone audiometry.[25] Thus, even though there is a long way to go to determine whether herbal medicines such as red ginseng and Gushen Pian could contribute meaningfully to the management of tinnitus, their initial results seem promising.

TRACE ELEMENTS
Zinc

Zinc can be found throughout the entire human body and participates in the function of more than 300 enzymes as well as several essential growth and maturation processes.[27-29] Animal studies have shown that the inner ear has the highest zinc content in a guinea pig,[30] which leads to the potential implication of inadequate levels of zinc in functional otologic disorders, such as tinnitus. Although studies have demonstrated a correlation between low zinc levels and tinnitus, the effects of zinc supplementation on tinnitus in general remain an item of debate.[31,32] A Cochrane review examining 3 studies found no improvements in tinnitus after supplementing with 50 to 66 mg zinc for 8 to 16 weeks.[33] Studies now, however, seem to be recognizing that treatments with zinc might have greater impacts on specific patient groups. First, zinc levels seem to decrease as age increases, potentially due to decreased oral intake and intestinal absorption, playing into the positive correlation of tinnitus and age.[34,35] In these older patients specifically, Yetiser and colleagues[28] reported 82% of elder patients indicating a better score following zinc supplementation for 8 weeks. Second, a large population including 2225 participants, among which 460 people suffered from tinnitus, concluded that serum zinc levels were only significantly lower in patients with extreme tinnitus.[36] Similarly, the fact that tinnitus loudness was significantly higher in patients with hypozincemia was determined by 2 additional studies.[30,34] Furthermore, Ochi and colleagues[30] found that particularly patients with tinnitus and normal hearing had significantly lower levels of zinc than healthy controls, as compared with patients with tinnitus and hearing loss who showed no significant difference in zinc levels to healthy controls. This is not to say that tinnitus patients with hearing loss might not benefit from zinc supplementation. On the contrary, 85% of patients participating in a trial on noise-induced hearing loss (NIHL)-associated tinnitus reported a statistically significant improvement in THI—emotional and catastrophic, but not functional—scores following 2 months of 40 mg zinc daily.[37] Although zinc supplementation was well tolerated in these studies, it needs to be noted that at a dose of 200 mg per day acute zinc toxicity may occur. Overall, despite an ongoing debate concerning the efficacy of zinc supplementation, studies are reporting some beneficial implementations of zinc, making a trial of this treatment option with appropriate dosing worthwhile.

Other Elements

Although zinc is the most commonly discussed trace element in terms of tinnitus cause and treatment, some investigators are turning their attention to other elements as well. Copper and zinc frequently act together as an enzyme called copper-zinc superoxide dismutase, which might lead to the consideration that in zinc-requiring processes, copper may be implicated as well.[38] Yasar and colleagues[38] measured the serum and hair levels of copper, zinc, and lead of 80 tinnitus patients compared with controls. Only serum copper was statistically significantly lower in the tinnitus group, with no statistically significant differences in the zinc or lead groups compared with controls. This could suggest another trace element that may be implicated in tinnitus. Unfortunately, copper and zinc compete during intestinal absorption, with the sole supplementation of one leading to a potential deficit of the other. Anecdotally, calcium and manganese may also reduce the symptoms of tinnitus after several months of supplementation.[27]

ANTIOXIDANT SUPPLEMENTS
B Vitamins

B-complex vitamins are necessary for the proper functioning of a healthy central nervous system, such as proper methylation relying on vitamin B12. Deficiencies in B vitamins may, therefore, lead to neuronal dysfunctions, followed by cochlear dysfunction and finally hearing loss and tinnitus.[27,39] A deficiency of vitamin B12 could furthermore result in an increase of oxygen and nitrogen free radicals due to the B12-dependent activity of methionine synthase.[40] Oxygen-free radicals, in turn, have been connected to age-related and noise-induced hearing loss through the loss of mitochondrial membrane potentials and cochlear hair cells.[41] B vitamins are thus a target of research in the potential treatment of tinnitus.

Shemesh and colleagues[42] first reported a significantly higher prevalence (47%) of vitamin B12 deficiency (<250 pg/mL) in patients with NIHL and tinnitus than in patients with NIHL alone or in controls, with some patients showing tinnitus symptom improvement following replacement therapy. Another study, however, found no significant difference in the prevalence of B12 deficiency (<180 pg/mL) between tinnitus patients and healthy controls, and although 8 patients reported some improvement after treatment, the difference was not significant.[43] In a more recent randomized, double-blind study, patients with chronic tinnitus were injected with 2500 mcg vitamin B12 weekly for 6 weeks. B12 deficiency was considered at less than 250 pg/mL,[39] and the prevalence of deficiency was similar to that found in Shemesh and colleagues' study (42.5%). Following vitamin B12 injections, initial B12-deficient tinnitus patients showed significant improvements in VAS and tinnitus severity index scores.[39] Thus, vitamin B12 may play a therapeutic role in patients with B12 deficiency, given a cutoff level of less than 250 pg/mL.

In addition, a Korean population survey of 1435 participants with tinnitus compared with 6186 without reported a significantly reduced intake and independent association of vitamin B2 with tinnitus.[44] Reduced intake of vitamin B3 was only associated with tinnitus annoyance in patients older than 66 years.[44] This contributes to the possibility that multiple B vitamins could be beneficial in the treatment of tinnitus. As such, a study administering vitamin B complex found a significant increase in OAE in patients with tinnitus.[45]

Other Antioxidants

As the thought of reactive oxygen species contributing to tinnitus continues, Ekinci and Kamaska actually determined that the total oxidant status and mean oxidative stress index were significantly higher in a group of patients with tinnitus compared with controls, supporting the therapeutic use of antioxidants.[46] Besides B vitamins, oral antioxidant therapy consisting of glycerophosphorylcholine, glycerophosphorylethanolamine, β-carotene, and vitamins C and E for 18 weeks showed a significant improvement in VAS and tinnitus loudness in patients with idiopathic tinnitus.[47] A more selective antioxidant therapy for 6 months, consisting of either α-lipoic acid and vitamin C or papaverine hydrochloride and vitamin E, however, resulted in no appreciable benefit for patients complaining of tinnitus associated with sensorineural hearing loss.[48] Lastly, the antioxidant coenzyme Q10 (CoQ10), which influences mitochondrial electron transport, has also been associated with a potential impact on tinnitus. A study showed that in patients with an initially low serum level of CoQ10, 12 weeks of 300 mg CoQ10 daily significantly improved their Tinnitus Questionnaire (TQ) and SF-36 scores.[49] Thus, although there is paucity of studies on the effect of various antioxidants on tinnitus, some patients may benefit from trial of supplementation with certain antioxidants.

CONSIDERATIONS OF TREATMENT COMPOSITION

Before administering the various herbs and supplements mentioned earlier, however, physicians need to consider differences in preparation of each treatment, so that patients can experience the greatest benefit possible. As such, some brands of Ginkgo supplements are, despite standardized compositions of 24% Gingko flavones and 6% terpenes, not highly purified and, as discussed, will not have the desired effect. Furthermore, minerals are most commonly supplied in their sulfate and carbonate form, which have significantly reduced absorption compared with minerals that are chelated or linked to an amino acid. Thus, zinc sulfate is significantly less absorbed than zinc monomethionate, and calcium carbonate is much less well absorbed compared with calcium glycinate. Similarly, the ubiquinone type of CoQ10 is much less absorbed than its ubiquinol type. Thus, it is important to remember that not all treatment preparations are created equal.

MELATONIN

Melatonin involved in sleep-wake cycles and produced by the pineal gland has been thought to favorably influence tinnitus through vasodilatory action by decreasing sympathetic tone to preserve labyrinthine perfusion, relaxation of muscular tone, antidepressive effects, and antioxidant effects.[50] In addition, melatonin may have a protective effect on vestibular hair cell loss following aminoglycoside and cisplatin therapy in animal models.[51] Analogous to results concerning zinc and vitamin B12, serum levels of melatonin may be significantly lower among elders suffering from tinnitus compared with those who are not.[52] A double-blind, placebo-controlled crossover study found that after 30 days of 3 mg melatonin daily with a 7-day washout period, the THI did not differ significantly from the placebo posttreatment scores.[53] Tinnitus-associated sleep disturbances, however, decreased significantly by nearly 50%.[53] A similar trial with the same treatment plan but a 30-day washout period, on the other hand, determined a significantly greater improvement in tinnitus matching and self-rated tinnitus scores following melatonin compared with placebo.[54] Thus, the shorter washout period may have influenced the results of the treatment crossover in the study by Rosenberg and colleagues.

Positive effects experienced by melatonin may actually last beyond its treatment duration as after 4 weeks of therapy with 3 mg melatonin daily the significant decrease in THI and Pittsburgh Sleep Quality Index was still present at 4 weeks posttreatment cessation.[55] Melatonin may even outperform guideline-recommended antidepressants,[35] as demonstrated by Abtahi and colleagues. Following 3 months of 3 mg melatonin daily compared with 50 mg sertraline daily, THI scores declined significantly for both groups; THI scores for melatonin, however, decreased significantly more than for sertraline.[56] Whether melatonin works for everyone, however, is questionable. Based on the results by Hurtuk and colleagues,[54] melatonin may be most efficacious in patients who are male, patients with severe bilateral tinnitus, patients with previous noise exposure, patients without a history of depression, and patients who have not tried any previous tinnitus treatment. Despite this plethora of positive results, systematic reviews cannot confirm the clinical efficiency of melatonin due to methodological weaknesses and investigators' potential exaggeration of treatment effect but recognize melatonin's potential usefulness in tinnitus and associated sleep disturbances depending on the patient.[57,58] No adverse effects of melatonin at a dose of 3 mg per day have been reported to date with the exception of an increase in vivid dreams or nightmares.

HYPNOSIS AND BIOFEEDBACK

Hypnosis and biofeedback, similarly to cognitive-behavioral therapy (CBT), aim at giving patients the power to control their conscious mind to bring about change. In the treatment of tinnitus, CBT is the only therapy recommended by the American Academy guideline, with hypnosis and biofeedback being commonly overlooked. During hypnosis and self-hypnosis, patients are guided to a state of deep relaxation while focusing their minds to allow increased control over their thoughts and behaviors.[59] Studies examining the effects of hypnosis on patients with tinnitus have been scarce since the late 1900s but generally report some benefit. Ericksonian hypnosis (EH) is the most commonly used technique, which begins with an exploration of the impact of tinnitus of the patient's life, followed by sessions focusing of relaxation and metal imagery.[59,60] The largest of such studies included 393 participants undergoing a 28-day course of inpatient therapy, evaluation by TQ and SF-36, and a 12-month follow-up.[61] Results were compared with controls on a waiting list. TQ scores decreased in nearly 90% of patients with subacute and chronic tinnitus, with the mean score decreasing significantly.[61] Other trials, using an outpatient approach, achieved comparable results after only 3 to 10 sessions of EH with statistically significant improvements in THI.[59,60] Although Maudoux and colleagues[60] invested additional sessions to teach patients self-hypnosis, only 3 sessions were necessary to attain improvements still present at 6-month follow-up.[59] Distinguishing between particular types of tinnitus, Mason and Rogerson found that although hypnosis has positive impacts in patients without hearing loss, patients with hearing loss did not benefit from therapy.[62] Although in all studies symptoms of tinnitus continued, the quality of life of patients improved dramatically. Thus, suggesting hypnosis as a noninvasive therapy, while potentially including instructions on self-hypnosis, may be a worthwhile treatment modality that could continue long beyond the actual treatment sessions. Because of the paucity and lack of comparability of data, however, no definitive statements can be made by current systematic reviews.[63]

Biofeedback includes learning to control autonomous physiologic processes through receiving immediate feedback while experiencing the physiologicchange.[64] Few studies investigating the usefulness of biofeedback in tinnitus treatment concluded that combining CBT with biofeedback displayed stable and highly effective improvements of psychophysiological interrelationships through psychological coping and physiologic control mechanisms; whether psychological and physiologic responses are depended on one another is unclear.[65,66] Alternatively, biofeedback-relaxation techniques seem to improve coping mechanisms, relief stress and muscle tension, and potentially reduce tinnitus intensity through increased peripheral vascular circulation.[67-69] Going along with these results, Haller and colleagues[64] demonstrated that biofeedback could help patients reduce activation of auditory brain areas through real-time functional MRI neurofeedback. Thus, the addition of biofeedback to other treatment modalities may aid improving patients' quality of life, but its value as a stand-alone therapy has not been substantiated.

ELECTRICAL STIMULATION
Nerve Stimulation

Transcutaneous electrical nerve stimulation is a noninvasive therapy used for tinnitus treatment during which patch electrodes are attached to the auricular area for low-intensity vagus nerve stimulation (VNS). It is hypothesized that this therapy decreases neuronal firing frequencies and sympathetic tone to potentially increase auditory circulation.[70,71] Studies investigating this treatment modality have thus far reported a more than 60% subjective improvement with statistically significant decreases in VAS and THI scores after 8 to 10 treatment sessions[70,72] and the ability to restore an autonomic nervous system imbalance in tinnitus patients with sympathetic predominance.[71]

Measuring brain activities, VNS has also been shown to suppress the auditory and limbic areas implicated in tinnitus etiology, which could potentially hamper tinnitus awareness.[73] None of the studies reported adverse events related to VNS, with one study stating that few patients have been using this technique every day for 3 years.[71,72]

Transcranial Magnetic Stimulation

Similar to VNS, transcranial magnetic stimulation (TMS) is a noninvasive treatment method with the capability of altering the excitability of brain cortices. During TMS for tinnitus, an electromagnet is positioned at the dorsolateral and temporoparietal cortices and stimulates at less than 1 Hz frequency to induce inhibition.[74] A previous review of TMS on chronic tinnitus concluded that most studies described little greater than 50% improvement rates but voiced criticism for small sample sizes and incomparable outcome measures.[75] More recent studies found that although TMS alone did not have significant effects on tinnitus perceptions,[74,76] TMS combined with low-level cochlear laser therapy or audio relaxation techniques did.[76] After 10 treatment sessions administered every other day over 3 weeks, both combination therapies reported significant decreases in THI, with the relaxation/TMS effect still present at 10 weeks post-treatment.[76,77] Nevertheless, electrical stimulation techniques for tinnitus treatment remain underresearched, which limits its use in everyday practice.

CANNABINOIDS

Since the approval of cannabinoids for the treatment of medical conditions, cannabinoids drugs have been readily used for chronic pain and epilepsy. The notion of cannabinoids having antiepileptic properties by decreasing neuronal hyperactivity could in theory imply that cannabinoids might have a similar effect on the CB1 receptors located in auditory brain areas, such as the cochlear nucleus, and therefore benefit the treatment of tinnitus.[78] Thus far, however, there have only been animal studies displaying an antiepileptiform effect. Similarly, there have been no studies on humans investigating the potential of cannabinoid drugs for tinnitus symptoms. Although neuronal inhibitory effects have been documented, they seem to be outweighed by simultaneously stronger excitatory effects, leading to net excitation of the auditory system and subsequent worsening of tinnitus.[79] Two studies examining the effects of selective as well as nonselective cannabinoid receptor agonists on salicylate-induced tinnitus in guinea pigs and rats, respectively, found that neither drug attenuated tinnitus perception based on tinnitus-related animal behavior but may actually intensify the symptom.[80,81] One of the problems in studying cannabinoids, however, is that Cannabis contains more than 400 chemicals, including 66 Cannabis-unique ones, with each different plant within the Cannabaceae family containing varying concentrations of said chemicals.[78] This alone leaves the question of whether some plants might have better efficacy than others. Based on anecdotal evidence, the potential for cannabinoids to improve tinnitus is quite variable and depends on the patient. Although some patients of the senior investigators as well as on Cannabis blogs online report relief of tinnitus or psychologically associated symptoms and sleep quality improvements, others describe a spiking in intensity.[82,83] Thus, cannabinoids may not be at a stage of recommended treatment of tinnitus, but should a patient take initiative in trying Cannabis with a successful outcome, it may be right for that person.

SUMMARY

Based on the evidence provided, complementary/integrative medicine poses viable options in the management of tinnitus. Although some physicians may be hesitant to use these treatment modalities, complementary/integrative medicine should not be looked upon as a last resort but as a complementary approach that might be less invasive and work for patients for whom conventional medicine does not. Especially, if patients are receptive to acupuncture, supplements, and herbal medicines, these options should be considered sooner rather than later during the course of treatment. Patients will communicate what works best for them and what does not, if they perceive their physician to be genuinely listening, emphasizing, and giving them hope. Sometimes, patients might even figure what works for them on their own, as in the case of cannabinoid usage.

In addition to patient preferences and trial and error, alternative treatment can be integrated in a more systematic approach to symptom improvement. Based on the presented research, patients' initial serum levels should be examined for the aforementioned possible deficiencies to further deduct if supplementation with B vitamin, zinc, and copper may be more or less helpful.

Considering many studies have come to contradictory results as to whether a treatment shows statistically significant improvements or not, it is obvious that not every treatment discussed will benefit every patient and that more double-blinded, placebo-controlled trials are needed. As described by the studies, some treatments may be more beneficial to certain patient populations, and just because one option might work for patient A does not mean it will work for patient B. Just as conventional medicine for the treatment of tinnitus, not every alternative treatment will work for everyone. Thus, these *Complementary Integrative Medicine* options should be in the repertoire of every physician taking care of patients with tinnitus, because the absence of trying is worse than failure in the face of giving everything.

DISCLOSURE

M.D.Seidman: Body Language Vitamins—Founder of nutritional supplement company; (7) patents—Intellectual property; Acclarent—Consultant; Auris Medical AM 101 &111—Clinical trials for tinnitus-noncompensated (Research); Envoy Medical—Assisting in postmarket studies-noncompensated (Research); NIH—Simulation Work/July 2012-June 2019 (Research); MicroTransponder, Inc—Vagal Nerve Stimulator Clinical Trial for tinnitus-non-compensated (Research).

REFERENCES

1. Seidman MD, Ahsan SF. Current opinion: the management of tinnitus. CurrOpinOtolaryngolHeadNeck Surg 2015;23(5):376–81.
2. Tunkel DE, Bauer CA, Sun GH, et al. Clinical practice guideline: tinnitus executive summary. OtolaryngolHeadNeck Surg 2014;151(4):533–41.
3. Kim JI, Choi JY, Lee DH, et al. Acupuncture for the treatment of tinnitus: a systematic review of randomized clinical trials. BMC Complement Altern Med 2012; 12:97.
4. Liu F, Han X, Li Y, et al. Acupuncture in the treatment of tinnitus: a systematic review and meta-analysis. Eur Arch Otorhinolaryngol 2016;273(2):285–94.
5. Wang K, Bugge J, Bugge S. A randomised, placebo-controlled trial of manual and electrical acupuncture for the treatment of tinnitus. Complement Ther Med 2010;18(6):249–55.
6. Low WK, Rangabashyam MS, Cui SL, et al. Is Electroacupuncture Treatment More Effective in Somatic Tinnitus Than in Nonsomatic Tinnitus? Med Acupunct 2017;29(3):138–44.

7. Cai W, Chen AW, Ding L, et al. Thermal effects of acupuncture by infrared thermography test in patients with tinnitus. J AcupunctMeridian Stud 2019. https://doi.org/10.1016/j.jams.2019.05.002.
8. Doi MY, Tano SS, Schultz AR, et al. Effectiveness of acupuncture therapy as treatment for tinnitus: a randomized controlled trial. Braz J Otorhinolaryngol 2016; 82(4):458–65.
9. Naderinabi B, Soltanipour S, Nemati S, et al. Acupuncture for chronic nonpulsatile tinnitus: A randomized clinical trial. Caspian J Intern Med 2018;9(1):38–45.
10. Rogha M, Rezvani M, Khodami AR. The effects of acupuncture on the inner ear originated tinnitus. J Res Med Sci 2011;16(9):1217–23.
11. Lin TY, Yang SW, Lee YS, et al. Analysis of Factors Influencing the Efficiency of Acupuncture in Tinnitus Patients. EvidBased Complement Alternat Med 2019; 2019:1318639.
12. Figueiredo RR, de Azevedo AA, de Mello Oliveira P. Correlation analysis of the visual-analogue scale and the Tinnitus Handicap Inventory in tinnitus patients. Braz J Otorhinolaryngol 2009;75(1):76–9.
13. de Azevedo RF, Chiari BM, Okada DM, et al. Impact of acupuncture on otoacoustic emissions in patients with tinnitus. Braz J Otorhinolaryngol 2007;73(5): 599–607.
14. Drew S, Davies E. Effectiveness of Ginkgo biloba in treating tinnitus: double blind, placebo controlled trial. BMJ 2001;322(7278):73.
15. Smith PF, Zheng Y, Darlington CL. Ginkgo biloba extracts for tinnitus: More hype than hope? J Ethnopharmacol 2005;100(1–2):95–9.
16. Mahmoudian-Sani MR, Hashemzadeh-Chaleshtori M, Asadi-Samani M, et al. Ginkgo biloba in the treatment of tinnitus: An updated literature review. IntTinnitus J 2017;21(1):58–62.
17. Holstein N. Ginkgo special extract EGb 761 in tinnitus therapy.An overview of results of completed clinical trials. Fortschr Med Orig 2001;118(4):157–64 [in German].
18. Ahsan SF, Seidman MD. Alternative medical management of tinnitus. BrainInj Prof 2016;13(1).
19. Rejali D, Sivakumar A, Balaji N. Ginkgo biloba does not benefit patients with tinnitus: a randomized placebo-controlled double-blind trial and meta-analysis of randomized trials. ClinOtolaryngolAllied Sci 2004;29(3):226–31.
20. von Boetticher A. Ginkgo biloba extract in the treatment of tinnitus: a systematic review. Neuropsychiatr Dis Treat 2011;7:441–7.
21. Morgenstern C, Biermann E. The efficacy of Ginkgo special extractEGb 761 in patients with tinnitus. Int J ClinPharmacolTher 2002;40(5):188–97.
22. Hilton MP, Zimmermann EF, Hunt WT. Ginkgo biloba for tinnitus. CochraneDatabaseSyst Rev 2013;(3):CD003852.
23. Kim TS, Lee HS, Chung JW. The Effect of Korean Red Ginseng on Symptoms and Quality of Life in Chronic Tinnitus: A Randomized, Open-Label Pilot Study. J AudiolOtol 2015;19(2):85–90.
24. Im GJ, Chang JW, Choi J, et al. Protective effect of Korean red ginseng extract on cisplatin ototoxicity in HEI-OC1 auditory cells. Phytother Res 2010;24(4):614–21.
25. Zhai S, Fang Y, Yang W, et al. Clinical investigation on the beneficial effects of the Chinese medicinal herb GushenPian on sensorineural deafness and tinnitus. Cell BiochemBiophys 2013;67(2):785–93.
26. Wang Z. Experimental study of Rhizomadrynariae (Gusuibu) in the treatment of streptomycin ototoxicity. ZhonghuaEr Bi Yan HouKeZaZhi 1989;24(2):79–81, 127. [in Chinese].

27. Seidman MD, Babu S. Alternative medications and other treatments for tinnitus: facts from fiction. OtolaryngolClin North Am 2003;36(2):359–81.
28. Yetiser S, Tosun F, Satar B, et al. The role of zinc in management of tinnitus. Auris-Nasus Larynx 2002;29(4):329–33.
29. Smith GS, Romanelli-Gobbi M, Gray-Karagrigoriou E, et al. Complementary and integrative treatments: tinnitus. OtolaryngolClin North Am 2013;46(3):389–408.
30. Ochi K, Kinoshita H, Kenmochi M, et al. Zinc deficiency and tinnitus. AurisNasus Larynx 2003;30(Suppl):S25–8.
31. Ochi K, Ohashi T, Kinoshita H, et al. The serum zinc level in patients with tinnitus and the effect of zinc treatment. Nihon JibiinkokaGakkaiKaiho 1997;100(9):915–9 [in Japanese].
32. Gersdorff M, Robillard T, Stein F, et al. A clinical correlation between hypozince-mia and tinnitus. Arch Otorhinolaryngol 1987;244(3):190–3.
33. Person OC, Puga ME, da Silva EM, et al. Zinc supplementation for tinnitus. Co-chraneDatabaseSyst Rev 2016;11:CD009832.
34. Berkiten G, Kumral TL, Yildirim G, et al. Effects of serum zinc level on tinnitus. Am J Otolaryngol 2015;36(2):230–4.
35. Seidman MD. Tinnitus.BMJ Best Practice 2018. Available at: https://bestpractice.bmj.com/topics/en-us/364. Accessed July 15, 2019.
36. Jun HJ, Ok S, Tyler R, et al. Is Hypozincemia Related to Tinnitus?: A Population Study Using Data From the Korea National Health and Nutrition Examination Survey. ClinExpOtorhinolaryngol 2015;8(4):335–8.
37. Yeh CW, Tseng LH, Yang CH, et al. Effects of oral zinc supplementation on patients with noise-induced hearing loss associated tinnitus: A clinical trial. Biomed J 2019;42(1):46–52.
38. Yasar M, Sahin MI, Karakukcu C, et al. The Role of Trace Elements in Tinnitus. BiolTrace Elem Res 2017;176(1):65–72.
39. Singh C, Kawatra R, Gupta J, et al. Therapeutic role of Vitamin B12 in patients of chronic tinnitus: A pilot study. Noise Health 2016;18(81):93–7.
40. Manzanares W, Hardy G. Vitamin B12: the forgotten micronutrient for critical care. CurrOpinClinNutrMetabCare 2010;13(6):662–8.
41. Darrat I, Ahmad N, Seidman K, et al. Auditory research involving antioxidants. CurrOpinOtolaryngolHeadNeck Surg 2007;15(5):358–63.
42. Shemesh Z, Attias J, Ornan M, et al. Vitamin B12 deficiency in patients with chronic-tinnitus and noise-induced hearing loss. Am J Otolaryngol 1993; 14(2):94–9.
43. Berkiten G, Yildirim G, Topaloglu I, et al. Vitamin B12 levels in patients with tinnitus and effectiveness of vitamin B12 treatment on hearing threshold and tinnitus. B-ENT 2013;9(2):111–6.
44. Lee DY, Kim YH. Relationship Between Diet and Tinnitus: Korea National Health and Nutrition Examination Survey. ClinExpOtorhinolaryngol 2018;11(3):158–65.
45. Hameed HM, Eleue AH, Al Mosawi AMT. The use of distortion product otoacoustic emissions (DPOAE) records to estimate effect of vitamin B complex on changing severity of tinnitus. Ann Med Surg(Lond) 2018;36:203–11.
46. Ekinci A, Kamasak K. Evaluation of serum prolidase enzyme activity and oxidative stress in patients with tinnitus. Braz J Otorhinolaryngol 2019. https://doi.org/10.1016/j.bjorl.2019.01.009.
47. Savastano M, Brescia G, Marioni G. Antioxidant therapy in idiopathic tinnitus: preliminary outcomes. Arch Med Res 2007;38(4):456–9.
48. Polanski JF, Soares AD, de Mendonca Cruz OL. Antioxidant therapy in the elderly with tinnitus. Braz J Otorhinolaryngol 2016;82(3):269–74.

49. Khan M, Gross J, Haupt H, et al. A pilot clinical trial of the effects of coenzyme Q10 on chronic tinnitus aurium. OtolaryngolHeadNeck Surg 2007;136(1):72–7.
50. Pirodda A, Raimondi MC, Ferri GG. Exploring the reasons why melatonin can improve tinnitus. Med Hypotheses 2010;75(2):190–1.
51. Reiter RJ, Tan DX, Korkmaz A, et al. Drug-mediated ototoxicity and tinnitus: alleviation with melatonin. J PhysiolPharmacol 2011;62(2):151–7.
52. Lasisi AO, Fehintola FA, Lasisi TJ. The role of plasma melatonin and vitamins C and B12 in the development of idiopathic tinnitus in the elderly. Ghana Med J 2012;46(3):152–7.
53. Rosenberg SI, Silverstein H, Rowan PT, et al. Effect of melatonin on tinnitus. Laryngoscope 1998;108(3):305–10.
54. Hurtuk A, Dome C, Holloman CH, et al. Melatonin: can it stop the ringing? Ann OtolRhinolLaryngol 2011;120(7):433–40.
55. Megwalu UC, Finnell JE, Piccirillo JF. The effects of melatonin on tinnitus and sleep. OtolaryngolHeadNeck Surg 2006;134(2):210–3.
56. Abtahi SH, Hashemi SM, Mahmoodi M, et al. Comparison of Melatonin and Sertraline Therapies on Tinnitus: A Randomized Clinical Trial. Int J Prev Med 2017; 8:61.
57. Merrick L, Youssef D, Tanner M, et al. Does melatonin have therapeutic use in tinnitus? South Med J 2014;107(6):362–6.
58. Miroddi M, Bruno R, Galletti F, et al. Clinical pharmacology of melatonin in the treatment of tinnitus: a review. Eur J ClinPharmacol 2015;71(3):263–70.
59. Yazici ZM, Sayin I, Gokkus G, et al. Effectiveness of Ericksonian hypnosis in tinnitus therapy: preliminary results. B-ENT 2012;8(1):7–12.
60. Maudoux A, Bonnet S, Lhonneux-Ledoux F, et al. Ericksonian hypnosis in tinnitus therapy. B-ENT 2007;3(Suppl 7):75–7.
61. Ross UH, Lange O, Unterrainer J, et al. Ericksonian hypnosis in tinnitus therapy: effects of a 28-day inpatient multimodal treatment concept measured by Tinnitus-Questionnaire and Health Survey SF-36. Eur Arch Otorhinolaryngol 2007;264(5): 483–8.
62. Mason J, Rogerson D. Client-centered hypnotherapy for tinnitus: who is likely to benefit? Am J ClinHypn 1995;37(4):294–9.
63. Cope TE. Clinical hypnosis for the alleviation of tinnitus. IntTinnitus J 2008;14(2): 135–8.
64. Haller S, Birbaumer N, Veit R. Real-time fMRI feedback training may improve chronic tinnitus. EurRadiol 2010;20(3):696–703.
65. Heinecke K, Weise C, Rief W. Psychophysiological effects of biofeedback treatment in tinnitus sufferers. Br J Clin Psychol 2009;48(Pt 3):223–39.
66. Weise C, Heinecke K, Rief W. Biofeedback-based behavioral treatment for chronic tinnitus: results of a randomized controlled trial. J ConsultClin Psychol 2008;76(6):1046–57.
67. Landis B, Landis E. Is biofeedback effective for chronic tinnitus? An intensive study with seven subjects. Am J Otolaryngol 1992;13(6):349–56.
68. Carmen R, Svihovec D. Relaxation-biofeedback in the treatment of tinnitus. Am J Otol 1984;5(5):376–81.
69. Walsh WM, Gerley PP. Thermal biofeedback and the treatment of tinnitus. Laryngoscope 1985;95(8):987–9.
70. Lee SK, Chung H, Chung JH, et al. Effectiveness of transcutaneous electrical stimulation for chronic tinnitus. ActaOtolaryngol 2014;134(2):159–67.

71. Ylikoski J, Lehtimaki J, Pirvola U, et al. Non-invasive vagus nerve stimulation reduces sympathetic preponderance in patients with tinnitus. ActaOtolaryngol 2017;137(4):426–31.
72. Shim HJ, Kwak MY, An YH, et al. Feasibility and Safety of Transcutaneous Vagus Nerve Stimulation Paired with Notched Music Therapy for the Treatment of Chronic Tinnitus. J AudiolOtol 2015;19(3):159–67.
73. Yakunina N, Kim SS, Nam EC. BOLD fMRI effects of transcutaneous vagus nerve stimulation in patients with chronic tinnitus. PLoS One 2018;13(11):e0207281.
74. Formanek M, Migalova P, Krulova P, et al. Combined transcranial magnetic stimulation in the treatment of chronic tinnitus. Ann ClinTransl Neurol 2018;5(7):857–64.
75. Theodoroff SM, Folmer RL. Repetitive transcranial magnetic stimulation as a treatment for chronic tinnitus: a critical review. OtolNeurotol 2013;34(2):199–208.
76. Thabit MN, Fouad N, Shahat B, et al. Combined central and peripheral stimulation for treatment of chronic tinnitus: a randomized pilot study. NeurorehabilNeuralRepair 2015;29(3):224–33.
77. Kreuzer PM, Poeppl TB, Bulla J, et al. A proof-of-concept study on the combination of repetitive transcranial magnetic stimulation and relaxation techniques in chronic tinnitus. J NeuralTransm(Vienna) 2016;123(10):1147–57.
78. Zheng Y, Smith PF. Cannabinoid drugs: will they relieve or exacerbate tinnitus? CurrOpin Neurol 2019;32(1):131–6.
79. Smith PF, Zheng Y. Cannabinoids, cannabinoid receptors and tinnitus. Hear Res 2016;332:210–6.
80. Berger JI, Coomber B, Hill S, et al. Effects of the cannabinoid CB1 agonist ACEA on salicylate ototoxicity, hyperacusis and tinnitus in guinea pigs. Hear Res 2017;356:51–62.
81. Zheng Y, Stiles L, Hamilton E, et al. The effects of the synthetic cannabinoid receptor agonists, WIN55,212-2 and CP55,940, on salicylate-induced tinnitus in rats. Hear Res 2010;268(1):145–50.
82. Ivanova A. Five people told us what they do for their tinnitus. 2018. Available at: https://www.vice.com/en_us/article/59qxkd/five-people-told-us-what-they-do-for-their-tinnitus. Accessed July 20, 2019.
83. Marijuana/Cannabis and Tinnitus. 2013. Available at: https://www.tinnitustalk.com/threads/marijuana-cannabis-and-tinnitus.1993/. Accessed July 20, 2019.

Current Clinical Trials for Tinnitus: Drugs and Biologics

Jonas Dyhrfjeld-Johnsen, PhD[a],*, Christopher R. Cederroth, PhD[b]

KEYWORDS

- Clinical trials • Preclinical development • Tinnitus • Hearing loss • NMDA
- Potassium • Glutamate • Calcium

KEY POINTS

- In spite of recent clinical trial failures, the tinnitus drug development remains active.
- Two ongoing clinical development programs for tinnitus drug candidates were identified—AM-101 (Auris Medical) in phase 2/3 and OTO-313 (Otonomy) in phase 1/2.
- Six preclinical programs were identified, focusing mainly on the modulation of different potassium channels.
- Lessons learnt from ongoing clinical studies for designing future trials include the importance of the definition of population, eligibility criteria, and the choice of primary endpoints.
- Key ongoing research directions include the development of novel compounds that are both safe and effective and the identification of objective outcome measures to facilitate clinical and translational research.

INTRODUCTION

With approximately 2% of the global population experiencing severe tinnitus seriously affecting quality of life and requiring medical intervention, effective therapeutic solutions are clearly needed.[1] Treatment of tinnitus has proved to be extremely challenging, and this disorder remains uncured. The only treatment currently recommended by the European Guideline is cognitive behavioral therapy.[2,3] Although several marketed drugs against tinnitus are available (eg, Tinnex, Adexor, Anginox, Angiozil Retard), their efficacy is not supported by strong evidence, and the tinnitus drug pipeline is concerningly lean.[4] Several reviews have covered the mixed successes in tinnitus treatment development[5] and the challenges faced in recent drug trials (AM-101 from Auris Medical and AUT00063 from Autifony Therapeutics).[6] However, the long-established positive effect of lidocaine on tinnitus supports the notion that it is a treatable disorder.[7,8]

a Research & Translational Development, Sensorion SA, 375 rue du Professeur Joseph Blayac, Montpellier, France; b Department of Physiology and Pharmacology, KarolinskaInstitutet, Solnavägen 9, Stockholm, Sweden
* Corresponding author.
E-mail address: jonas.dyhrfjeld-johnsen@sensorion-pharma.com

Otolaryngol Clin N Am 53 (2020) 651–666
https://doi.org/10.1016/j.otc.2020.03.012
0030-6665/20/© 2020 Elsevier Inc. All rights reserved.

List of specific abbreviations	
CAP	Compound Action Potential
EudraCT	European Union Drug Regulating Authorities Clinical Trials Database
GPIAS	Gap Prepulse Inhibition of Acoustic Startle
ISSHNL	Idiopathic Sudden Sensorineural Hearing Loss
PRO	Patient Reported Outcome
SBAD	Sound-Based Avoidance Detection
SIPAC	Schedule Induced Polydipsia Avoidance Conditioning
TFI	Tinnitus Functional Index
THI	Tinnitus Handicap Inventory
TLQ	Tinnitus Loudness Questionnaire
VAS	Visual Analog Scale

The large number of factors contributing to tinnitus (aging, hearing loss, conductive hearing loss, thyroid disorders, etc.) has led to the proposal that the poor response to existing treatments is due to extensive heterogeneity.[9] Multiple preclinical models are now converging toward a theory that tinnitus may be a maladaptive compensatory response to diminished sensory input.[10] This leads to increased spontaneous firing rates and increased neural synchrony along the auditory pathway, involving, at least in part, KCNQ2/3 potassium channels and hyperpolarization-activated cyclic nucleotide-gated channels in the midbrain,[11] as well as perturbed homeostatic plasticity in the auditory cortex due to lower GABAergic control.[12] Nonauditory brain regions have been linked to tinnitus in humans and animals, showing that the limbic system also interacts with auditory structures and contributes to the pathophysiology of tinnitus.[13,14] In humans, studies have demonstrated cortical coupling (functional connectivity) as well as specific patterns of thalamocortical dysrhythmia in individuals suffering from tinnitus, revealing further complexity in the neural network involved in tinnitus.[15,16] These studies have focused research efforts for drug candidates in new directions.

Peripherally, damage in the ear due to noise or medications involves N-methyl-D-aspartate (NMDA) receptors, and their blockade abolishes behavioral evidence of tinnitus in animal models.[17,18] Early research identified the role of NMDA receptors in excitatory synaptic transmission between inner hair cells and spiral ganglion neurons in the cochlea[19,20] and implicated these receptors in pathophysiologic processes of excitotoxicity and ischemia.[21–24] This highlighted their potential as therapeutic targets for pharmacological intervention in auditive pathologies such as hearing loss and tinnitus. Experiments using preclinical in vivo rodent models of tinnitus induced by salicylate administration or noise trauma exposure demonstrated a reduction of tinnitus symptom measures following local administration of NMDA receptor antagonists such as ketamine, esketamine (the S-enantiomer of ketamine), and ifenprodil,[17,18,25] although with a potentially clinically limiting parameter of an apparent treatment initiation window of up to 4 days following tinnitus induction.[25]

There is currently a paucity of approved effective drugs, biological agents, and promising clinical leads, and treatment of tinnitus is largely restricted to cognitive therapies and the management of associated symptoms (hearing loss, depression etc.). Given the difficulties experienced with the drug candidates evaluated clinically to date, and available evidence from preclinical models revealing new potential clinical avenues, targeting both the ear and/or the brain is a rational clinical tactic for treating tinnitus. This article presents the results of a review of published data sources to identify drugs in development; the status of a limited number of identified drugs in the clinic is described and supplemented with preclinical programs holding promise for the clinic.

APPROACH

Current development programs of drug candidates for the treatment of tinnitus (where "in development" is defined as at a minimum, a disclosed, identified target in active development) were identified by cross-referencing a recent review by Schilder and colleagues[26] (2019) of emerging therapeutics for inner ear and central hearing disorders (June 2018 cutoff), with clinical trial registries (such as clinicaltrials.gov and EudraCT) and the Drugs Database of Global Data (December 2019 cutoff).[27] This was supplemented with information from the Websites and press releases of the identified biotechs and pharmaceutical companies in question. Because no development programs of biologics for tinnitus treatment were identified, the following sections only cover small molecule approaches.

CLINICAL STAGE PROGRAMS

Only 2 active clinical development programs for the pharmacologic treatment of tinnitus were identified through the review (**Table 1**). Both of these programs (detailed in **Table 2**), from Auris Medical (phase 2/3) and Otonomy (phase 1/2), are based on antagonizing excitatory, glutamatergic NMDA receptors in the auditory periphery via local, transtympanic administration of the active principle in a gel formulation for slow, sustained release from the middle ear to the inner ear.

AM-101: N-Methyl-D-Aspartate Receptor Antagonist

The most advanced clinical program in active development is AM-101 (Keyzilen, esketamine hydrochloride) from Auris Medical, an NMDA receptor antagonist administered intratympanically in a slow-release gel formulation). An initial double-blind, randomized, single-ascending dose, phase 1/2 trial in 24 patients suffering from tinnitus with onset within 3 months after noise trauma or from sudden deafness reported a good safety profile and apparent benefits on tinnitus loudness (visual analogue scale [VAS]) and minimum masking level compared with placebo.[27,28] The 2 highest dose levels in the phase 1/2 trial, 0.27 mg/mL and 0.81 mg/mL injections of 0.25 mL AM-101, were retained for further testing in phase 2 clinical trials.

The phase 2 clinical program for AM-101 consisted of 2 randomized, double-blind trials, TACTT0 and TACTT1. TACTT0 (NCT00860808) enrolled 248 patients suffering from tinnitus following acute acoustic trauma, idiopathic sudden sensorineural hearing loss (ISSNHL), or otitis media, randomized to receive 3 intratympanic doses of either placebo, 0.27, or 0.81 mg/mL AM-101 over 3 consecutive days.[29] No significant effect was found on minimal masking level (primary endpoint), but a dose-dependent effect improvement was demonstrated in the subgroup of acute acoustic trauma and otitis media combined, on tinnitus loudness (coprimary endpoint), annoyance (coprimary endpoint), sleep difficulties, and impact of tinnitus (assessed using the tinnitus handicap inventory 12, THI-12). The highest AM-101 dose maintained statistically significant improvement for all measures when assessed 90 days after the initial administration. However, no benefits were reported for the ISSNHL subgroup. Subsequent randomized comparison of a single dose of 0.81 mg/mL AM-101 versus 3 doses of 0.81 mg/mL AM-101 over the course of 2 weeks and matched placebo regimens in the TACTT1 study (NCT01270282) in 85 patients suffering from tinnitus after documented acute acoustic trauma, inner ear barotrauma, middle ear surgery, or acute otitis media found no difference between the 2 AM-101 dosing schedules but

Table 1
Active clinical development programs for the treatment of tinnitus

Company	Therapeutic Target	Mechanism of Action	Drug Candidate	Route of Administration	Stage of Development
Auris Medical	NMDA receptor	Antagonist	Keyzilen (AM-101)	Transtympanic injection	Phase 2/3
Otonomy	NMDA receptor	Antagonist	Gacyclidine (OTO-313)	Transtympanic injection	Phase 1/2
Canbex	BKCa (calcium-activated potassium channel)	Activator	VSN16 R	Oral	Preclinical
Knopp Biosciences	KCNQ2 potassium channel	Modulators	Not available	-	Preclinical
Autifony Therapeutics Ltd	Kv3.1 potassium channel	Modulator	Not available	Oral	Preclinical
AudioCure Pharma GmbH	Not available	Betacarboline	AC-102	Transtympanic	Preclinical
Gateway Biotechnology	Calcium channel and oxidation and inflammatory pathways	Calcium channel blocker acting on oxidation and inflammatory pathways	GW-201	-	Preclinical
Pragma Therapeutics	mGluR7 metabotropic glutamate receptor	Antagonist	Not available	Oral	Preclinical

Table 2
Detailed overview of clinical trial programs for tinnitus treatment using N-methyl-D-aspartate receptor antagonists

Development Program (Company)	Clinical Phase	Trial Identifier	Trial Population	Treatment Design	Clinical Endpoints
AM-101 (Auris Medical)	Phase 1/2	EudraCT2006-002692-41	24 patients w. tinnitus with onset within 3 mo after noise trauma or from sudden deafness	Single ascending dose	• Safety • Pharmacokinetics • Tinnitus severity (TBF-12) • Tinnitus loudness (TLQ) • Minimum masking level (MML)
	Phase 2	TACTT0 NCT00860808	48 patients w. tinnitus following acute acoustic trauma, idiopathic sudden sensorineural hearing loss (ISSNHL) or otitis media	Three doses of either placebo, 0.27, or 0.81 mg/mL AM-101 over 3 consecutive days	• Safety • MML • Tinnitus loudness (TLQ) • Tinnitus annoyance (TAQ) • Sleep difficulties • Tinnitus severity (THI-12)
	Phase 2	TACTT1 NCT01270282	85 patients w. tinnitus after documented acute acoustic trauma, inner ear barotrauma, middle ear surgery, or acute otitis media	Single dose of 0.81 mg/mL AM-101 vs 3 doses of 0.81 mg/mL AM-101 over 2 wk and matched placebo	• Safety • Pharmacokinetics • Tinnitus loudness (loudness matching) • Tinnitus severity (THQ, THI-12) • Tinnitus annoyance (TAQ) • Patient global impression of change (PGIC) in tinnitus severity • MML
	Phase 3	TACTT2 NCT01803646	343 patients within 3 mo of tinnitus onset following traumatic cochlear injury (acute acoustic trauma, blast trauma, middle ear surgery, inner ear barotrauma, tympanic membrane trauma) or otitis media	Three intratympanic injections of 0.87 mg/mL AM-101 over the course of 3 d vs placebo	• Safety • Tinnitus loudness (TLQ) • Tinnitus severity (TFI)

(continued on next page)

Table 2
(continued)

Development Program (Company)	Clinical Phase	Trial Identifier	Trial Population	Treatment Design	Clinical Endpoints
	Phase 3	TACTT3 NCT02040194	893 patients within 3 mo of tinnitus onset following traumatic cochlear injury (acute acoustic trauma, blast trauma, middle ear surgery, inner ear barotrauma, tympanic membrane trauma) or otitis media	Three intratympanic injections of 0.87 mg/mL AM-101 over the course of 3 d vs placebo	• Safety • Tinnitus loudness (TLQ) • Tinnitus severity (TFI) • Tinnitus annoyance (TAQ) • PGIC in tinnitus severity
OTO-313 (Otonomy)	Phase 1	Not available	Healthy volunteers	Single ascending dose	• Safety • Pharmacokinetics
	Phase 1/2	NCT03918109	58 patients w. subjective unilateral tinnitus of cochlear origin (eg, associated with sensorineural hearing loss: acute hearing loss from noise trauma, barotrauma, acute acoustic trauma, blast trauma, middle ear surgery, inner ear barotrauma, as well as age-related hearing loss; resolved otitis media; ototoxic drug exposure)	Single intratympanic injection of OTO-313 vs placebo	• Safety • Pharmacokinetics • Tinnitus severity (TFI) • Tinnitus annoyance (VAS) • Tinnitus loudness (VAS) • PGIC

concluded that 3 doses of 0.81 mg/mL AM-101 over 3 consecutive days (TACTT0) was superior to both TACTT1 regimens.[30]

In late 2019, the AM-101 phase 3 clinical program consisted of 2 primary trials in acute tinnitus (TACTT2 and TACTT3), along with their respective open-label extension studies (AMPACT1/NCT01934010 and AMPACT2/NCT02040207) in postacute tinnitus. Here the authors focus on the acute tinnitus trials, building on the prior phase 1/2 and phase 2 learnings. The TACTT2 (NCT01803646) double-blind, placebo-controlled trial randomized 343 patients who were within 3 months of tinnitus onset following traumatic cochlear injury (acute acoustic trauma, blast trauma, middle ear surgery, inner ear barotrauma, tympanic membrane trauma) or otitis media. Patients were randomized to 2 arms in a 3:2 ratio, receiving either 3 intratympanic injections of 0.87 mg/mL AM-101 over the course of 3 days or placebo. The study failed to show an overall statistically significant treatment effect of AM-101 versus placebo on the primary endpoint (tinnitus loudness questionnaire [TLQ], numerical rating scale from 0–100) or on the co-primary endpoint (Tinnitus Functional Index [TFI]) at day 84 after inclusion; however, the safety and tolerability were considered good.[27,31] Pre-specified subgroup analysis subsequently reported a statistically significant improvement of TFI in patients suffering from tinnitus following otitis media, as well as trends toward improvement of TFI in the traumatic cochlear insult subgroup (acute noise trauma, barotrauma, surgery trauma) and in patients with severe to extreme tinnitus.[32] The TLQ however showed lower sensitivity than the TFI, perhaps due to frequently repeated assessments. This knowledge led to a protocol amendment to the ongoing TACTT3 (NCT02040194) trial, to reduce the frequency of TLQ assessments and elevate the TFI from a key secondary to an alternate primary efficacy endpoint. The sample size was also increased to allow for an additional 120 patients to sufficiently power the statistical analysis of potential efficacy in the subgroups identified in TACTT2.[32] Unfortunately, despite the protocol amendment, the TACTT3 trial failed to show efficacy overall or in any of the prespecified subgroups, for either of the primary endpoints.[33] Auris Medical is currently planning the execution of a newly designed phase 2/3 clinical trial for AM-101, incorporating the learnings from the previously executed late-stage clinical trials.[34]

OTO-313: N-Methyl-D-Aspartate Receptor Antagonist

The second active clinical development program by Otonomy is developing the noncompetitive NMDA-antagonist gacyclidine for local intratympanic administration as a gel for the treatment of tinnitus. Initially code-named OTO-311, the drug candidate name was changed to OTO-313 after a reformulation of the gel carrier.[35] No additional preclinical data have been published for this drug candidate in tinnitus, and the rationale is based on the original research on the role of NMDA receptors in cochlear excitotoxicity and tinnitus models presented in the introduction. Early clinical research at an academic center in Germany tested the local, sustained administration of gacyclidine solution into the round window niche via a catheter as a compassionate use treatment of sensorineural tinnitus.[36] In a case series of 6 patients, 4 patients experienced temporary tinnitus relief after 36- to 63-hour infusions of up to 0.075 mg/kg gacyclidine/day, as evaluated by VAS for tinnitus intensity, tinnitus annoyance, and subjective disability.

An initial single-ascending-dose phase 1 study of OTO-311 in healthy volunteers did not raise any safety or tolerability concerns.[27,37] A randomized, double-blind, placebo-controlled phase 1/2 trial of OTO-313 is ongoing for patients suffering subjective unilateral tinnitus of cochlear origin (eg, associated with sensorineural hearing loss: acute hearing loss from noise trauma, barotrauma, acute acoustic trauma, blast trauma, middle ear surgery, inner ear barotrauma, as well as age-related hearing loss; resolved otitis media; ototoxic drug exposure) (NCT03918109[27]). The study is scheduled to enroll 58 patients in 1:1 ratio to receive a single intratympanic injection of OTO-313 or placebo after a 14-day lead-in period and will evaluate effects according to the TFI, tinnitus annoyance (VAS), tinnitus loudness (VAS), and global impression of change, in addition to safety and pharmacokinetics. The projected completion date is May 2020.

PRECLINICAL STAGE PROGRAMS

Several companies with active preclinical drug development programs for the treatment of tinnitus were identified from the search (**Table 3**): Canbex Therapeutics, Knopp Biosciences, Autifony Therapeutics, AudioCure Pharma, Gateway Biotechnology, and Pragma Therapeutics. Because it is not mandatory to register details of preclinical development programs in public databases (unlike for clinical trials), and disclosure of detailed information is often limited for competitive and strategic reasons, information on these programs is sparse and accuracy may be limited, notably when scientific studies have not yet been published.

Potassium Channel Modulators

Several programs within the field (Canbex Therapeutics, Knopp Biosciences, Autifony Therapeutics) target the modulation of various types of potassium channels. Hyperexcitability and hypersynchrony are generally considered an underlying pathophysiologic mechanism of tinnitus.[38,39] Potassium channels are the largest and most diverse ion channel family, with defined tissue distributions. They play a clear role in stabilizing neuronal resting membrane potentials and controlling neuronal activity levels and patterns, making them an attractive—but complex—therapeutic target.[40]

The most advanced development program targeting potassium channels is that of Canbex Therapeutics, a spin-off from University College London. The lead oral drug candidate VSN16R is an activator of neuronal calcium-activated potassium channels (BK channels), primarily developed for the nonsedative treatment of spasticity in multiple sclerosis,[41] for which it failed to show significant effects in a phase 2 clinical trial (NCT02542787) after successfully completing a phase 1 study in healthy volunteers.[27,42] Although no specific data in tinnitus models are available, VSN16R has demonstrated the ability to modulate CNS neuronal activity in vitro,[43] and BK-channel activators have been suggested as potential therapeutic agents for the treatment of tinnitus.[44]

The potassium channel modulator opener program from Knopp Biosciences targeting tinnitus and hearing disorders is currently still in the preclinical discovery stage, aiming to modulate ion channels of the KCNQ2-KCNQ5 families.[26,27,45] A lead drug candidate has yet to be named, but effects of reference compounds such as Maxipost (BMS-204352) and Retigabine in tinnitus models has previously been reported.[46–48] In in-vivo models of either noise- or salicylate-induced tinnitus, systemic administration of Maxipost or Retigabine before or immediately after tinnitus induction, protected against reduction of auditory compound action potential amplitudes and reduced the number of animals that developed tinnitus as evaluated by Gap Prepulse Inhibition of Auditory Startle (GPIAS) testing or Schedule-Induced Polydipsia Avoidance Conditioning testing. However, as the R-enantiomer of Maxipost (which negatively modulates KCNQ2-KNCQ5 channel opening, contrary to its racemate) also dose-dependently abolished behavioral evidence of tinnitus, it was speculated that perhaps other common mechanisms of action such as KCNQ1 inhibition or BK-channel

Table 3
Active preclinical development programs for the treatment of tinnitus

Company	Therapeutic Target	Mechanism of Action	Drug Candidate	Route of Administration	Stage of Development
Canbex	BKCa (calcium activated potassium channel)	Activator	VSN16R	Oral	Preclinical
Knopp Biosciences	KCNQ2 potassium channel	Modulators	Not available	-	Preclinical
Autifony Therapeutics Ltd	Kv3.1 potassium channel	Modulator	Not available	Oral	Preclinical
AudioCure Pharma GmbH	Not available	Betacarboline	AC-102	Transtympanic	Preclinical
Gateway Biotechnology	Calcium channel and oxidation and inflammatory pathways	Calcium channel blocker acting on oxidation and inflammatory pathways	GW-201	-	Preclinical
Pragma Therapeutics	mGluR7 metabotropic glutamate receptor	Antagonist	Not available	Oral	Preclinical

activation could be responsible for the determined therapeutic potential.[47] The latter would suggest an overlap in the mechanism of action with the above-mentioned Canbex Therapeutics program.

The Autifony Therapeutics program targets the high-threshold delayed rectifier channel Kv3.1 that is widely expressed in fast-spiking neurons throughout the auditory brainstem. In preclinical models, an earlier AutifonyKv3.1 modulator AUT00063 reduced hyperactivity in the inferior colliculus, dorsal cochlear nucleus, and auditory cortex after cochlear ouabain lesions[49] or noise trauma.[50,51] AUT00063 was found to be safe with a good pharmacokinetic profile following oral administration in a first-in-human, phase 1 double-blind, randomized, single and repeat dose escalating trial in healthy volunteers but subsequently failed to demonstrate efficacy in terms of TFI or tinnitus loudness in the QUIET-1 phase 2a randomized placebo-controlled trial enrolling patients with subjective tinnitus lasting between 6 and 18 months (NCT02315508).[52] The Kv3.1 program remains active but is now exploring new candidate compounds in the preclinical discovery stage.[27]

Other Molecular Targets

In addition to potassium channel modulators, the companies AudioCure Pharma, Gateway Biotechnology, and Pragma Therapeutics are pursuing different mechanisms of action for early stage programs listed as targeting the development of therapeutics for tinnitus.

AC-102, developed by AudioCure Pharma is a compound from the beta-carboline family suggested to have protective and/or reparative properties against inner ear cellular damage through the upregulation of neurotrophic factor expression and the enhancement of neurite extension.[27,53] Although AC-102 is listed as being in development either broadly for hearing disorders in general or specifically for hearing loss or tinnitus, it seems from the company's description of its mechanisms of action that it acts on inner and outer hair cells, as well as on spiral ganglion neurons, to "protect them from further damage or restore already damaged cells."[54] Thus, the potential effect on tinnitus would likely be indirect through the reduction of auditory deficits. No data have been published in either hearing loss or tinnitus models; however, the interpretation of the mechanism of action as being mainly otoprotective is supported by the orphan drug designation granted by the European Medicines Agency for AC-102 for the treatment of sudden sensorineural hearing loss.[55]

GateWay Biotechnology is developing GW-201 for the treatment of tinnitus.[27,56] Although the mechanism of action is undisclosed, the compound in question is presumably the T-type calcium channel blocker tetrandrine, which also demonstrates antioxidant and immunomodulating properties.[27,57] After systemic administration, GW-102 demonstrated dose-dependent reduction of tinnituslike behaviors in both salicylate- and noise-induced tinnitus models using a sound-based avoidance detection paradigm. As is the case for AC-102 from AudioCure Pharma, GW-201 also demonstrated otoprotective properties and, as the timing of administration relative to salicylate- or noise-induction of tinnitus is not clearly reported, it is again unclear whether treatment effects on tinnitus symptoms are direct or rather an indirect consequence of otoprotection.[57]

The preclinical stage development program from Pragma Therapeutics targets the metabotropic glutamate receptor mGluR7.[26,27] Metabotropic glutamate receptors are expressed throughout peripheral and central auditory structures and have been implicated in controlling both peripheral and central auditory spontaneous activities.[58–60] Specific alleles of the *GRM7* gene encoding the mGluR7 receptor were suggested to be associated with tinnitus severity in an aging Portuguese population.[61] The company Website does not explicitly list tinnitus as a target indication but focuses on hearing loss and posttraumatic stress disorder.[62] Similarly, recent presentations of data around the negative allosteric mGluR7 modulator PGT-117 have focused uniquely on otoprotective properties after oral administration in a rodent model of acute acoustic trauma.[63] Thus, as for AC-102 (AudioCure Pharma) and GW-201 (Gateway Biotechnology), it is unclear whether Pragma Therapeutics are targeting a direct treatment effect on tinnitus through mGluR7 modulation or an indirect effect through otoprotection potentially combined with reduction of tinnitus-associated stress and anxiety.

DISCUSSION

Despite the recent negative late clinical stage results communicated by Auris Medical (AM-101) and Autifony Therapeutics (AUT-00063), several diverse clinical and preclinical development programs for the treatment of tinnitus are still active. Notably, despite both companies suffering late-stage failures in the clinic, neither has been sufficiently discouraged to abandon the therapeutic field and are either revising the clinical trial design or developing new chemical entities for the same target. Overall, this is positive news for patients with an unmet and debilitating medical need and as well for clinicians who care for them. Nonetheless based on the experience in the field to date, several conclusions can be drawn that caution patience.

The lack of translationally and clinically validated endpoints for clinical trials noted in recent reviews[6,64] is clearly hampering progress, in terms of both preclinical selection and characterization of drug candidates, as well as the ability to evaluate efficacy at the clinical level. Preclinically, tinnitus-like symptoms and cellular/network level activity in animal models are evaluated by methods ranging from single-unit electrophysiology over GPIAS reflex testing to sound-associated avoidance or reward paradigms.[65] Notably, none of these clearly evaluate the actual presence of subjectively experienced sound, reported as the root of all comorbidities for patients with tinnitus. Conversely, these preclinical paradigms are generally more objective and (semi-) quantitative than clinical level assessments of tinnitus, which is generally based on subjective questionnaires, rating scales, and psychoacoustic tests with questions around sensitivity.[66] These clinical measures are based on diagnostic tests and are not yet well established as clinical trial endpoints for evaluating treatment-related effects. Combined with the frequent inclusion of patients with highly variable tinnitus subtypes/causes in the clinical trial populations, which may respond differently to the tested drug candidate and have heterogeneous comorbidities affecting questionnaire and rating scale scores, the lack of sensitivity and interindividual variabilities renders clinical evaluation of treatment-induced change complex. Evidence for this can be seen throughout the clinical development program of AM-101, with changes in patient populations, primary clinical trial endpoints, and etiologic subtype analysis as a function of knowledge gained from previous and ongoing clinical trials. Ideally, quantitative, objective pharmacodynamic clinical endpoints will be developed, along with well-correlated patient-reported outcomes such as questionnaires and rating scales. Such measures could then be back-translated to the preclinical setting and used to robustly select characterize drug candidates ahead of clinical testing, thus reducing the difficulties in evaluating clinical efficacy due to potential lack of relevant mechanisms of action or semiarbitrary selection of doses to test. This would furthermore allow us to solidify and validate preclinical animal models of tinnitus, as well as facilitate preclinical and clinical trial designs in terms of optimal timing of efficacy evaluations.

Several preclinical stage development programs have emerged, targeting modulation of potassium channels, initially based as a relevant target and mechanism of action for other pathologies involving neural hyperactivity and hypersynchrony, such as spasticity in multiple sclerosis and epilepsy.[41,67] Because of the diversity of potassium channels, this rationale remains strong despite clinical stage failures such as AUT-00063 targeting Kv3.1 channels (Autifony Therapeutics) in phase 2 studies[52] and SF0034 targeting KCNQ2/3 channels (SciFluor Life Sciences) in a phase 1 context,[68] particularly because the latter program was terminated due to a metabolic safety signal likely to be compound specific and not target specific.[27] These approaches typically target oral administration with general systemic drug exposure and are likely to be relevant for chronic types of tinnitus, which may involve both the inner ear and central auditory structures.[38]

Contrary to programs targeting modulation of potassium channels, most of the active drug development programs in tinnitus seem to target early stage tinnitus where peripheral mechanisms in the cochlea are likely to play the largest role after damage, before central auditory plasticity responses dominate.[38] Current clinical stage programs from both Auris Medical and Otonomy are based on NMDA receptor antagonism with local intratympanic delivery to the cochlea, thus targeting early stage, peripheral excitotoxic hyperactivity/damage mechanisms following various types of hearing loss. Similarly, the development programs of AudioCure Pharma, Gateway Biotechnology, and Pragma Therapeutics seem to predominantly target otoprotection through different mechanisms. Although the mGluR7 antagonism approach of Pragma Therapeutics uses oral administration to target central CNS structures and has demonstrated protective effects on central auditory structures in acoustic trauma models,[67] reported experiments have so far been carried out with drug administration early after insult and no effects have been reported on tinnituslike symptoms in what could be considered chronic/centralized tinnitus models.

Taken together, this suggests that the patients with tinnitus most likely to benefit from the first targeted treatments to emerge will be those at early stage after onset, still likely having a major cochlear component, whereas treatment of chronic tinnitus may be further away on therapeutic horizon. Such treatments could, to some extent, be classified as "tinnitus preventive" or "otoprotective" as opposed to treatment of established and/or chronic tinnitus. With this in mind, patients and clinicians alike would be well advised to also be aware of the much larger number of active otoprotective and hearing reparative/restorative development programs (recently reviewed by Schilder and colleagues,[26] 2019), attempting to reduce the sensorineural hearing loss generally considered a trigger for subjective tinnitus.

The current limited drug pipeline for the treatment of tinnitus also urges for research programs aimed at increasing fundamental knowledge on the mechanisms involved in tinnitus.[64] This can involve preclinical research, which is often more hypothesis driven, as exemplified by recent findings showing the involvement of neuroinflammation in the auditory cortex of mice with noise-induced tinnitus.[69] Complementary to this, data-driven clinical research may also help identify new drug targets that can be back-translated and validated in animal models.[70] This could potentially involve large-scale genetic studies such as genome-wide association studies, in light of recent evidence in twins and adoptees that tinnitus is influenced by genetics.[71,72] Given the importance of human genetic studies in increasing the likelihood of success in clinical trials,[73,74] genetic studies in humans will be indispensable along the route toward effective drug treatments of tinnitus.

DISCLOSURE

J. Dyhrfjeld-Johnsen is an employee of Sensorion and has stock options in the company.

REFERENCES

1. Langguth B, Kreuzer PM, Kleinjung T, et al. Tinnitus: causes and clinical management. Lancet Neurol 2013;12(9):920–30.
2. Cima RFF, Maes IH, Joore MA, et al. Specialised treatment based on cognitive behaviour therapy versus usual care for tinnitus: a randomised controlled trial. Lancet 2012;379(9830):1951–9.
3. Cima RFF, Mazurek B, Haider H, et al. A multidisciplinary European guideline for tinnitus: diagnostics, assessment, and treatment. HNO 2019;67(Suppl 1):10–42.
4. Cederroth CR, Canlon B, Langguth B. Hearing loss and tinnitus–are funders and industry listening? Nat Biotechnol 2013;31(11):972–4.
5. Langguth B, Elgoyhen AB, Cederroth CR. Therapeutic approaches to the treatment of tinnitus. Annu Rev PharmacolToxicol 2019;59:291–313.
6. Cederroth CR, Dyhrfjeld-Johnsen J, Langguth B. An update: emerging drugs for tinnitus. ExpertOpinEmergDrugs 2018;23(4):251–60.
7. Israel JM, Connelly JS, McTigue ST, et al. Lidocaine in the treatment of tinnitus aurium.A double-blind study. Arch Otolaryngol 1982;108(8):471–3.
8. Trellakis S, Lautermann J, Lehnerdt G. Lidocaine: neurobiological targets and effects on the auditory system. ProgBrain Res 2007;166:303–22.
9. Cederroth CR, Gallus S, Hall DA, et al. Editorial: towards an understanding of tinnitus heterogeneity. Front AgingNeurosci 2019;11:53.
10. Shore SE, Roberts LE, Langguth B. Maladaptive plasticity in tinnitus–triggers, mechanisms and treatment. Nat Rev Neurol 2016;12(3):150–60.
11. Li S, Kalappa BI, Tzounopoulos T. Noise-induced plasticity of KCNQ2/3 and HCN channels underlies vulnerability and resilience to tinnitus. Elife 2015;4. https://doi.org/10.7554/eLife.07242.
12. Yang S, Weiner BD, Zhang LS, et al. Homeostatic plasticity drives tinnitus perception in an animal model. ProcNatlAcadSci U S A 2011;108(36):14974–9.
13. Chen Y-C, Li X, Liu L, et al. Tinnitus and hyperacusis involve hyperactivity and enhanced connectivity in auditory-limbic-arousal-cerebellar network. Elife 2015;4:e06576.
14. Leaver AM, Renier L, Chevillet MA, et al. Dysregulation of limbic and auditory networks in tinnitus. Neuron 2011;69(1):33–43.
15. Schlee W, Weisz N, Bertrand O, et al. Using auditory steady state responses to outline the functional connectivity in the tinnitus brain. PLoSOne 2008;3(11):e3720.
16. Vanneste S, Song J-J, De Ridder D. Thalamocortical dysrhythmia detected by machine learning. Nat Commun 2018;9(1):1103.
17. Bing D, Lee SC, Campanelli D, et al. Cochlear NMDA receptors as a therapeutic target of noise-induced tinnitus. Cell PhysiolBiochem 2015;35(5):1905–23.
18. Guitton MJ, Caston J, Ruel J, et al. Salicylate induces tinnitus through activation of cochlear NMDA receptors. J Neurosci 2003;23(9):3944–52.
19. Puel JL, Ladrech S, Chabert R, et al. Electrophysiological evidence for the presence of NMDA receptors in the guinea pig cochlea. Hear Res 1991;51(2):255–64.
20. Ehrenberger K, Felix D. Glutamate receptors in afferent cochlear neurotransmission in guinea pigs. Hear Res 1991;52(1):73–80.

21. Lefebvre PP, Weber T, Leprince P, et al. Kainate and NMDA toxicity for cultured developing and adult rat spiral ganglion neurons: further evidence for a glutamatergic excitatory neurotransmission at the inner hair cell synapse. Brain Res 1991; 555(1):75–83.
22. Pujol R, Puel JL, Eybalin M. Implication of non-NMDA and NMDA receptors in cochlear ischemia. Neuroreport 1992;3(4):299–302.
23. Puel JL, Pujol R, Tribillac F, et al. Excitatory amino acid antagonists protect cochlear auditory neurons from excitotoxicity. J Comp Neurol 1994;341(2): 241–56.
24. Pujol R, Puel JL, Gervaisd'Aldin C, et al. Pathophysiology of the glutamatergic synapses in the cochlea. ActaOtolaryngol 1993;113(3):330–4.
25. Guitton MJ, Dudai Y. Blockade of cochlear NMDA receptors prevents long-term tinnitus during a brief consolidation window after acoustic trauma. NeuralPlast 2007;2007:80904.
26. Schilder AGM, Su MP, Blackshaw H, et al. Hearing protection, restoration, and regeneration: an overview of emerging therapeutics for inner ear and central hearing disorders. OtolNeurotol 2019;40(5):559–70.
27. GlobalData. Available at: https://www.globaldata.com/. Accessed December 18, 2019.
28. EudraCT Number 2006-002692-41 - Clinical trial results - EU Clinical Trials Register. Available at: https://www.clinicaltrialsregister.eu/ctr-search/trial/2006-002692-41/results. Accessed December 18, 2019.
29. van de Heyning P, Muehlmeier G, Cox T, et al. Efficacy and safety of AM-101 in the treatment of acute inner ear tinnitus–a double-blind, randomized, placebo-controlled phase II study. OtolNeurotol 2014;35(4):589–97.
30. Staecker H, Maxwell KS, Morris JR, et al. Selecting appropriate dose regimens for AM-101 in the intratympanic treatment of acute inner ear tinnitus. AudiolNeurootol 2015;20(3):172–82.
31. Staecker H, Morelock M, Kramer T, et al. Safety of repeated-dose intratympanic injections with AM-101 in acute inner ear tinnitus. OtolaryngolHeadNeck Surg 2017;157(3):478–87.
32. Auris Medical. Innovative treatments for inner ear disorders.Keyzilen TM program update 2016. Available at:https://ir.aurismedical.com/static-files/3242fda3-4830-4b34-aabf-98c725b1cc5e. Accessed November 1, 2019.
33. Press release. Auris Medical Provides Business Update. Available at: https://ir.aurismedical.com/news-releases/news-release-details/auris-medical-provides-business-update. Accessed November 1, 2019.
34. Press Release. Auris medical provides update on tinnitus drug development strategy. Auris Medical Holding Ltd.. Available at: https://ir.aurismedical.com/news-releases/news-release-details/auris-medical-provides-update-tinnitus-drug-development-strategy. Accessed November 1, 2019.
35. Press release. Otonomy Provides Corporate and Product Pipeline Update. Available at: https://investors.otonomy.com/news-releases/news-release-details/otonomy-provides-corporate-and-product-pipeline-update-2. Accessed November 1, 2019.
36. Wenzel GI, Warnecke A, Stöver T, et al. Effects of extracochleargacyclidine perfusion on tinnitus in humans: a case series. Eur Arch Otorhinolaryngol 2010;267(5): 691–9.
37. Press Release. Otonomy Reports First Quarter 2017 Financial Results and Provides Corporate Update. Available at: https://investors.otonomy.com/news-releases/news-release-details/otonomy-reports-first-quarter-2017-financial-results-and. Accessed November 1, 2019.

38. Noreña AJ. Revisiting the cochlear and central mechanisms of tinnitus and therapeutic approaches. AudiolNeurootol 2015;20(Suppl 1):53–9.
39. Noreña AJ, Farley BJ. Tinnitus-related neural activity: theories of generation, propagation, and centralization. Hear Res 2013;295:161–71.
40. Humphries ESA, Dart C. Neuronal and cardiovascular potassium channels as therapeutic drug targets: promise and pitfalls. J Biomol Screen 2015;20(9):1055–73.
41. Baker D, Pryce G, Visintin C, et al. Big conductance calcium-activated potassium channel openers control spasticity without sedation. Br J Pharmacol 2017;174(16):2662–81.
42. Farrell R, Selwood D, Baker D, CanbexVSN16R Spasticity Study Group. P1797 - Results from a phase II proof of concept trial of VSN16R to treat multiple sclerosis related spasticity. 34th Congres of the European Committee for Treatment and Research in Multiple Sclerosis. 10-12 October 2018. Berlin. Germany. Available at: http://www.professionalabstracts.com/ectrims2018/iplanner/#/presentation/2371. Accessed December 20, 2019.
43. Tabatabaee S, Baker D, Selwood DL, et al. The cannabinoid-like compound, VSN16R, acts on large conductance, Ca2+-activated K+ channels to modulate hippocampal CA1pyramidal neuron firing. Pharmaceuticals (Basel) 2019;12(3). https://doi.org/10.3390/ph12030104.
44. Wu C, V Gopal K, Lukas TJ, et al. Pharmacodynamics of potassium channel openers in cultured neuronal networks. Eur J Pharmacol 2014;732:68–75.
45. Knopp Biosciences.Pursuing novel drug treatments. Available at: https://knoppbio.com/pipeline. Accessed December, 2019.
46. Li S, Choi V, Tzounopoulos T. Pathogenic plasticity of Kv7.2/3 channel activity is essential for the induction of tinnitus. ProcNatlAcadSci U S A 2013;110(24):9980–5.
47. Lobarinas E, Dalby-Brown W, Stolzberg D, et al. Effects of the potassium ion channel modulators BMS-204352 Maxipost and its R-enantiomer on salicylate-induced tinnitus in rats. PhysiolBehav 2011;104(5):873–9.
48. Sheppard AM, Chen G-D, Salvi R. Potassium ion channel openers, Maxipost and Retigabine, protect against peripheral salicylate ototoxicity in rats. Hear Res 2015;327:1–8.
49. Chambers AR, Pilati N, Balaram P, et al. Pharmacological modulation of Kv3.1 mitigates auditory midbrain temporal processing deficits following auditory nerve damage. Sci Rep 2017;7(1):17496.
50. Anderson LA, Hesse LL, Pilati N, et al. Increased spontaneous firing rates in auditory midbrain following noise exposure are specifically abolished by a Kv3 channel modulator. Hear Res 2018;365:77–89.
51. Glait L, Fan W, Stillitano G, et al. Effects of AUT00063, a Kv3.1 channel modulator, on noise-induced hyperactivity in the dorsal cochlear nucleus. Hear Res 2018;361:36–44.
52. Hall DA, Ray J, Watson J, et al. A balanced randomised placebo controlled blinded phase IIa multi-centre study to investigate the efficacy and safety of AUT00063 versus placebo in subjective tinnitus: The QUIET-1 trial. Hear Res 2019;377:153–66.
53. Patent. Beta-carbolines for use in the treatment of hearing loss and vertigo.US20130028958A1. Available at: https://patents.google.com/patent/US20130028958. Accessed November 1, 2019.
54. AudioCurePharma. Our technology: AC102. Available at: https://www.audiocure.com/our-technology/ac102/. Accessed November 1, 2019.

55. Press Release. AudioCurePharma'sAC102 receives EMAorphan drug designation for the treatment of sudden sensorineural hearing loss (SSNHL). Available at: https://www.audiocure.com/wp-content/uploads/2019/01/AudioCure_PressRelease_20190129_AC102_receives_EMA_orphan_drug.pdf. Accessed November 1, 2019.

56. Gateway Biotechnology Inc. Product pipelines. Available at: http://www.gatewaybiotechnology.com/#team-skills. Accessed November 1, 2019.

57. Patent. Methods and compositions for treating hearing disorders.US10434097B1. Available at: https://patents.google.com/patent/US10434097B1/en. Accessed November 1, 2019.

58. Galazyuk AV, Longenecker RJ, Voytenko SV, et al. Residual inhibition: From the putative mechanisms to potential tinnitus treatment. Hear Res 2019;375:1–13.

59. Lu Y. Metabotropic glutamate receptors in auditory processing. Neuroscience 2014;274:429–45.

60. Ye Z, Goutman JD, Pyott SJ, et al. mGluR1 enhances efferent inhibition of inner hair cells in the developing rat cochlea. J Physiol 2017;595(11):3483–95.

61. Haider HF, Flook M, Aparicio M, et al. Biomarkers of presbycusis and tinnitus in a Portuguese older population. Front AgingNeurosci 2017;9:346.

62. Pragma Therapeutics website. Available at: http://pragmatherapeutics.com/. Accessed December 18, 2019.

63. Amanipour R, Zhu X, Ding B, et al. Preclinical evaluation of a novel mGluR7 negative allosteric modulator in a noise-induced hearing loss mouse model.-Poster 060.13.Society for Neuroscience Annual Meeting, October 19-23, 2019. Available at: https://eventpilotadmin.com/web/page.php?page=Session&project=SFN19&id=P44568. Accessed December 18, 2019.

64. McFerran DJ, Stockdale D, Holme R, et al. Why is there no cure for tinnitus? Front Neurosci 2019;13:802.

65. von der Behrens W. Animal models of subjective tinnitus. NeuralPlast 2014;2014:741452.

66. Hall DA, Haider H, Szczepek AJ, et al. Systematic review of outcome domains and instruments used in clinical trials of tinnitus treatments in adults. Trials 2016;17(1):270.

67. N'Gouemo P. BKCa channel dysfunction in neurological diseases. Front Physiol 2014;5:373.

68. Kalappa BI, Soh H, Duignan KM, et al. Potent KCNQ2/3-specific channel activator suppresses in vivo epileptic activity and prevents the development of tinnitus. J Neurosci 2015;35(23):8829–42.

69. Wang W, Zhang LS, Zinsmaier AK, et al. Neuroinflammation mediates noise-induced synaptic imbalance and tinnitus in rodent models. PLoS Biol 2019;17(6):e3000307.

70. Lopez-Escamez JA, Bibas T, Cima RFF, et al. Genetics of tinnitus: an emerging area for molecular diagnosis and drug development. Front Neurosci 2016;10:377.

71. Cederroth CR, PirouziFard M, Trpchevska N, et al. Association of genetic vs environmental factors in swedish adoptees with clinically significant tinnitus. JAMAOtolaryngolHeadNeck Surg 2019;145(3):222–9.

72. Maas IL, Brüggemann P, Requena T, et al. Genetic susceptibility to bilateral tinnitus in a Swedish twin cohort. Genet Med 2017;19(9):1007–12.

73. Cook D, Brown D, Alexander R, et al. Lessons learned from the fate of AstraZeneca's drug pipeline: a five-dimensional framework. Nat Rev DrugDiscov 2014;13(6):419–31.

74. Morgan P, Brown DG, Lennard S, et al. Impact of a five-dimensional framework on R&D productivity at AstraZeneca. Nat Rev DrugDiscov 2018;17(3):167–81.

Avenue for Future Tinnitus Treatments

Tobias Kleinjung, MD[a],*, Berthold Langguth, MD[b]

KEYWORDS

- Tinnitus • Neuromodulation • Novel approaches • Tinnitus pathophysiology
- Tinnitus models

KEY POINTS

- Current challenges in the development of new treatments for tinnitus.
- Neuromodulation approaches for tinnitus treatment.
- New drug targets for tinnitus treatment.
- The importance of clinical tinnitus databases.
- Lack of funding in tinnitus research.

INTRODUCTION

With prevalence rates of 10% to 20% of the population, tinnitus represents a major global burden.[1,2] Tinnitus prevalence grows with age and has increased in the past decades,[3] presumably owing to an increased exposure to loud sounds. Although most patients can cope adequately with their tinnitus, nearly 1 out of 10 (ie, in 2%–3% of the total population) experiences severe tinnitus[4] that can be accompanied by frustration, annoyance, anxiety, depression, cognitive dysfunction, insomnia, stress, and emotional exhaustion—all of which lead to a substantial decrease in quality of life[5,6] and an enormous socioeconomic burden.[7]

The available treatment options for tinnitus are limited. Cognitive behavioral therapy (CBT) is helpful for reducing tinnitus annoyance and tinnitus handicap, but there exists no established treatment that has shown evidence in randomized controlled studies to reduce tinnitus loudness. Thus, given the high prevalence and the enormous socioeconomic relevance, there is an urgent need to develop better treatment options for tinnitus.

This article first provides a short overview about recent advances in the understanding of the pathophysiology of tinnitus, because this provides the basis for the

a Department of Otorhinolaryngology and Head and Neck Surgery, University Hospital Zurich, University of Zurich, Frauenklinikstrasse 24, Zurich CH 8091, Switzerland; b Department of Psychiatry and Psychotherapy, Interdisciplinary Tinnitus Center, University of Regensburg, Universitätsstrasse 84, Regensburg D 93053, Germany
* Corresponding author.
E-mail address: tobias.kleinjung@usz.ch

Otolaryngol Clin N Am 53 (2020) 667–683
https://doi.org/10.1016/j.otc.2020.03.013
0030-6665/20/© 2020 The Authors. Published by Elsevier Inc. This is an open access article under the CC BY-NC-ND license (http://creativecommons.org/licenses/by-nc-nd/4.0/).

development of new treatments. There exist several challenges in the development of new treatments, and how these can be addressed is discussed. Then, current research activities in neuromodulation, auditory treatments, pharmacotherapy, eHealth, and patient involvement are summarized before what might be needed to attract more private and public funding in the tinnitus field is discussed.

CURRENT KNOWLEDGE OF THE PATHOPHYSIOLOGY OF TINNITUS

In recent decades, knowledge about the pathogenesis of tinnitus has increased massively. Although there is no complete consensus among experts, the dominant opinion is that tinnitus is preceded by peripheral hearing loss. Often the affected person describes a hearing sensation that lies in a frequency range that is congruent with the frequency range of the hearing loss.[8] After peripheral hearing loss due to partial damage of the hair cells in the inner ear, the transmission of stimuli from the cochlea to the auditory cortex in the brain is interrupted.[9] Because of this sensory deprivation, an increased synchronicity of the spontaneous activity of the neurons in the auditory cortex, which represents the corresponding frequency ranges, is observed.[10] A weakening of the intracortical balance of excitation and inhibition leads to a reorganization of the architecture of the auditory cortex, resulting in new ensembles of nerve cells that have changed their frequency specificity.[11] If the synchronous activity of these nerve cell clusters continues undiminished for some time, the affected persons may perceive an ear noise with different characteristics and variable loudness and duration. Whether this maladaptive phenomenon leads to tinnitus perception at all and to what extent it is pronounced in terms of personal aversiveness, loudness, or accompanying symptoms, such as sleep disorders, anxiety, panic, and stress, depend on coactivation of nonauditory brain networks.[12,13] These networks include limbic, insular, parahippocampal, frontal, and parietal structures.[14] In the context of this more generally formulated idea on the pathogenesis of tinnitus, several models exist that give more or less weight to certain aspects of network theory.[11,15–17] These are not discussed in detail. It must be seen as a decisive moment of the modern models for the genesis of tinnitus that it is no longer the periphery with the ear structures or the auditory nerve that is in the foreground but the neuroplastic changes in central nervous structures that occur as a consequence of peripheral deafferentation. Furthermore, it has been shown that neural connections between the auditory and somatosensory systems located at the dorsal cochlear nucleus play a role in tinnitus perception as well.[18] In particular, the ability of some affected individuals to modulate the tinnitus sound through somatic maneuvers is at stake.

All these new insights have changed the focus with regard to potential therapies. For 2 decades, methods have been under discussion in research, which take into account the central aspects of tinnitus genesis, such as neuromodulation, the neural connections between the somatosensory and auditory systems, and pharmacotherapy of centrally acting neurotransmitters.

CURRENT CHALLENGES IN THE DEVELOPMENT OF NEW TREATMENTS

Based on current knowledge, that tinnitus results from functional changes of neuronal activity, there exists no reason to believe that tinnitus cannot be efficiently treated either by neuromodulation or by pharmacotherapy. But why do effective treatments for tinnitus not exist?

There are several reasons that can explain why the development of effective treatments for tinnitus is so difficult.[19]

From a historical perspective, the development of treatments for brain disorders was driven by serendipitous discoveries. Apart from lidocaine, such serendipitous discoveries are lacking in the tinnitus field, and lidocaine cannot be applied regularly because of its side effects nor can other drugs with a comparable effect be identified. Moreover, because no exact drug target is known that reliably reduces tinnitus, there also do not exist in vitro bioassays for high-throughput screening of pharmacologic compounds.[20]

Animal models have been developed but have limitations.[21] Further challenges for the development of new compounds are the heterogeneity of tinnitus and its subjective nature, which make tinnitus assessment difficult.

Limitations of Available Animal Models of Tinnitus

For the development of a valid animal model of tinnitus, it is necessary to develop methods for both reliable tinnitus induction and assessment. Two different approaches are used to generate tinnitus: first, the systemic administration of ototoxic drugs, such as salicylate or quinine; and second, the exposure to loud noise. These two methods induce tinnitus via different mechanisms, with the latter probably more similar to the clinical situation.

Assessment of tinnitus typically has been performed indirectly by measuring behavioral reactions to silence. These behavioral tests require months to train the animals and, to circumvent this problem, another animal model of tinnitus exploits the acoustic startle response, which is based on an objective reflex response that does not require lengthy training sessions.[22] The magnitude of the startle reflex in response to, for example, a loud sound, is reduced when the startling stimulus is preceded by a silent gap in an otherwise continuous acoustic background. In animals that are noise-traumatized or salicylate-treated, the inhibition of the startle reflex by the gap is reduced and this is interpreted as an indication of tinnitus. What exactly is assessed by these behavioral tests and what modulates the startle response, however, are matters of debate. The magnitude of the startle response itself can be influenced by hearing loss, hyperacusis, and anxiety. The degree of inhibition caused by gaps also varies considerably between rodent species. Nevertheless, among animals that all have been exposed to a similar noise trauma, those that demonstrate behavioral evidence of tinnitus, as assessed with the Gap-Prepulse Inhibition of the Acoustic Startle Reflex, show consistent neurophysiologic alterations compared with those that do not.[18] An additional challenge to the use of tinnitus animal models is that, in humans, the phantom sound frequently is accompanied by emotional and cognitive symptoms,[14,23] which still are not recapitulated in available animal models.[24,25]

Challenges in Translating Animal Findings to Humans

The usefulness of available animal models for testing tinnitus treatments is still a matter of debate, because some treatments, which were successful in animal studies, failed to show positive effects in humans. For instance, carbamazepine seems to be efficacious in rats[26] but not in humans,[27] and the same is true for ginkgo biloba.[28] An enriched acoustic environment seems to ameliorate tinnitus in animals[29] but not as much in humans.[30] The reported discrepancies between the results from animal models and human treatment studies do not necessarily mean that animal models of tinnitus have no predictive value, because inconsistencies also may be related to limitations in both animal and human studies (eg, methodology, outcome measure, etiology, comorbidities, time and duration of the treatment, and sample size). Caution is warranted, however, in the direct translation of tinnitus animal research to humans, especially research into novel treatments.

Tinnitus Heterogeneity

Tinnitus differs across patients in its perceptual characteristics (eg, frequency and intensity), in its time course (constant, fluctuating, and intermittent), response to interventions (eg, masking sounds and somatic maneuvers), etiologic factors, and comorbidities. This heterogeneity of tinnitus is reflected by a substantial variability in tinnitus pathophysiology.[13] This means that probably many different forms of tinnitus exist, which vary in their pathophysiology and their response to a specific treatment intervention. If patients with different subtypes are included in a clinical trial, a high variability in the treatment outcome has to be expected. Therefore, a major challenge in clinical tinnitus research is the identification of reliable subtypes or the identification of relevant criteria for subtyping patients.[31,32] One approach is the development of large clinical databases for disentangling subgroups of tinnitus.[33]

Measurement of Tinnitus in Humans

Outcome measurement in clinical trials is complicated by the fact that tinnitus is a purely subjective phenomenon, for which objective measurements are still missing.

A further difficulty is that perceptual aspects of tinnitus (eg, loudness) do not explain the subjectively perceived severity of the symptom. Thus, a comprehensive evaluation of tinnitus has to include the assessment of both perceptual aspects of tinnitus (eg, loudness and pitch) and of subjective tinnitus severity (eg, tinnitus related functional impairment or tinnitus handicap). Perceptual aspects can be assessed by psychoacoustic methods and subjective rating scales (eg, visual analog scales or numeric rating scales); tinnitus impairment can be quantified by various validated questionnaires.[34,35] Because the different measurements provide complementary information, current best practice is the use of several outcome measurements in parallel for the evaluation of treatment-induced changes.[36–38] A recent analysis revealed a high variability in the outcome instruments used in clinical trials,[35] indicating the need to standardize outcome measurement.[36,39,40] This is important particularly because regulatory agencies, such as the Food and Drug Administration (FDA) or European Medicines Agency lack standardized protocols for their approval process.

NEUROMODULATION

As a consequence of the models for the pathogenesis of tinnitus, described previously, it seems reasonable to consider a modification of neuronal activity in the areas of the brain involved in the neuronal circuits responsible for tinnitus. In this way, both auditory and nonauditory areas can be reached. Essentially, a distinction is made between invasive and noninvasive neuromodulation. The aim of any method is to normalize the tinnitus-related brain activity. The increasing improvement of structural and functional neuroimaging techniques made it possible to more precisely target those areas of the brain that are mainly responsible for tinnitus perception or the tinnitus-related distress. Over the past 2 decades, many different methods of neuromodulation have been evaluated for their effectiveness in tinnitus control. Noninvasive methods included repetitive transcranial magnetic stimulation,[41–43] transcranial electric stimulation,[44–46] transcutaneous electric nerve stimulation,[47,48] and neurofeedback.[49–51] All techniques have been tested at different institutions and with different approaches in various studies.[52] In the meantime, standardized reviews for the individual techniques are available.[45,53,54] It could be shown that the targeted neuromodulation of brain activity leads in certain cases to a reduction of tinnitus or tinnitus-related complaints.The data regarding long-term effects and complete elimination of tinnitus by noninvasive neuromodulation have not been achieved. Thus, all of these techniques are experimental at this time.[52] In this context, it seems of great importance to make further progress in the better phenotyping of tinnitus and to better understand which changes in the neuronal networks are the most important in individual cases. The general trend in noninvasive neuromodulation certainly is also in the direction of simplifying procedures. Therefore, strategies that could be carried out by those affected without dependence on complex equipment or a clinical institution, for example, at home, also are regarded as ideal procedures. First experiments with mobile electroencephalogram systems will focus on, in particular, neurofeedback or transcranial electric stimulation and transcutaneous electric nerve stimulation procedures for the future.[55,56]

Invasive neuromodulation procedures involve implanting electrodes extradurally (epidural), cortically (subdural), or for deep brain stimulation.[57] These procedures were applied experimentally in tinnitus patients, or had effects on tinnitus in patients undergoing deep brain stimulation for treatment of movement disorders (eg, Parkinson disease).[58–62] In particular, with regard to deep brain stimulation of the auditory system (inferior colliculus and medial geniculate body), animal studies currently are under way to evaluate the significance of direct electrostimulation of the structures, described previously.[63–65] Case reports exist on the use of brain stem implants in humans, suggesting a positive effect on tinnitus-related complaints.[66,67] Due to the significantly greater invasiveness, the data on invasive neuromodulation are limited.. Nevertheless, there also are reviews that attempt to evaluate the previous studies as a whole.[52,68] The quality of the studies, however, which generally do not exceed the level of case reports or case series, does not permit a final evaluation at this point in time. The significant invasiveness of the procedures, however, in conjunction with a considerable side-effect profile, suggest that such procedures will be considered for only a very small subgroup of tinnitus patients in the future, if at all.[69]

In this context of invasive neuromodulation techniques, two procedures that directly stimulate nerve structures through implanted electrodes, cochlear implantation and vagus nerve stimulation, should be discussed. In particular, cochlear implantation is a routine procedure that is used for bilateral and now also single-sided deafness. Multiple studies and reviews have shown that cochlear implantation not only improves hearing but also reduces tinnitus perception in the recipients.[70,71] The high suppression rates of tinnitus when the implant is switched on must be interpreted as an outstanding tinnitus therapy that can certainly surpass the effect of standard procedures. The indication reduced to severe hearing loss and deafness is considered a limitation. This success suggests, however, that electric stimulation of peripheral auditory structures can improve tinnitus. The exact mechanism of action has not yet been clarified. Tinnitus suppression might be discussed as a direct effect of electric stimulation or as an indirect consequence in the sense of masking with improved hearing. For future scientific approaches, this represents an approach that already has been applied in experimental form to single subjects with tinnitus who have normal hearing in the sense of stimulation of the external auditory canal, the promotorium, or the round window.[72,73] There is great potential for future studies. Because vagus nerve stimulation in tinnitus is applied in clinical studies in terms of bimodal or multimodal stimulation, it is discussed subsequently in more detail.

SOMATOSENSORY STIMULATION

An interaction between the auditory and somatosensory system has been demonstrated on different levels. Auditory and somatosensory input converges already at the level of the dorsal cochlear nucleus.[18] Further interactions occur at higher brain levels.[74] Clinical reflections of these interactions are the onset of tinnitus after neck trauma,[75] the comorbidity of tinnitus with neck pain and temporomandibular disorder,[76] and the observation that tinnitus can be modulated by head or neck movements in a majority of cases.[77]

These phenomena are summarized by the term, *somatosensory tinnitus*, but it is important to note that this term does not describe a clearly defined subtype of tinnitus but rather the degree of involvement of the somatosensory system in an individual's tinnitus. Therefore, somatosensory tinnitus should be viewed as a dimensional rather than categorical term.[78]

The involvement of the somatosensory system is the basis for several treatment approaches. First, if there exist pathologies in the neck area or in the temporomandibular system, they should be treated, because a normalization of these pathologies can improve tinnitus.[79] Second, treatments, such as transcutaneous electrical stimulation,[80] acupuncture, neural therapy, and muscle relaxation,[81] have shown promising results in subgroups of patients.

BIMODAL OR MULTIMODAL STIMULATION

Bimodal or multimodal stimulation presumably is more effective for the induction of neuroplastic effects than unimodal stimulation. Recently, different approaches of bimodal or multimodal stimulation have been proposed for the treatment of tinnitus.

A combination of auditory stimulation with vagal stimulation has demonstrated highly impressive results in an animal model of tinnitus.[82] Based on the rationale that vagal stimulation renders the simultaneously presented sounds more salient, the combined treatment almost completely reversed neurophysiologic and behavioral signs of tinnitus, which was not the case with auditory stimulation alone. In subsequent human pilot studies, the efficacy of the treatment could be confirmed albeit the effects were clearly less pronounced than in animals.[83]

Another approach explored transcranial direct current stimulation of cortical areas to facilitate the effects of masking sounds and notched music with only limited success.[84,85]

In a recent pilot study, a combination of sounds with transcutaneous electrical stimulation to the neck or the temporomandibular area yielded impressive results. The somatosensory and auditory stimuli were presented at specific intervals that were derived from basic neurophysiologic studies describing stimulus timing–dependent plasticity in the dorsal cochlear nucleus.[86]

A combined application of sounds and electrical stimulation of the tongue was investigated in 2 large trials with results not yet published.[87,88] Simultaneous application of sounds and electrical stimulation of the tongue afferents may reduce tinnitus by providing a compensatory input to the partly deafferented central auditory system.

CLINICAL DATABASES

A major limitation with regard to finding a causal therapy for tinnitus lies in the heterogeneity of the symptom.[32] Thus, the phenomenon of therapeutic procedures that help 1 person but do not work for others reflects a repeated finding. Therefore, it is a great challenge for a therapist to find out which is the most promising procedure for a specific patient. Unfortunately, there are no reliable clinical predictors for most procedures that could predict the success of a therapy from the outset. An additional complicating factor is that most studies evaluating a specific method to improve tinnitus involve only a small number of cases. The comparability between studies is hampered by different methods in tinnitus assessment and in the determination of therapy outcome. Thus, most standardized reviews come to the conclusion that a concrete statement on the value of a therapy is difficult or that the quality of the data is so limited that certain approaches cannot be recommended.[19]

In order to address these shortcomings, it makes sense that generally accepted methodological measures are taken into account in studies to improve the comparability of the studies afterward. One possibility is that there would be international databases in which both data on tinnitus assessment and data on responsiveness to certain therapies would be entered according to the same pattern. An attempt in this respect is the database of the Tinnitus Research Initiative.[33] The database is open to all interested therapists and scientists who are willing to contribute patient data according to the guidelines. After corresponding consensus conferences,[36] it was agreed that certain guidelines should be followed when entering data, such as the primary tinnitus assessment, using a standardized case report form, or a standardized recording of the success of therapy. In addition, data on hearing ability (pure tone audiometry), tinnitus matching, or tinnitus severity can be entered according to questionnaires validated in different languages. This project, established in 2008, currently comprises more than 4000 data sets on tinnitus patients from more than 10 different countries (https://www.tinnitusresearch.net/index.php/for-clinicians/database). In this way it is possible to improve the subtyping of tinnitus by cluster analyses, to identify subgroups that could respond particularly well to certain treatments, to answer epidemiologic questions, or to improve the statistical power for certain questions by pooling data. Such projects are indispensable for future genetic research. Legal and data privacy issues have to be considered in such projects. Cooperation within the framework of major research projects financed by the European Union could play an important pioneering role. In the future, it can be assumed that such database projects will represent an important step with regard to personalized medicine in the care of tinnitus patients.

eHealth (APPS AND OTHERS)

eHealth is a highly dynamic research area in medicine and refers to the use of electronic information and communication technologies for health management. In recent years, there has been an increasing interest in eHealth technologies for the support of tinnitus patients. These include tools for patient communication and information, ecological momentary assessment of tinnitus symptoms, smartphone-based auditory treatments, Internet-based CBT (iCBT), serious games, and virtual reality applications. Similar to other medical fields, within a short time a large number of electronic tools have been developed and are offered in app stores. Most of these tools, however, have no regulatory approval and a vast majority are not scientifically evaluated.

Counseling is considered the basis of every tinnitus treatment. A majority of tinnitus patients worldwide, however, do not receive structured counseling according to modern standards. Thus, information about tinnitus and counseling via the Internet or a smartphone app represents a feasible and cost-effective option to reach many tinnitus patients who currently are lacking adequate counseling. An example represents the Tinnitus E-Programme, which is an Internet-based intervention program that consists of mainly educational content (ie, about tinnitus or "the role of psychological mechanisms in tinnitus") and relaxation-focused and attentional-focused exercises.[89] The program has been evaluated and all of the files are accessible for free on a Web site created for this intervention program [http://www.tinnituseprogramme.org/].[90] Several smartphone apps for tinnitus counseling currently are under development.

eHealth tools also have been developed for assisting diagnosis and assessment of tinnitus patients. These include Internet-based hearing tests,[91,92] tinnitus matching tools,[93,94] and tools for ecological momentary assessment.[95,96] Internet-based or app-based hearing tests and tinnitus matching tools aim at offering audiological measurements for tinnitus patients at low cost, easy availability, and sufficient quality. This approach is important especially in the context of therapeutic auditory stimulation, because many innovative auditory stimulation approaches are individualized according to a person's hearing function and tinnitus pitch.

Ecological momentary assessment in contrast opens up a new quality in tinnitus assessment, because it enables to record fluctuations in tinnitus perception and annoyance in real time.[95] This is important because the retrospective assessment of tinnitus fluctuations is only of limited reliability, for example, due to a recall bias. By assessing tinnitus by repeated assessment in normal life conditions, these ecological momentary assessment apps enable real-time assessment of tinnitus fluctuations under normal life conditions. This information can be used for diagnostic purpose, for counseling, and for CBT. Moreover, it represents the basis for the development of a closed-loop system that offers therapeutic interventions exactly at the moment when they are needed or most effective.

iCBT is an approach that delivers CBT via the Internet, either only online-based or in a blended fashion, that integrates face-to-face and online therapy. Available studies have demonstrated that its efficacy is in a similar range to that of conventional CBT. An online version of acceptance and commitment therapy (ACT) for tinnitus has been developed as well.[97] A comparison between Internet-based ACT (iACT), iCBT, and a moderated online discussion forum revealed substantial improvements for both iCBT and iACT, with no significant difference between the 2 treatments.[98]

With technological advances in the development of smartphones, sound therapy is an easily accessible treatment option. There are smartphone applications that claim to reduce tinnitus loudness by the usage of tailor-made notched music (eg, Tinnitracks [www.tinnitracks.com] or Tinnitus Pro: Music Therapy [https://tinnitus-pro-music-therapy-ios.soft112.com]).[99] One study provided the patients with tinnitus masking technologies.[100] The efficacy of none of these approaches has yet been evaluated.

Further eHealth-based approaches that have been proposed are serious games and virtual reality.[101–103]

POTENTIAL NEW DRUG TARGETS

Although many different drugs with different mechanisms of action have been investigated in the past decades, no drug target could be identified for alleviating either tinnitus loudness, tinnitus-related distress, or both. Moreover, because there are no approved drugs for the treatment of tinnitus, there also are no examples of a successful pharmacologic development program that could provide a blueprint for the development of a new compound.

Based on an increasing understanding of the pathophysiology of tinnitus, new potential target structures emerged and several candidate drugs for the treatment of tinnitus have been identified in past years.

Recent clinical research programs that targeted N-methyl-D-aspartate receptor (NMDA) receptors, α-amino-3-hydroxy-5-methyl-4-isoxazolepropionic acid (AMPA) receptors, and potassium channels are summarized.

In animal experiments NMDA receptors have been identified to pay a critical role in the development of salicylate-induced tinnitus.[104,105] These findings formed the basis for the clinical development of the NMDA receptor antagonist Keyzilen (AM-101), esketamine hydrochloride, by Auris Medical (Basel, Switzerland).

The intratympanic delivery of a gel formulation of Keyzilen (AM-101) was investigated in patients with acute tinnitus caused by acoustic trauma, idiopathic sudden sensorineural hearing loss, or otitis media.[106] This phase 2 clinical trial failed to achieve the primary endpoint of improving minimum masking level; however, statistical significant improvement was demonstrated for tinnitus loudness, annoyance, sleep difficulties, and tinnitus impact in the high-dose Keyzilen (AM-101) patient groups with tinnitus after noise trauma or otitis media.[106] Based on these findings, a phase 3 program was initiated, which unfortunately could not confirm the data from the phase 2 trial.[107,108]

Another pharmacologic compound, that has been investigated recently (2011–2012), is BGG492 (selurampanel), which is an orally active AMPA/kainate receptor antagonist.[109] The AMPA receptor has been chosen as target as the main excitatory activity in both cochlea and the central auditory pathways is AMPA mediated.[110] BGG492 was evaluated in patients with moderate to catastrophic chronic subjective tinnitus. After a 2-week treatment with BGG492, significantly greater proportion of patients showed response (improvement of ≥ 4 points from baseline in Tinnitus Beeinträchtigungs Fragebogen (TBF-12), a German short version of the Tinnitus Handicap Inventory) compared with placebo (26.7% vs 14%).[111] Due to an unfavorable side-effect profile, however, BGG492 has not been further developed.

Targeting the central nervous system also has been the focus of AUT00063, a Kv3.1 channel inhibitor. This compound has been investigated in a phase 2a study but was not superior to placebo in reducing the score of the Tinnitus Functional index.[112]

Also, Kv7.2/3, another potassium channel, has been proposed as a potential target for tinnitus treatment. It has been shown that application of the Kv7.2/3 opener retigabine prevents behavioral signs of tinnitus in mice.[113] Retigabine was approved in 2011 by the FDA as an adjunctive treatment of partial epilepsies, but the clinical use of retigabine is limited by its side effects. This may explain why this compound has not yet been investigated in a clinical trial for tinnitus. The promising findings from animal studies and its availability as an approved drug for epilepsy, however, have motivated patients to try this potassium channel modulator for tinnitus treatment. Moreover, some of the patients shared their experiences with this drug via an Internet-based tinnitus forum.[114]

An improved Kv7.2/3 activator, the compound SF0034, has been shown to act more specifically and more potently on Kv7.2/3 channels and to prevent the development of tinnitus in mice after noise trauma.[115] Because SF0034 is less toxic than retigabine, it might represent a candidate for tinnitus treatment with a more favorable side effect profile.

Thus, in summary, four different new drug targets have been explored in recent years. Two studies failed; in 1 case, the development of the compound has not been continued and a further drug has demonstrated promising results in animal studies but has not yet been investigated in humans. This illustrates the difficulty in the development of pharmacologic treatments of tinnitus. A more and more detailed knowledge about the pathophysiology of tinnitus enables the identification of new potential targets for pharmacologic treatment. With the lack of valid preclinical screening methods, however, potential new compounds still have to be tested in human pilot trials. The design of human pilot trials for screening promising compounds is not trivial. First, the definition of inclusion and exclusion criteria is of particular relevance because of the clinical heterogeneity of tinnitus. Second, the correct estimation of the dose range and the duration of the treatment is challenging, especially when knowledge about pharmacokinetics and pharmacodynamics is limited. Third, a sufficiently sensitive instrument for outcome measurement has to be chosen. Therefore, preclinical endpoints with validated translation into clinical application would be highly desirable to improve the risk/benefit balance of preclinical and clinical development of new compounds for tinnitus treatment.

In summary, despite huge advances in pathophysiologic knowledge and research methodology in the past decades, pharmaceutical research in tinnitus still represents a high-risk field. On the other hand, if there were a drug for which a robust effect could be demonstrated, such a drug would have a huge impact on the field, even if the effect were small and occurred only in a subgroup of tinnitus patients.

PATIENT INVOLVEMENT

A recent development in tinnitus research is the increasing involvement of tinnitus patients. Patient representatives were critically involved in recent approaches to identify patient-relevant outcome measurements.[116]

Moreover, patient self-organization via the Internet opens up entire new possibilities compared with traditional patient organizations, because it speeds up interactions between patients, researchers, and clinicians across borders. For example, the Internet-based tinnitus forum (tinnitus talk) reaches many thousand patients; via this forum, patients are informed about newest developments in the field, but they also can contribute to research, by participating in surveys or by providing the database for trend analyses of current hot topics.

Recently, the results of a patient survey from tinnitus talk, with more than 5000 participants, provided the first empirical confirmation that there exist different tinnitus subtypes that vary in their response to different therapeutic interventions.[31]

Finally, in the competition for research money with other research areas, the close and active interaction between researchers and patients is of utmost importance, because patient involvement is an increasingly important requirement at more and more grant agencies.

GRANTS AND FUNDING

Despite the increasing incidence of hearing impairment, funding for research in this area appears to be significantly under-represented compared with other health problems of similar relevance.[117] If searching specifically for the promotion of tinnitus in the complex of hearing disorders, a further imbalance becomes apparent. Obviously, a larger part of the money is spent on research and improvement of technical approaches, such as cochlear implants and hearing aids. In relation to the large number of people affected, too little funding remains for tinnitus. This may be explained to a large extent by the fact that tinnitus is a complex disorder whose exact pathophysiology is not yet clarified in detail and for which there is no causal therapy in most cases. For the pharmaceutical industry, in particular, these facts seem to represent a too great risk for large-scale research campaigns. The few pharmaceutical studies carried out in recent years essentially have been initiated by small companies and have largely ended with a negative result without corresponding marketing approval, so that risk appetite will tend to decline. Other funding opportunities are provided by large self-help institutions, such as the American Tinnitus Association, the British Tinnitus Association, and the UK Action on Hearing Loss Campaign. In recent years, a gradual increase in funding has been recorded by these institutions. The funding provided by state institutions in Europe (German Research Foundation in Germany, Wellcome Trust in the United Kingdom, and Swiss National Science Foundation in Switzerland) appears to be lower than in the United States (eg, National Institute on Deafness and Other Communication Disorders). It can be seen, however, that in the

United States, primarily basic research projects in animal research are funded, whereas in Europe the focus is on clinical research in tinnitus.[117] Thanks to private investors (often suffering from tinnitus themselves), significant progress has been made in recent years. Specific funding programs have improved the networking and collaboration of scientists in the field of tinnitus. This has led to an enormous increase in publications in the field of tinnitus, which in turn has improved public perception by funding institutions. As a result of this development, 2 major projects on tinnitus have been funded by the European Union in recent years, with a total investment of approximately $10 million. Within the Innovative Training Networks, including the European School for Interdisciplinary Tinnitus Research (https://esit.tinnitusresearch.net)[118] and Tinnitus Assessment Causes Treatment [https://tinact.eu/]), 30 PhD students are being trained in tinnitus research. In the future, an important input into tinnitus research in general can be expected from this.

Together, the efforts of recent years have increased the funding volume in tinnitus research. In comparison to the frequency of the symptom and the amount of severely impaired individuals with resulting high socioeconomic burden, however, the investment for research still seems low.

SUMMARY

In the past decade, various efforts have been made to identify potential new targets[20] and to develop innovative auditory, behavioral, pharmacologic, and neuromodulatory interventions. Moreover, there are ongoing research efforts to refine and validate animal models further,[22,119] to develop large clinical databases to address the heterogeneity of tinnitus, and to optimize and standardize clinical trial design[39] and outcome measurement tools.[36,40] Recently the growing possibilities of eHealth have been explored for their use in tinnitus, and new media facilitate interaction between patients, researchers, and clinicians of different disciplines. With all these developments, tinnitus research has reached a state of increasing activity and diversity reflected by a growing number of publications. It is hoped that these developments soon will lead to more efficient treatment options for the many patients who currently still suffer from tinnitus.

DISCLOSURE

The authors declare that they have nothing to disclose.

REFERENCES

1. Gallus S, Lugo A, Garavello W, et al. Prevalence and determinants of tinnitus in the Italian adult population. Neuroepidemiology 2015;45(1):12–9.
2. McCormack A, Edmondson-Jones M, Somerset S, et al. A systematic review of the reporting of tinnitus prevalence and severity. Hear Res 2016;337:70–9.
3. Nondahl DM, Cruickshanks KJ, Huang GH, et al. Generational differences in the reporting of tinnitus. Ear Hear 2012;33(5):640–4.
4. Axelsson A, Ringdahl A. Tinnitus–a study of its prevalence and characteristics. Br J Audiol 1989;23(1):53–62.
5. Langguth B. A review of tinnitus symptoms beyond 'ringing in the ears': a call to action. Curr Med Res Opin 2011;27(8):1635–43.
6. Hebert S, Canlon B, Hasson D. Emotional exhaustion as a predictor of tinnitus. Psychother Psychosom 2012;81(5):324–6.

7. Friberg E, Jansson C, Mittendorfer-Rutz E, et al. Sickness absence due to otoaudiological diagnoses and risk of disability pension: a nationwide Swedish prospective cohort study. PLoS One 2012;7(1):e29966.

8. Schecklmann M, Vielsmeier V, Steffens T, et al. Relationship between Audiometric slope and tinnitus pitch in tinnitus patients: insights into the mechanisms of tinnitus generation. PLoS One 2012;7(4):e34878.

9. Norena AJ, Eggermont JJ. Changes in spontaneous neural activity immediately after an acoustic trauma: implications for neural correlates of tinnitus. Hear Res 2003;183(1–2):137–53.

10. Eggermont JJ. The auditory cortex and tinnitus - a review of animal and human studies. Eur J Neurosci 2015;41(5):665–76.

11. De Ridder D, Vanneste S, Langguth B, et al. Thalamocortical dysrhythmia: a theoretical update in tinnitus. Front Neurol 2015;6:124.

12. De Ridder D, Elgoyhen AB, Romo R, et al. Phantom percepts: tinnitus and pain as persisting aversive memory networks. Proc Natl Acad Sci U S A 2011; 108(20):8075–80.

13. Elgoyhen AB, Langguth B, De Ridder D, et al. Tinnitus: perspectives from human neuroimaging. Nat Rev Neurosci 2015;16(10):632–42.

14. Langguth B, Kreuzer PM, Kleinjung T, et al. Tinnitus: causes and clinical management. Lancet Neurol 2013;12(9):920–30.

15. Sedley W, Friston KJ, Gander PE, et al. An integrative tinnitus model based on sensory precision. Trends Neurosci 2016;39(12):799–812.

16. De Ridder D, Vanneste S, Weisz N, et al. An integrative model of auditory phantom perception: tinnitus as a unified percept of interacting separable subnetworks. Neurosci Biobehav Rev 2014;44:16–32.

17. Rauschecker JP, May ES, Maudoux A, et al. Frontostriatal gating of tinnitus and chronic pain. Trends Cogn Sci 2015;19(10):567–78.

18. Shore SE, Roberts LE, Langguth B. Maladaptive plasticity in tinnitus–triggers, mechanisms and treatment. Nat Rev Neurol 2016;12(3):150–60.

19. McFerran DJ, Stockdale D, Holme R, et al. Why is there no cure for tinnitus? Front Neurosci 2019;13:802.

20. Langguth B, Elgoyhen AB, Cederroth CR. Therapeutic approaches to the treatment of tinnitus. Annu Rev Pharmacol Toxicol 2019;59:291–313.

21. Eggermont JJ. Can animal models contribute to understanding tinnitus heterogeneity in humans? Front Aging Neurosci 2016;8:265.

22. Turner JG. Behavioral measures of tinnitus in laboratory animals. Prog Brain Res 2007;166:147–56.

23. Jastreboff PJ. Phantom auditory perception (tinnitus): mechanisms of generation and perception. Neurosci Res 1990;8(4):221–54.

24. Zheng Y, Hamilton E, McNamara E, et al. The effects of chronic tinnitus caused by acoustic trauma on social behaviour and anxiety in rats. Neuroscience 2011; 193:143–53.

25. Hayes SH, Radziwon KE, Stolzberg DJ, et al. Behavioral models of tinnitus and hyperacusis in animals. Front Neurol 2014;5:179.

26. Zheng Y, Hooton K, Smith PF, et al. Carbamazepine reduces the behavioural manifestations of tinnitus following salicylate treatment in rats. Acta Otolaryngol 2008;128(1):48–52.

27. Hoekstra CE, Rynja SP, van Zanten, et al. Anticonvulsants for tinnitus. Cochrane Database Syst Rev 2011;(7):CD007960.

28. Hilton MP, Zimmermann EF, Hunt WT. Ginkgo biloba for tinnitus. Cochrane Database Syst Rev 2013;(3):CD003852.

29. Norena AJ, Eggermont JJ. Enriched acoustic environment after noise trauma abolishes neural signs of tinnitus. Neuroreport 2006;17(6):559–63.

30. Vanneste S, van Dongen M, De Vree B, et al. Does enriched acoustic environment in humans abolish chronic tinnitus clinically and electrophysiologically? A double blind placebo controlled study. Hear Res 2013;296:141–8.

31. Simoes J, Neff P, Schoisswohl S, et al. Toward personalized tinnitus treatment: an exploratory study based on internet crowdsensing. Front Public Health 2019;7:157.

32. Cederroth CR, Gallus S, Hall DA, et al. Editorial: towards an understanding of tinnitus heterogeneity. Front Aging Neurosci 2019;11:53.

33. Landgrebe M, Zeman F, Koller M, et al. The Tinnitus Research Initiative (TRI) database: a new approach for delineation of tinnitus subtypes and generation of predictors for treatment outcome. BMC Med Inform Decis Mak 2010;10:42.

34. Adamchic I, Langguth B, Hauptmann C, et al. Psychometric evaluation of Visual Analog Scale for the assessment of chronic tinnitus. Am J Audiol 2012;21(2):215–25.

35. Hall DA, Haider H, Szczepek AJ, et al. Systematic review of outcome domains and instruments used in clinical trials of tinnitus treatments in adults. Trials 2016;17(1):270.

36. Langguth B, Goodey R, Azevedo A, et al. Consensus for tinnitus patient assessment and treatment outcome measurement: Tinnitus Research Initiative meeting, Regensburg, July 2006. Prog Brain Res 2007;166:525–36.

37. Milerova J, Anders M, Dvorak T, et al. The influence of psychological factors on tinnitus severity. Gen Hosp Psychiatry 2013;35(4):412–6.

38. Schlee W, Hall DA, Edvall NK, et al. Visualization of global disease burden for the optimization of patient management and treatment. Front Med (Lausanne) 2017;4:86.

39. Landgrebe M, Azevedo A, Baguley D, et al. Methodological aspects of clinical trials in tinnitus: a proposal for an international standard. J Psychosom Res 2012;73(2):112–21.

40. Londero A, Hall DA. Call for an evidence-based consensus on outcome reporting in tinnitus intervention studies. Front Med (Lausanne) 2017;4:42.

41. Londero A, Bonfils P, Lefaucheur JP. Transcranial magnetic stimulation and subjective tinnitus. A review of the literature, 2014-2016. Eur Ann Otorhinolaryngol Head Neck Dis 2018;135(1):51–8.

42. Landgrebe M, Hajak G, Wolf S, et al. 1-Hz rTMS in the treatment of tinnitus: A sham-controlled, randomized multicenter trial. Brain Stimul 2017;10(6):1112–20.

43. Soleimani R, Jalali MM, Hasandokht T. Therapeutic impact of repetitive transcranial magnetic stimulation (rTMS) on tinnitus: a systematic review and meta-analysis. Eur Arch Otorhinolaryngol 2016;273(7):1663–75.

44. Yuan T, Yadollahpour A, Salgado-Ramirez J, et al. Transcranial direct current stimulation for the treatment of tinnitus: a review of clinical trials and mechanisms of action. BMC Neurosci 2018;19(1):66.

45. Wang TC, Tyler RS, Chang TY, et al. Effect of transcranial direct current stimulation in patients with tinnitus: a meta-analysis and systematic review. Ann Otol Rhinol Laryngol 2018;127(2):79–88.

46. Vanneste S, Fregni F, De Ridder D. Head-to-head comparison of transcranial random noise stimulation, transcranial AC stimulation, and transcranial DC stimulation for tinnitus. Front Psychiatry 2013;4:158.

47. Tutar B, Atar S, Berkiten G, et al. The effect of transcutaneous electrical nerve stimulation (TENS) on chronic subjective tinnitus. Am J Otolaryngol 2020; 41(1):102326.
48. Vanneste S, Plazier M, Van de Heyning P, et al. Transcutaneous electrical nerve stimulation (TENS) of upper cervical nerve (C2) for the treatment of somatic tinnitus. Exp Brain Res 2010;204(2):283–7.
49. Guntensperger D, Thuring C, Kleinjung T, et al. Investigating the efficacy of an individualized alpha/delta neurofeedback protocol in the treatment of chronic tinnitus. Neural Plast 2019;2019:3540898.
50. Dohrmann K, Weisz N, Schlee W, et al. Neurofeedback for treating tinnitus. Prog Brain Res 2007;166:473–85.
51. Guntensperger D, Thuring C, Meyer M, et al. Neurofeedback for tinnitus treatment - review and current concepts. Front Aging Neurosci 2017;9:386.
52. Peter N, Kleinjung T. Neuromodulation for tinnitus treatment: an overview of invasive and non-invasive techniques. J Zhejiang Univ Sci B 2019;20(2):116–30.
53. Meng Z, Liu S, Zheng Y, et al. Repetitive transcranial magnetic stimulation for tinnitus. Cochrane Database Syst Rev 2011;(10):CD007946.
54. He M, Li X, Liu Y, et al. Electroacupuncture for tinnitus: a systematic review. PLoS One 2016;11(3):e0150600.
55. Elbogen EB, Alsobrooks A, Battles S, et al. Mobile neurofeedback for pain management in veterans with TBI and PTSD. Pain Med 2019. https://doi.org/10.1093/pm/pnz269.
56. O'Neill F, Sacco P, Nurmikko T. Evaluation of a home-based transcranial direct current stimulation (tDCS) treatment device for chronic pain: study protocol for a randomised controlled trial. Trials 2015;16:186.
57. De Ridder D, Vanneste S, Menovsky T, et al. Surgical brain modulation for tinnitus: the past, present and future. J Neurosurg Sci 2012;56(4):323–40.
58. Langguth B, De Ridder D. Tinnitus: therapeutic use of superficial brain stimulation. Handb Clin Neurol 2013;116:441–67.
59. De Ridder D, De Mulder G, Walsh V, et al. Magnetic and electrical stimulation of the auditory cortex for intractable tinnitus. Case report. J Neurosurg 2004; 100(3):560–4.
60. De Ridder D, De Mulder G, Verstraeten E, et al. Auditory cortex stimulation for tinnitus. Acta Neurochir Suppl 2007;97(Pt 2):451–62.
61. Cheung SW, Racine CA, Henderson-Sabes J, et al. Phase I trial of caudate deep brain stimulation for treatment-resistant tinnitus. J Neurosurg 2019;1–10. https://doi.org/10.3171/2019.4.JNS19347.
62. Larson PS, Cheung SW. A stroke of silence: tinnitus suppression following placement of a deep brain stimulation electrode with infarction in area LC. J Neurosurg 2013;118(1):192–4.
63. Smit JV, Janssen ML, van Zwieten G, et al. Deep brain stimulation of the inferior colliculus in the rodent suppresses tinnitus. Brain Res 2016;1650:118–24.
64. Offutt SJ, Ryan KJ, Konop AE, et al. Suppression and facilitation of auditory neurons through coordinated acoustic and midbrain stimulation: investigating a deep brain stimulator for tinnitus. J Neural Eng 2014;11(6):066001.
65. van Zwieten G, Janssen MLF, Smit JV, et al. Inhibition of experimental tinnitus with high frequency stimulation of the rat medial geniculate body. Neuromodulation 2019;22(4):416–24.
66. Roberts DS, Otto S, Chen B, et al. Tinnitus suppression after auditory brainstem implantation in patients with neurofibromatosis type-2. Otol Neurotol 2017;38(1): 118–22.

67. Gilles A, Song JJ, Hofkens-Van den Brandt A, et al. Neural substrates of tinnitus in an auditory brainstem implant patient: a preliminary molecular imaging study using H2 15 O-PET including a 5-year follow-up of auditory performance and tinnitus perception. Otol Neurotol 2020;41(1):e15–20.

68. Deklerck AN, Marechal C, Perez Fernandez AM, et al. Invasive neuromodulation as a treatment for tinnitus: a systematic review. Neuromodulation 2019. https://doi.org/10.1111/ner.13042.

69. Smit JV, Pielkenrood BJ, Arts R, et al. Patient acceptance of invasive treatments for tinnitus. Am J Audiol 2018;27(2):184–96.

70. Peter N, Liyanage N, Pfiffner F, et al. The influence of cochlear implantation on tinnitus in patients with single-sided deafness: a systematic review. Otolaryngol Head Neck Surg 2019;161(4):576–88.

71. Ramakers GG, van Zon A, Stegeman I, et al. The effect of cochlear implantation on tinnitus in patients with bilateral hearing loss: a systematic review. Laryngoscope 2015;125(11):2584–92.

72. Zeng FG, Richardson M, Tran P, et al. Tinnitus treatment using noninvasive and minimally invasive electric stimulation: experimental design and feasibility. Trends Hear 2019;23. 2331216518821449.

73. Wenzel GI, Sarnes P, Warnecke A, et al. Non-penetrating round window electrode stimulation for tinnitus therapy followed by cochlear implantation. Eur Arch Otorhinolaryngol 2015;272(11):3283–93.

74. Moller AR. Tinnitus and pain. Prog Brain Res 2007;166:47–53.

75. Kreuzer PM, Landgrebe M, Vielsmeier V, et al. Trauma-associated tinnitus. J Head Trauma Rehabil 2014;29(5):432–42.

76. Vielsmeier V, Strutz J, Kleinjung T, et al. Temporomandibular joint disorder complaints in tinnitus: further hints for a putative tinnitus subtype. PLoS One 2012; 7(6):e38887.

77. Sanchez TG, Rocha CB. Diagnosis and management of somatosensory tinnitus: review article. Clinics (Sao Paulo) 2011;66(6):1089–94.

78. Michiels S, Ganz Sanchez T, Oron Y, et al. Diagnostic criteria for somatosensory tinnitus: a delphi process and face-to-face meeting to establish consensus. Trends Hear 2018;22. 2331216518796403.

79. Michiels S, van der Wal AC, Nieste F, et al. Conservative therapy for the treatment of patients with somatic tinnitus attributed to temporomandibular dysfunction: study protocol of a randomised controlled trial. Trials 2018;19(1):554.

80. Moller AR, Moller MB, Yokota M. Some forms of tinnitus may involve the extralemniscal auditory pathway. Laryngoscope 1992;102(10):1165–71.

81. Biesinger E, Kipman U, Schatz S, et al. Qigong for the treatment of tinnitus: a prospective randomized controlled study. J Psychosom Res 2010;69(3): 299–304.

82. Engineer ND, Riley JR, Seale JD, et al. Reversing pathological neural activity using targeted plasticity. Nature 2011;470(7332):101–4.

83. Tyler R, Cacace A, Stocking C, et al. Vagus nerve stimulation paired with tones for the treatment of tinnitus: a prospective randomized double-blind controlled pilot study in humans. Sci Rep 2017;7(1):11960.

84. Shekhawat GS, Searchfield GD, Stinear CM. Randomized trial of transcranial direct current stimulation and hearing aids for tinnitus management. Neurorehabil Neural Repair 2014;28(5):410–9.

85. Teismann H, Wollbrink A, Okamoto H, et al. Combining transcranial direct current stimulation and tailor-made notched music training to decrease tinnitus-related distress–a pilot study. PLoS One 2014;9(2):e89904.

86. Marks KL, Martel DT, Wu C, et al. Auditory-somatosensory bimodal stimulation desynchronizes brain circuitry to reduce tinnitus in guinea pigs and humans. Sci Transl Med 2018;10(422) [pii:eaal3175].

87. Conlon B, Hamilton C, Hughes S, et al. Noninvasive bimodal neuromodulation for the treatment of tinnitus: protocol for a second large-scale double-blind randomized clinical trial to optimize stimulation parameters. JMIR Res Protoc 2019; 8(9):e13176.

88. D'Arcy S, Hamilton C, Hughes S, et al. Bi-modal stimulation in the treatment of tinnitus: a study protocol for an exploratory trial to optimise stimulation parameters and patient subtyping. BMJ Open 2017;7(10):e018465.

89. Greenwell K, Featherstone D, Hoare DJ. The application of intervention coding methodology to describe the tinnitus E-programme, an internet-delivered self-help intervention for tinnitus. Am J Audiol 2015;24(3):311–5.

90. Greenwell K, Sereda M, Coulson N, et al. Understanding user reactions and interactions with an internet-based intervention for tinnitus self-management: mixed-methods process evaluation protocol. JMIR Res Protoc 2016;5(1):e49.

91. Sheikh Rashid M, Dreschler WA. Accuracy of an internet-based speech-in-noise hearing screening test for high-frequency hearing loss: incorporating automatic conditional rescreening. Int Arch Occup Environ Health 2018;91(7):877–85.

92. Rothpletz AM, Moore AN, Preminger JE. Acceptance of internet-based hearing healthcare among adults who fail a hearing screening. Int J Audiol 2016;55(9): 483–90.

93. Mahboubi H, Ziai K, Brunworth J, et al. Accuracy of tinnitus pitch matching using a web-based protocol. Ann Otol Rhinol Laryngol 2012;121(10):671–4.

94. Wunderlich R, Stein A, Engell A, et al. Evaluation of iPod-based automated tinnitus pitch matching. J Am Acad Audiol 2015;26(2):205–12.

95. Schlee W, Pryss RC, Probst T, et al. Measuring the moment-to-moment variability of tinnitus: the TrackYourTinnitus smart phone app. Front Aging Neurosci 2016; 8:294.

96. Wilson MB, Kallogjeri D, Joplin CN, et al. Ecological momentary assessment of tinnitus using smartphone technology: a pilot study. Otolaryngol Head Neck Surg 2015;152(5):897–903.

97. Westin VZ, Schulin M, Hesser H, et al. Acceptance and commitment therapy versus tinnitus retraining therapy in the treatment of tinnitus: a randomised controlled trial. Behav Res Ther 2011;49(11):737–47.

98. Hesser H, Gustafsson T, Lunden C, et al. A randomized controlled trial of Internet-delivered cognitive behavior therapy and acceptance and commitment therapy in the treatment of tinnitus. J Consult Clin Psychol 2012;80(4):649–61.

99. Kim SY, Chang MY, Hong M, et al. Tinnitus therapy using tailor-made notched music delivered via a smartphone application and Ginko combined treatment: A pilot study. Auris Nasus Larynx 2017;44(5):528–33.

100. Mahboubi H, Ziai K, Djalilian HR. Customized web-based sound therapy for tinnitus. Int Tinnitus J 2012;17(1):26–30.

101. Malinvaud D, Londero A, Niarra R, et al. Auditory and visual 3D virtual reality therapy as a new treatment for chronic subjective tinnitus: Results of a randomized controlled trial. Hear Res 2016;333:127–35.

102. Schickler M, Pryss R, Reichert M, et al. Using mobile serious games in the context of chronic disorders a mobile game concept for the treatment of tinnitus. Comp Med Sy 2016;343–8.

103. Wise K, Kobayashi K, Searchfield GD. Feasibility study of a game integrating assessment and therapy of tinnitus. J Neurosci Methods 2015;249:1–7.

104. Guitton MJ, Caston J, Ruel J, et al. Salicylate induces tinnitus through activation of cochlear NMDA receptors. J Neurosci 2003;23(9):3944–52.
105. Ruel J, Chabbert C, Nouvian R, et al. Salicylate enables cochlear arachidonic-acid-sensitive NMDA receptor responses. J Neurosci 2008;28(29):7313–23.
106. van de Heyning P, Muehlmeier G, Cox T, et al. Efficacy and safety of AM-101 in the treatment of acute inner ear tinnitus–a double-blind, randomized, placebo-controlled phase II study. Otol Neurotol 2014;35(4):589–97.
107. Auris-Medical. AM-101 in the Treatment of Acute Tinnitus 2 2018. Available at: https://clinicaltrials.gov/ct2/show/NCT01803646?term=AM-101&rank=4. Accessed December 19, 2019.
108. Auris-Medical. AM-101 in the Treatment of Acute Tinnitus 3; 2018. Available at: https://clinicaltrials.gov/ct2/show/NCT02040194?term=AM-101&rank=3. Accessed December 19, 2019.
109. Faught E. BGG492 (selurampanel), an AMPA/kainate receptor antagonist drug for epilepsy. Expert Opin Investig Drugs 2014;23(1):107–13.
110. Lee AC, Godfrey DA. Cochlear damage affects neurotransmitter chemistry in the central auditory system. Front Neurol 2014;5:227.
111. Novartis. Available at: https://www.novctrd.com/CtrdWeb/displaypdf.nov?trial resultid=12123. Accessed December 19, 2019.
112. Autifony. 2016. Available at: https://www.clinicaltrialsregister.eu/ctr-search/trial/2014-002179-27/results. Accessed December 19, 2019.
113. Li S, Choi V, Tzounopoulos T. Pathogenic plasticity of Kv7.2/3 channel activity is essential for the induction of tinnitus. Proc Natl Acad Sci U S A 2013;110(24):9980–5.
114. Cederroth CR, Dyhrfjeld-Johnsen J, Langguth B. An update: emerging drugs for tinnitus. Expert Opin Emerg Drugs 2018;23(4):251–60.
115. Kalappa BI, Soh H, Duignan KM, et al. Potent KCNQ2/3-specific channel activator suppresses in vivo epileptic activity and prevents the development of tinnitus. J Neurosci 2015;35(23):8829–42.
116. Hall DA, Smith H, Hibbert A, et al. The COMiT'ID study: developing core outcome domains sets for clinical trials of sound-, psychology-, and pharmacology-based interventions for chronic subjective tinnitus in adults. Trends Hear 2018;22. 2331216518814384.
117. Cederroth CR, Canlon B, Langguth B. Hearing loss and tinnitus–are funders and industry listening? Nat Biotechnol 2013;31(11):972–4.
118. Schlee W, Hall DA, Canlon B, et al. Innovations in doctoral training and research on tinnitus: the European School on Interdisciplinary Tinnitus Research (ESIT) perspective. Front Aging Neurosci 2017;9:447.
119. Turner J, Larsen D, Hughes L, et al. Time course of tinnitus development following noise exposure in mice. J Neurosci Res 2012;90(7):1480–8.

Special Article Series: Intentionally Shaping the Future of Otolaryngology

Editor

JENNIFER A. VILLWOCK

OTOLARYNGOLOGIC CLINICS OF NORTH AMERICA

www.oto.theclinics.com

Consulting Editor
SUJANA S. CHANDRASEKHAR

August 2020 • Volume 53 • Number 4

Foreword

Spreading Our Wings: Leadership and Personal Growth in Otolaryngology

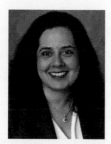

Sujana S. Chandrasekhar, MD, FACS, FAAOHNS
Consulting Editor

Although disorders and treatments of the ears, nose, and throat (ENT) were described in ancient Indian, Chinese, and Greek texts, otolaryngology–head and neck surgery as a specialty began in the Western world in the nineteenth century, when doctors figured out that the ears, the nose, and the throat are closely connected by a system of tubes and passages. An important new medical specialty was thus born. ENT problems are the most common reasons for physician visits around the world, both in developing and developed countries and in rural and urban communities. As such, most people have interacted with an otolaryngologist. In addition to guiding, mentoring, and sponsoring younger ENTs, we are uniquely poised to lead, not just in our field but also in the greater House of Medicine and in society.

"Intentionally Shaping the Future of Otolaryngology" is a special section of *Otolaryngologic Clinics of North America* featuring a series of articles authored by leaders in our field and curated by Jennifer Villwock, MD. Two articles from this series will be published in every issue of *Otolaryngologic Clinics of North America*, starting with this one, covering the breadth of opportunities and possibilities. The topics range from mentorship and sponsorship, to strategies for achieving leadership positions in societies and in various types of practice settings, to the importance of thoughtful diversity and inclusion in keeping our field strong, and opportunities for personal and professional growth that may not be obvious to the practicing otolaryngologist.

The first 2 articles of this series are by 2 past presidents of the American Academy of Otolaryngology–Head and Neck Surgery. Dr. K.J. Lee has held high leadership positions in our field and has advised several presidents of the United States. His article chronicles his leadership experiences at the highest levels and demonstrates how we can affect meaningful change in our communities, large and small. My article,

Otolaryngol Clin N Am 53 (2020) xix–xx
https://doi.org/10.1016/j.otc.2020.04.005
0030-6665/20/© 2020 Published by Elsevier Inc.

initially published in *Otology and Neurotology* and reprinted here with permission, looks at the importance of diversity and inclusion within our scientific societies, so that our field continues to grow and appropriately represents our membership and our patients.

I commend Dr Villwock on spearheading the creation of this special section and for guest-editing it. Singer and humanitarian Dolly Parton says, "I'm not going to limit myself just because people won't accept the fact that I can do something else." I hope that the articles in Intentionally Shaping the Future of Otolaryngology" inspire you to spread your wings.

Sujana S. Chandrasekhar, MD, FACS, FAAOHNS
Consulting Editor, Otolaryngologic Clinics of North America

Past President, American Academy of Otolaryngology-Head and Neck Surgery

Secretary-Treasurer, American Otological Society

Partner, ENT & Allergy Associates LLP
18 East 48th Street, 2nd Floor, New York, NY 10017, USA

Clinical Professor, Department of Otolaryngology-Head and Neck Surgery
Zucker School of Medicine at Hofstra-Northwell, Hempstead, NY, USA

Clinical Associate Professor, Department of Otolaryngology-Head and Neck Surgery
Icahn School of Medicine at Mount Sinai, New York, NY, USA

E-mail address:
ssc@nyotology.com

Preface

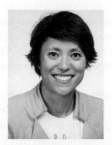

Jennifer A. Villwock, MD
Editor

Multigenerational, multicultural, multiethnic. These words describe our increasingly global society as well as many of our organizations, colleagues, communities, and patients. "Intentionally Shaping the Future of Otolaryngology" seeks to provide evidence and insight and to provoke critical thought and conversations regarding issues facing the future of our field.

Dr K.J. Lee begins the dialogue with his reflection on being both a physician and an advocate in "Otolaryngologist as a Political Leader?" The arc of Dr Lee's career spans continents, communities, and presidential candidates. He astutely notes that "as physicians, we serve" and that there are many ways to do so that go beyond patient care. As we think about the future, no one is better equipped to enact the future we envision, and need, than us.

I sincerely applaud and thank Dr Lee for his fearlessness and steadfastness in his eloquent efforts to advocate for patients and physicians. For example, in communications with presidential administrations, he presents key points including that "Health care is a right, a commodity, and a service. We have to balance these three concepts" and that health care reform will struggle to be successful until there is a system in place that rewards "good outcomes rendered with great compassionate care" *and* "being a good steward of the health care dollar." Dr Lee also provides a wealth of evidence and perspective to support these calls to action. I also greatly appreciated the honesty woven into this article. The authors note that being a leader and an advocate is often a difficult and frustrating endeavor. Nonetheless, the work must be done; one voice can make a difference.

Dr Sujana Chandrasekhar is no stranger to being that single voice. I first met her at a conference when I was a junior resident. While I had incredible mentors in my residency program, the academic faculty at that time was all male. It was striking for me to see Dr Chandrasekhar meaningfully contribute on panels and ask insightful questions at scientific sessions. Having experienced that "it's hard to be what you can't see," this was the first time I viscerally felt the opposite. It is experiences like this that reinforce the importance of inclusion and representation within our specialty.

Otolaryngol Clin N Am 53 (2020) xxi–xxii
https://doi.org/10.1016/j.otc.2020.04.006
0030-6665/20/© 2020 Published by Elsevier Inc.

oto.theclinics.com

In her article "Strengthening Our Societies with Diversity and Inclusion," Dr Chandrasekhar combines her wealth of experience, including her tenure as president of the American Academy of Otolaryngology–Head and Neck Surgery Foundation, with the available data. She describes her experience in publicly calling out a "manel" or all-male panel at a national meeting in a room filled with equally, or more, qualified women. She also presents data from her review of the gender composition at national conferences of presented papers versus invited presentations and panels. I will let Dr Chandrasekhar's words speak for themselves, but the data reveal significant room for improvement.

Representation matters, whether it's physicians in politics and advocacy as Dr Lee's piece highlights or in professional society membership and engagement as Dr Chandrasekhar illustrates. The ramifications of who we recruit, retain, and engage will shape the future of both medicine and otolaryngology.

Jennifer A. Villwock, MD
Department of Otolaryngology
Head and Neck Surgery
Kansas University
University of Kansas Medical Center
3901 Rainbow Boulevard, MS 3010
Kansas City, KS 66160, USA

E-mail address:
jvillwock@kumc.edu

Otolaryngologist as a Political Leader?

K.J. Lee, MD[a,b,c],*, Mark E. Lee, MBA[d,1]

KEYWORDS

- Health care reform • Pay for performance • Pay for value • Hybrid payment • EHR
- AAO-HNS

KEY POINTS

- Otolaryngologists can advocate and thus be a "political" leader for our specialty and the house of medicine.
- Unless an otolaryngologist runs for a state or federal office, he or she is not really a political leader.
- To be taken seriously by those in power, we need to advocate the skills to treat and the heart to care at a sensible cost.

I was asked to write on "Otolaryngologist as Political Leader." As a doctor, it is not easy to be a "political leader." We are more often an unpaid advisor, consultant, or an advocate. It is even harder for an otolaryngologist to be a political leader. We are a small specialty by numbers. The powers that be prefer to rely on advice from the numerous primary care, internists, and perhaps general surgeons. However, otolaryngologists are civic minded. We are more active than some of the larger specialties. We work hard. Over the past decades, we have transformed our specialty to more depths and breadths. Please keep up the great work.

One way for an otolaryngologist to be a political leader is to run for public office. Federal office is a full-time position. State or local officers can serve part time. Both are demanding of time and focus. Politicians originate policies, which can be molded by party politics and external forces.[1–8]

The world of politics often seems unrelated to health care; as physicians, our attention tends to remain firmly focused on our diligent work to take care of our patients, ideally as if we were the patient. As physicians, we serve. We serve our patients; we advocate for health care guidelines and protocols that keep our patients safe, and

[a] Hofstra University Donald and Barbara Zucker School of Medicine; [b] Quinnipiac University Frank H. Netter MD School of Medicine; [c] Yale University School of Medicine; [d] Halo Media Group
[1] Present address: 4533 Vista Del Monte Avenue #405, Sherman Oaks, CA 91403.
* Corresponding author. 669 Boston Post Road, Suite 8, Guilford, CT 06437.
E-mail address: kjleemd@aol.com

Otolaryngol Clin N Am 53 (2020) 685–699
https://doi.org/10.1016/j.otc.2020.03.014
0030-6665/20/© 2020 Elsevier Inc. All rights reserved.

we put our patients first. In my personal experience, which has stretched across many presidential administrations, one need not be in politics to be a "political" leader. Understanding the following may help us. Effective leaders know that they first have to touch the people's hearts before they ask them for a hand. People usually buy into the leader first, then the leader's vision. The best leaders are servants. They appreciate and nurture the talents of an individual and manage the limitations of an individual. The greatest accomplishments happen when the leaders give others credit and believe that people are the greatest asset. Leaders have the abilities to recognize problems before they become an emergency, and they are seldom blindsided. Most great leaders have experienced failures and learn from their failures. Life is better when you are happy, and life is best when other people are happy because of you.

I have never run for political office, but I have worked behind the scenes advising candidates for public office and holders of public office. I have spent untold hours developing policies, advocating, and advising many politicians at the state and federal levels.

My colleague and I worked diligently with 2 US presidential candidates. We very strongly advocated that (a) health care information and data needed to be digitized; (b) with proper privacy control, the medical records needed to be available, efficiently within seconds, for the patients and all their doctors; and (c) the technologies have to be intuitive, user-friendly, and following the doctors' workflow, allowing the doctors to focus on the patients and not on the computer screen and keyboard.

The administration did digitize medical records, but huge outside forces beyond physicians' control created a system that interferes with the day-to-day practice of medicine, the interactions between patients and doctors. Today's electronic health record (EHR) disrupts the doctor-patient encounter. However, we cannot give up, but continue to advise the government and the health care industry to make EHR very intuitive, user friendly, and with the patient's approval, have the ability to quickly interconnect with other EHR products ("interoperability in real life and in real time").

Besides working on the above, we advocated for "no preexisting disease exclusion." We also realized that to make the industry financially sustainable, the healthy and the young have to participate in such a health care scenario. Otherwise, there will be an adverse selection and the "arithmetic does not add up" for a financially viable health care system. We also advocated to streamline the billing, claims filing, and reimbursement system. In one of my discussions with President Clinton, he mentioned that the "paperwork and the bureaucracy" wasted 30% of the overall health care dollar. We demonstrated that streamlining the business processes and decreasing the duplication and unnecessary tests and procedures could save 28% of the health care dollar while increasing satisfaction among patients and doctors.

In our submission to 1 administration, we outlined the following:

- Health care is a right, a commodity, and a service. We have to balance these 3 concepts.
- Coverage for all; no preexisting disease exclusion. (Avoid the term "universal health care." It has been misconstrued as socialized medicine, big government.)
- Health care reform is about collaborating among stakeholders, not winning by a stakeholder.
- It should be a private system offering choices of doctors, hospitals, and insurance carriers.
- Decisions on patient care are made between the providers and the patients with certain guidelines and not in the halls of Congress or the corporate offices of insurance companies.

- It is a private system with government oversight on cost, improving quality and efficiency.
- No health care reform can be successful unless it also addresses the fee-for-service compensation system for providers, which rewards volume of services (utilization), as opposed to a system that rewards good outcomes rendered with great compassionate care and being a good steward of the health care dollar.

When the current administration was attempting to repeal the so-called Obamacare, we submitted the following to the decision makers:

"Here's how to reduce healthcare costs, May 09, 2017.

The recent White House-Congressional fiasco epitomizes the lack of basic understanding regarding healthcare and healthcare reform.

Obamacare (ACA [Affordable Care Act]) and the Republicans' AHCA (American Health Care Act), each with its pros and cons, are more like "health insurance coverage reform" or "healthcare payers reform" rather than healthcare reform for patients. Offering "coverage" is different than offering "real access" to receive efficient, quality, compassionate healthcare in a timely manner. Just because someone has an insurance, Medicare or Medicaid card, does not necessarily help him or her get an appointment for treatment in an efficient, timely manner. In addition, it does not guarantee the patient can afford the co-pay or deductible required before he or she is examined. The goal of our healthcare solution is to offer access at a sensible price.

In 2004, the United States spent $1.7 trillion on healthcare. In 2008, we spent $2.3 trillion, or 16% of Gross Domestic Product (GDP). In 2016, we spent more than $3 trillion. It is not that we are not spending enough money on healthcare, the problem is that we are not spending the money wisely. There is wastage, redundancy, inefficiency, bureaucracy, and perhaps, even charging more than necessary in some sectors. We have to align the long-term incentives of insurers, payers, providers and patients. We need to restore trust between parties. Otherwise, we shall continue to be in chaos regardless of how much money we spend in healthcare. We are reshuffling the deck chairs on the sinking Titanic. This skyrocketing cost has already made us less competitive in the world economy. It is not necessary for finger pointing. If we all collaborate, it can be achieved without too much sacrifice from each sector of the healthcare industry.

The following is a plan to reduce healthcare cost by 28%, making it much more affordable. This will make "healthcare insurance coverage reform" and "healthcare payers reform" easier. Thus, a "replacement" or "improvement" of ACA can be achieved less acrimoniously.

I. *Streamline the current manner in which providers bill insurance companies, Medicare, Medicaid or patients. It is a very convoluted and expensive system. To illustrate simply: A $100 item is billed out between $400 and $1200 or sometimes more. After months of back and forth and mountains of paperwork, consuming millions of hours of computer time, the bill is settled for $125.32, part of which is paid by the insurance carrier or Medicare and part of it by the patient's co-pay or deductible. There is a simpler way.*

Simplifying the medical billing system would save at least 20% of the healthcare dollar, bringing relief to both the payers and the providers...a win-win situation.

II. *The surge of hospitals charging very high "facility fees" for routine office visits has exacerbated the skyrocketing cost of healthcare. It is not uncommon that the facility fee is 2 to 5 times the fee charged by the doctor for an office visit, which does not require the use of an operating room, emergency room, intensive care unit or an admission for an overnight stay in the hospital.*

III. *A certain percentage of non-cosmetic elective surgeries, not tests, may be unnecessary. This amount is considered enough not only to raise the cost of healthcare, but also causes pain and suffering, potential complications and absenteeism from work. I realize each surgeon believes that she or he does not perform such unnecessary surgery, it is the other guy. Medical Societies have started to produce evidence-based clinical guidelines for surgeries and certain diagnostic tests and procedures. Introducing appropriate common sense, non-draconian "pay for value" instead of "pay for volume" reimbursement could be the first step to decrease healthcare costs, or perhaps, a hybrid of the two payment methods. At the same time, we need to diminish the cumbersome and unnecessary mandates imposed by the government such as Meaningful Use, MACRA and MIPS. As one national leader advocates, too much regulation stifles productivity. There is a simple way to achieve value.*

IV. *A pill produced by the same company is sold in the U.S. at a price multiple times of the same pill being sold in other countries. We understand fully that the cost of developing a new drug is prohibitive. Is there a solution for all parties if we all work together? We should take a good look at the arduous process of developing a new drug. Will the application of a modified "favorite nation clause" help? We need Solomon's wisdom to create a win-win for industry and patients. (As we write this article in January 2020, Democratic presidential candidates as well as President Trump, attorney-generals and members of Congress are seeking a solution to reduce prescription drugs without stifling the discovery of new drugs.)*

V. *Expanding Medicare for younger and healthier people to buy into it will help to sustain and stabilize Medicare. We are not proposing free healthcare for all. Medicare has an adverse selection actuarially of its members, old and disabled. Insurance companies, experts on actuarial science, are needed at the table to decrease healthcare costs.*

VI. *Rather than allocating different budgets for Medicaid, block grants, debating whether it is federally or state funded, could we explore the mechanism for all licensed providers to donate a percentage of their time to take care of the less privileged, the way it was done in the '50s and '60s? It would also eliminate the labor-intensive billing for Medicaid whose reimbursement could be less than the overhead to render such services, according to some doctors.*

We could expand the system to encourage more recently qualified doctors to serve in the U.S. HealthCorps for 2 years, caring for the less privileged and in areas having insufficient doctors. In return, these doctors could get their student loan forgiven. If history is any indication, the experiences will give these doctors great satisfaction and experience like those who served in the armed forces or U.S. public health services prior to the 1970s.

VII. *Deploy telemedicine. The current sporadic practice of medicine through e-mails and text messages can create slipshod medicine leading to errors. Both patients and providers can be distracted while e-mailing or texting and there is no opportunity to dialogue properly. Instead, introduce a new method, deploying virtual visits via Skype or FaceTime at an appointed time so that both patients and providers are concentrating. This also creates the appropriate medical record keeping. The provider should be compensated but at a more cost-effective rate, as overhead may be lower. This will decrease healthcare cost and make it more convenient for both providers and patients. Furthermore, the patients do not have to miss work.*

VIII. *We should also deploy more nurse practitioners and physician assistants who are well trained in the specialty in which they practice. It has been pointed out that a generalized nurse practitioner or physician assistant can lower the quality of healthcare. A well supervised specialty trained nurse practitioner or physician assistant can lower the total healthcare cost for the country and at the same time maintain quality of care as well as improve access. Another win-win.*

The above is not a panacea to completely cure our healthcare chaos. It took us decades to get here, but if we all collaborate, we can reduce healthcare costs by at least 28% of over $3 trillion without significantly compromising care, instead increasing the quality of healthcare.

Simplifying the medical billing alone can save 20% of healthcare cost, helping payers and providers achieve a win-win. The above could be a first step to bring parties together in a round table to improve healthcare for the patients. We are all patients, whether in the past, present or in the future. Once Democrats and Republicans, conservatives and liberals, work together on the above eight points for the common good, the debate on ACA and AHCA will hopefully be more cordial."

In most walks of life, people are evaluated for their performance and, oftentimes, compensation is linked to such evaluation. In most industries, there are standardized, acceptable ways, or a range of ways to perform a job well. Clinical guidelines are being developed at a steady rate by academic institutions and organized medicine, including the American Academy of Otolaryngology–Head and Neck Surgery. If we do not craft these guidelines, nonmedical entities will impose their guidelines upon us. Much as we prefer not to have cookbook medicine, we can embrace well-crafted guidelines that also allow for legitimate deviation from the guidelines.

It is the consensus among medical economists that a "fee-for-service" or "pay-for-volume" model is not sustainable in health care. "Fee for Service" works in other industries because the consumer can judge better whether to purchase the service or not as well as judge the quality of the service or goods. In other industries, the consumer is not in pain or afraid of dying or being disabled. Capitation, Accountable Care Organization, and similar solutions being proposed do not solve the problem; in fact, they can create new problems. I was asked to develop a physician reimbursement model that incorporates the positive aspects of "pay for volume" and "pay for value," almost finding the Holy Grail. We welcome any comment or advice.

The closest model is the so-called Hybrid Payment System ("HPS"). HPS takes into account human nature. It incentivizes the providers to be accessible on 1 hand and good stewards of the health care dollar on the other hand. As consumers, we all want quality, customer service, and "bang for our buck." The HPS comes the closest to fulfilling the consumer's wish. Besides, we are patients, or, someday, we will be patients, consumers of health care. The HPS incorporates the use of good clinical guidelines. As a collateral benefit, we can slowly affect tort reform. If the provider follows the guideline and an untoward event happens, the filing of a suit should not be permitted, or following acceptable guidelines should at least be a powerful aid in the defense.

The HPS keeps the fee-for-service payment system; however, instead of paying 100% of the claims, X% of the claims, which can range from 70% to 99%, is paid within 1 week from the date of claim, with no denial and no hassles. This system will decrease unnecessary administrative costs on the payers' side and on the providers' side. Every quarter, the payer and the provider will review online the electronic medical records of a small but statistically valid number of the provider's patients to measure the provider's performance based on how he or she follows the practice guidelines. It is not cookbook medicine. Current technology allows physicians to deviate from the guidelines, documenting the good reasons for the deviation to avoid a bad score. Depending on the results of this evaluation, the provider will get Y% of the claims or part of Y%.

Once we decide what X% is, we can decide what Y% of the claims will be. If X% is 70%, Y% can range from 40% to 0%. X% + Y% can be equal to 110% or less. A quality, cost-effective doctor who does not underutilize or overutilize will get paid 110% of the maximum allowable fee. He or she will not only get the full value of the claims, but also a 10% bonus can be added. Those who score lower will get paid a total of between 70% and 100% of the claims.

HPS also borrows but modifies the principle of "HMOs withholding" of a prior era. In the 1980s, the return of the "withhold" depended on the total performance of all the providers in the network and how the administrators manage the health maintenance organization (HMO). In this new HPS, each provider is measured according to his or her own performance. Hence, we are holding each provider accountable for his or her actions according to the criteria set by pay for performance. His or her compensation is thus not dependent on the performances of other physicians or the administrators.

The old "capitation model" or putting providers on salary without incentive will lead to less "access" for the patients, encouraging underutilization as well as making the provider want to pass the patient with more ailments on to another provider (or refer to another specialty) to take care of.

This HPS methodology is not ideal but it is hoped will decrease cost without compromising quality and access. Once rational payment systems are adopted, providers will have no conflict with their conscience to overutilize and upcode, or underutilize or limit patient access. HPS is not going to be perfect at the beginning, but once we work with it, we can amend and improve it.

I was interviewed by the George W. Bush Administration to be head of Medicare (Centers for Medicare and Medicaid Services). The interview went well until the last question. At that period, the Bush Administration was introducing Medicare Part D for drug coverage. In the proposal, there was a clause that prohibited Medicare from negotiating prices with pharmaceutical companies. I was asked, if appointed, could I unequivocally support Medicare Part D. I mentioned that covering the drugs for seniors and the disabled is noble, but I did not understand the rationale to prohibit Medicare from bargaining for lower pharmaceutical cost. Instead of being diplomatic and perhaps even ducking the question, I started to "debate" the topic. Obviously, I was not invited back for the second round of interviews.

If otolaryngologists are interested in becoming political leaders or advisors, we suggest they volunteer to participate in the county or state medical societies and definitely join the advocacy team of the American Academy of Otolaryngology–Head and Neck Surgery and the ENT-PAC (Ear, Nose, Throat Political Action Committee). If possible, involve the politicians early in their career. First, genuinely get to know them as a person, their likes and dislikes, and their background before discussing specific policies. Be a friend, a person they can trust to be unbiased and analytical. When Senator Joe Lieberman was Attorney General of Connecticut, the incumbent US Senator was running for another term. When Linda and I were having dinner with Mr and Mrs Lieberman, I suggested that he run for the US Senate. In fact, I placed a wager that Joe would win. Sure enough, Joe became Senator Joe Lieberman. Soon after Barack Obama became Senator Obama, I sat next to him at dinner. I suggested he should run for president. He said not so soon because he just became senator. At a dinner with Mr Warren Buffett arranged by President Obama's office, I asked Mr Buffett if the administration could not fix the escalating cost of health care, could he. To paraphrase Mr Buffett, he said, "[n]o industry or profession come to Washington asking to be paid less, everyone comes asking to get paid more. No, I can't fix it." Nevertheless, later when he, Amazon, and J.P. Morgan were forming a new health care company, I submitted to him excerpts from "Here's how to reduce healthcare costs, May 9, 2017." Another avenue is to write an op-ed in a national or local newspaper such as the following:

Kinder and gentler

New Haven Register (Sunday) (New Haven, CT) · 22 Mar 2020

With the onslaught of coronavirus upon humanity, perhaps we can create a silver lining. In this day and age of fear, can we as humans reenergize ourselves to be more compassionate to each other? When another shopping cart bumped into us at the supermarket, we utter: "not a problem, you go ahead" with a genuine smile. Likewise, on the highway, lining up at the post office, work place and at home, etc. Be more tolerant of our fellow human beings. There are good aspects in everyone. Republican have good and poor ideas. Similarly Democrats have good points and not-so-good ones. When one party does something good, the other party should acknowledge the good points when criticizing the other's flawed policies. May this coronavirus crisis teach us to be a kinder and gentler nation, thus a kinder and more gentle world. Dr. KJ Lee Guilford

---

Is it a satisfactory endeavor for me to be involved in health care politics over the past decades? I am not sure. At times, I feel like I am "fighting city hall, banging my head against the wall." At other times, I feel elated. One voice is heard, perhaps, slowly but surely, perhaps part of it or not at all. If caregivers and patients do not advocate and be leaders, what would happen?

Any questions or advice can be sent to the authors at kjleemd@aol.com (www.kjlee.world) or mlee@halomediagroup.com.

DISCLOSURE

The authors have nothing to disclose.

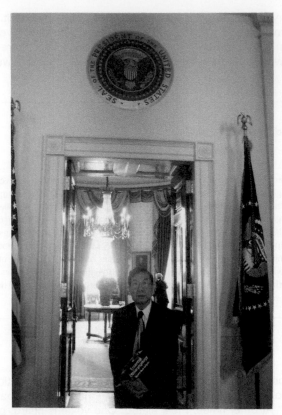

Fig. 1. At the White House with K.J. Lee's Essential Otolaryngology-Head and Neck Surgery.

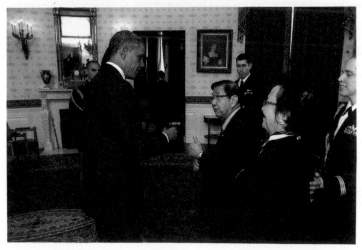

All the best,

Fig. 2. At the White House.

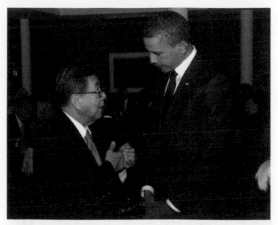

Fig. 3. Discussing health care.

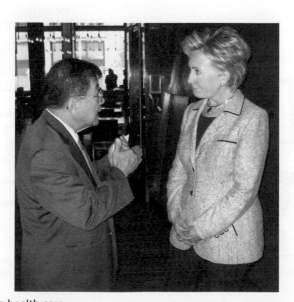

Fig. 4. Discussing health care.

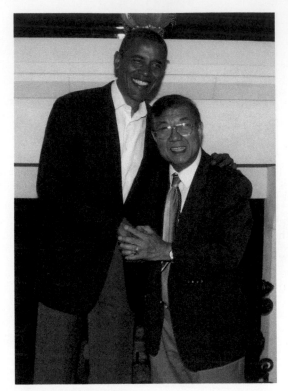

Fig. 5. When Barack Obama was a senator.

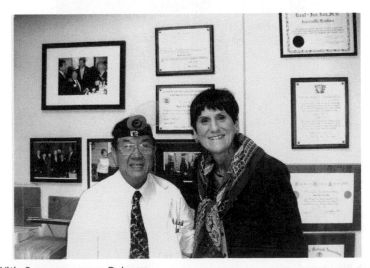

Fig. 6. With Congresswoman DeLauro.

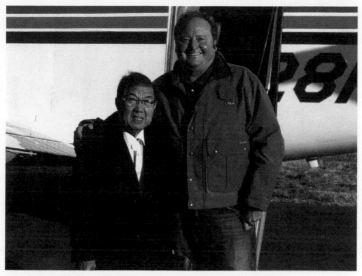

Fig. 7. With Governor Schweitzer touring the Montana coal mines.

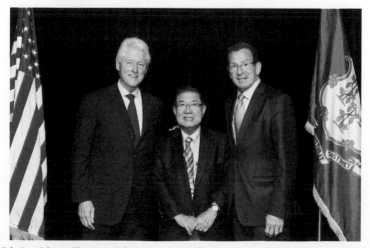

Fig. 8. With President Clinton and Governor Malloy.

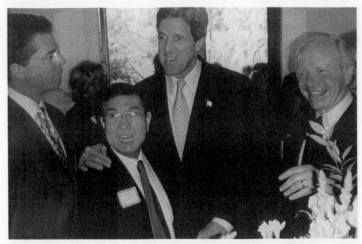

Fig. 9. With Presidential candidate John Kerry, Senator Lieberman, and Kevin Powell.

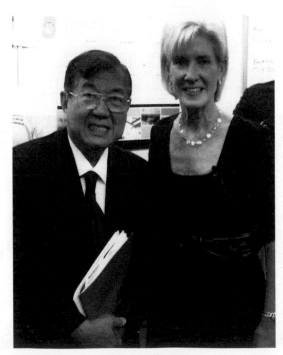

Fig. 10. With Secretary Sebelius discussing health care.

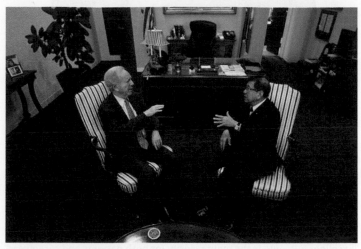

Fig. 11. With Senator Lieberman.

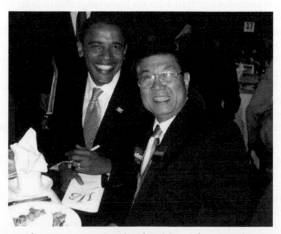

Fig. 12. With Senator Obama, suggesting he should run for president.

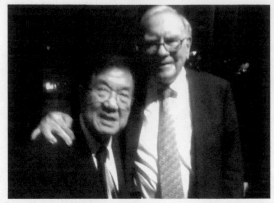

Fig. 13. Dinner meeting with Mr Warren Buffett.

THE PATIENT IS U FOUNDATION, INC.

A 501(c)(3) nonprofit organization dedicated to promote
SKILLS TO TREAT and the HEART TO CARE at a SENSIBLE COST

"Excellent outcome is the main priority for both patients and caregivers"

TPIU encourages all those who come into contact with patients to interact as if they are, in fact, the patient.

Research has demonstrated that compassionate care and great patient experience lead to better outcome.

To enhance patient experience, we believe that patients very much appreciate:

- Being greeted by a user-friendly phone system including a helpful person with whom to speak;
- Not having to wait a long period of time to get an appointment for a visit, test or procedure;
- Receiving clear and understandable directions to the office building as well as directions to the office within the building;
- Having convenient and inexpensive parking with compassionate attendants;
- Having open and available lines of communication between the patient and all the caregivers, including the patient's Attending Doctor;
- All caregivers for any patient communicate with each other;
- Doctors' representatives or staff who are knowledgeable in their specialty and well versed in the patient's case;
- Obtaining test results and the Doctor's interpretation of those results promptly;
- Being informed of the pros and cons of the recommended tests, treatment(s), including the preoperative, operative and postoperative care and possible side effects thereof;
- Being informed of possible alternative tests or treatments and an explanation of the pros and cons of those tests and treatments;
- Making electronic health record user friendly and eliminate unnecessary government or insurance mandates so that the doctors can once again focus on patients.

It is helpful for the patients to prepare a written summary of their ailment and a list of questions before seeing the doctor

TPIU will also outline steps to eliminate stress among caregivers in this day and age of a fast paced medical industry

www.TPIU.org

Fig. 14. Pamphlet submitted to legislature.

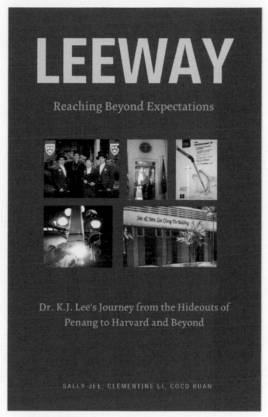

Fig. 15. Cover of K.J. Lee's memoir.

REFERENCES

1. Lee KJ. The impact of health care reform on providers (doctors). In: Chan Y, editor. Healthcare reform through practical clinical guidelines ear nose throat, chapter 1. San Diego (CA): Plural Publishing, Inc; 2010. p. 3–8.
2. Lee KJ. Usable EMRs and you. American Academy of Otolaryngology – Head and Neck Surgery Bulletin 2010.
3. Lee KJ. What to look for in an EMR. Med Econ 2010.
4. Lee KJ. Healthcare: affordable quality coverage for all. Otolaryngol Head Neck Surg 2009;140(6):775–81.
5. Lee KJ. Electronic medical records (EMR)–the train has left the station. ENTNews 2007;16(3):45–6.
6. Lee KJ, Lee M. Universal healthcare: a bold proposal. Conn Med 2000;64(8): 485–91.
7. Mujtaba F, Sullivan E, Lee KJ. A method for detecting errors in discounted fee-for-service payments by insurance companies. Ear Nose Throat J 2000;79(3):148–52.
8. Lee KJ, Cobert-Alvarez J, Lee ME. Survival in the era of managed care. In: Advances in otolaryngology—head and neck surgery, vol. XIII. Saint Louis (MO): Mosby, Inc; 1999. p. 357–65. Chapter 15.

Strengthening Our Societies with Diversity and Inclusion

Sujana S. Chandrasekhar, MD, FACS, FAAOHNS[a,b,c,d,]*

KEYWORDS

- Diversity • Inclusion • Gender • Leadership • Manels

KEY POINTS

- US medical societies have historically excluded women and other underrepresented minorities (URM) from serving as guests of honor and from moderating or serving on panels.
- This exclusion weakens both the society and the member, as the society fails to represent its membership, and the contributions of a significant swath of the membership are not recognized.
- Despite increasing percentages of women and URM members, with ascending experience and seniority, there was notable exclusion from these visible positions even in the modern era.
- Starting in the autumn of 2017, otolaryngology societies in the United States began deliberately including women and URM, some even going so far in 2018 as to establish a "no more manels" rule for all society meetings.

In 2018, the Joint Councils of the American Otological Society (AOS) and the American Neurotology Society (ANS) adopted a statement on diversity and inclusion for programs henceforth. That statement is published on their Web sites and in this edition of *Otology & Neurotology*. I think that it will stand as a landmark touch point in our societies that heralds the engagement of all our members as we all work to advance knowledge and skills in otology and neurotology. I am honored to be asked to write this piece explaining how and why we came to this point and to this decision.

During the 2017 fall meeting of the ANS, at the conclusion of the Middle Fossa Craniotomy: Spectrum of Application and Technical Pearls panel, I stood at the

Actively working towards diversity and inclusion in organized medicine is challenging. The American Otological and Neurotology Societies acted by adopting a landmark statement in 2018. This article, which first appeared in Otology and Neurotology, establishes a baseline understanding of the historical limitations in organized otolaryngology and the willingness of societies to adapt and lead in shaping our profession's future.

Footnote: This article was republished with permission from Chandrasekhar S. Strengthening our societies with diversity and inclusion [editorial]. Otol Neurotol. 2018;40(1):1–5.
[a] ENT and Allergy Associates, LLP, 18 East 48th Street 2nd Floor, New York, NY 10017, USA;
[b] American Academy of Otolaryngology-Head and Neck Surgery, Alexandria, VA, USA;
[c] Otolaryngology-HNS, Zucker School of Medicine at Hofstra-Northwell, Hempstead, NY, USA;
[d] Otolaryngology-HNS, Icahn School of Medicine at Mount Sinai, New York, NY, USA
* 18 East 48th Street 2nd Floor, New York, NY 10017.
E-mail address: ssc@nyotology.com

microphone and "complimented" the society for organizing an excellent "manel." I explained that a manel is a new term for an all-male (and usually all-white) panel.[1] The middle fossa craniotomy manel had a male moderator and 7 male panelists, of whom 2 were Asian American. I went on to say that I felt it was disrespectful of our society to disregard the diversity among its membership. I was rebuked from the podium by the president of the society and informed that there were plenty of women on the program.

Review of the program shows that there was 1 woman panelist of a total of 10 panelists and she presented a nonsurgical topic, 3 of 4 moderators were men, the 1 named speaker was a non-MD woman, and on the other ANS panel there was a male panelist who was presenting the work of a senior female member of our societies, work he had not participated in developing, as she sat in the audience next to me. When I asked her why she was not presenting her own work, she pointed out that ideally her post-doc should have been asked to present that work, as a way to mentor him up. In the audience were a host of woman at least as qualified, if not more so, to present at the only surgical panel, the one with 8 men on it. The 1 female comoderator was for the Fellows video competition, which can be classified as less surgical than educational.

It was difficult to stand at that microphone and give voice to the pain of being regarded as either invisible, second-class, or a token. It has been difficult to be made to feel this way for my entire career in medicine in general and otolaryngology in particular, and, of course, in my chosen niche in otology and neurotology. I have literally (used correctly, by the way) written some variation of "where are the women?" on every single program evaluation form since I began attending ENT (ear, nose, and throat) meetings. It has been some source of bemused amusement to the program committees at the AOS and ANS, as members have joked with me later that they read my (deidentified) comments. The first time I was asked to be a panelist, at the AOS in 2006, I remember that then-administrator Mrs Shirley Gossard called me to congratulate me that my comments had finally been paid attention to! I hadn't written them for myself, but for my gender and for my societies, but if this was the way to pave the path, so be it. Knowing that Shirley, and later Kristen Bordignon and Ashley Westbrook, had our backs has always given me great strength.

Several years ago, the guest of honor speaker at the Triological Society at the Combined Otolaryngology Spring Meetings (COSM), a respected senior otolaryngologist in charge of a residency program, essentially told the audience that the ENT physician shortage in the United States was directly attributable to the presence of women in our field, who, naturally and/or by his reckoning, work less. The late, brave Dr Linda Brodsky stood up at the microphone that time and told off the speaker and the leaders of Trio for propagating this nonsense. I remember us senior women counseling a large group of younger women outside the room who were horrified and felt entirely unwelcome in that Society, of which I am a proud member as well. I imagine that the senior women had heard such sentiments so often that, hurtful though they were, were not permitted to penetrate our psyches.

In June 2003, the Association of American Medical Colleges Executive Council adopted the use of the term "underrepresented in medicine (UIM), which is different from society's underrepresented minority (URM)."[2] The Association of American Medical Colleges states, "'Underrepresented in medicine' means those racial and ethnic populations that are underrepresented in the medical profession relative to their numbers in the general population." Why is it important for women and other UIM to be seen at the podium as moderators, panelists, and invited lecturers? Because that status provides the society's imprimatur on those individuals as leaders. Having only white men up there sends a strong message that nonwhite, nonmales are welcome only to learn and not to teach.

In 2017, the ANS membership survey[3] revealed that 10% of the society's membership was female, with a median female membership year of 2011 versus 1995 for men. Women make up 30% of ANS's Young Members Group. Membership in ANS is possible after being 5 years out of neurotology training and taking the board examination in neurotology. This means that in 2018 the median woman neurotologist is 7 to 12 or more years out of training and at the peak of her clinical and academic productivity. In 2007, the ratio of men to women members was 18 to 1; in 2017, it was 9 to 1. In the history of the ANS, 2 women have served as secretary-treasurer, and they both went on to be president; 19 men have been secretary-treasurer, and 47 have been president. Since 2002, committee chairships have been held by 29 men and 2 women. Just as with the men, nearly all women physicians in the ANS perform otologic and lateral skull base surgery.

Nine percent of the active membership of AOS, the more "senior" of the 2 societies, is female. There have been 25 male secretary-treasurers of AOS; the current one is the first woman to hold that position. There have been 120 presidents of the AOS. The first woman president served in 2001, the second in 2016, and the third holds the office currently. There have been 2 presidents of Hispanic heritage; the remainder have been white. Similar to our male colleagues, all women physicians in the AOS perform otologic surgery, with rare exceptions. We are not the "medical" (read "tinnitus, dizziness, sensorineural hearing loss, education") arm of our societies or our profession.

To clarify the representation of women and other UIM at meetings of the AOS and ANS, I assessed the makeup of the invited lecturers and panels. Free papers are chosen on merit and should not carry potential for discrimination. Invited and/or named lecturers are chosen by the president of the society with input from other leaders. Panels are a way to highlight present and future key opinion leaders in any field. Panel topics and moderators are chosen by the leadership/program committee; moderators are asked to choose their panelists. I recall being at an ANS program committee meeting when the only other woman member presented a thoroughly thought-out and well-crafted idea for a panel, addressing educational needs expressed by the membership. Once we decided to proceed with that idea, the chair looked around the table and asked who should moderate it and another member of the committee immediately volunteered himself. When I pointed out that it was HER idea and SHE should be the moderator, the "compromise" reached was comoderation by both of them. It is clear, therefore, that this process may permit the exercise of both conscious and unconscious bias in the selection of speakers. What has the recent history of our society meetings been? Well, not good, in terms of diversity. Here are some facts and figures.

THE AMERICAN OTOLOGICAL SOCIETY

From 1993 to 2018 there were 44 invited and/or named lecturers. Two of the 26 guest of honor (GOH) lectures were delivered by women. The first was in 1999 and was a basic science talk given by a PhD. The second occurred just this year, delivered by an MD, PhD surgeon. Of these 26 GOH lectures, 2 were delivered by a speaker of Hispanic heritage, 1 by a speaker of Asian heritage, and the rest were delivered by whites. Twenty-three of the 26 GOH lectures have been given by otologic surgeons; the remainder were by PhDs. Of the MD lecturers, 19 of the 22 men had "only" an MD degree. The other 3 men and the 1 woman surgeon GOH lecturers held both MD and PhD degrees. This is shown in **Fig. 1**.

There have been 18 basic science lecturers at the AOS meetings, from 2006 onward, with a new category, the Clinician-Scientist Award Lecture, added in 2018. In

AOS Guest Of Honor Speakers, 1993-2018

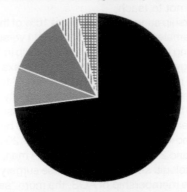

■ Male MD   ■ Male PhD   ■ Male MD-PhD   ▓ Female MD   ⌷ Female PhD   ⌷ Female MD-PhD

Fig. 1. AOS guest of honor speakers, 1993 to 2018. There have been 2 female speakers: 1 PhD and 1 MD-PhD. There have been no female speakers who hold only an MD. There have been 19 male speakers with only an MD, 2 male PhDs, and 3 male MD-PhDs.

2015, the Basic Science Lecture was renamed the Saumil N. Merchant Memorial Lecture, after the untimely death of our well-respected and well-beloved colleague, who happened to be Indian-American. Of these 18 individuals, 2 were women, 1 with a PhD and 1 with an MD. The PhD shared billing on her talk with 2 other (male) presenters, a PhD and an MD. That male MD has the distinct honor of being the only person to have been invited to give 2 different AOS Basic Science/Merchant lectures, 12 years apart, and is also the only non-white to have been invited: he is an Asian American. The one woman MD invited to give an AOS basic science talk did so in 2012.

Panel composition at AOS meetings was reviewed for 2010 to 2018. In this period, there were 14 panel moderators, 8 men and 1 woman on surgical topics and 4 men and 1 woman on nonsurgical topics. There were 28 men and 8 women MD panelists on surgical topics and 8 men and 4 women MD panelists on nonsurgical topics. Three non-MD men and 3 non-MD women served as panelists. There were a total of 3 Hispanic and African American individuals as moderators or panelists. The non-white group that had more prominent representation was Asian American, including both East and South Asians.

THE AMERICAN NEUROTOLOGY SOCIETY

The programs of the 2 meetings per year for the ANS were reviewed from 2010 to 2018 (spring meeting only for 2018). Of the 9 William F. House Memorial Lecturers, the 2011 lecturer was a woman. Of the 7 William E. Hitselberger Memorial Lecturers, the 2013 lecturer was a woman, a PhD. Of the 7 Franklin M. Rizer Memorial Lecturers, 2 were women and both were PhDs. This results in only 4 of 23 invited speakers in the past 8 years being women, and, in a surgical society in which 10% of the membership is female (and in a country in which 50% of the population is female), only 1 of 23 (4%) named lecture speakers was a woman.

Because the ANS has 2 meetings per year, there are a larger number of ANS than AOS panels. In the same 8-year period from 2010 to 2018, men were moderators for 22 surgical and 12 nonsurgical panels, and women were moderators for 4 and 8, respectively. For the surgical topics, 88 panelists were male MDs, 3 were male non-MDs, and 6 were female MDs. For the nonsurgical topics, 31 panelists were male

MDs (one of whom was not an otologist), 6 were male non-MDs, 5 were female MD otologists, 2 were female non-MDs, and 1 was a female non-otologist MD. Of note, 6 panels had 5 or more panelists (not including the moderators, who were all male) in which all panelists were men. Five of these panels were on surgical topics. One additional panel of 6 had the only woman on the panel giving one of the only 2 nonsurgical talks. The infrequent female moderator was only more likely than the men to have selected women panelists for the nonsurgical panels.

The panels presented at ANS (spring and fall) number a total of 47 since 2010. One was the combined AOS-ANS panel on superior semicircular canal dehiscence that was discussed previously. Of the remaining 46 panels, 12 were moderated by a woman neurotologist, either solely or shared with a man. One male moderator is of African American heritage; 3 of the women are of Asian heritage (2 were the same woman: me). Twenty-six panels were surgical either in part or in toto. One of those was moderated by a woman and 3 more had both a male and female moderator. One surgical session included in the panel count comoderated by a woman was a Fellows Surgical Video competition and, therefore, although it was surgical in nature, it was primarily about education. Of the 12 panels comoderated or moderated by a woman, 8 were on nonsurgical topics, including vestibular disorders, health care reform, pediatric unilateral hearing loss, and pediatric vertigo and tinnitus.

The panel data from both societies have been combined in **Fig. 2**. The data are clear that not only are women and other UIM not asked to moderate or serve on panels at anything approaching an equitable rate, the women in particular are assigned nonsurgical topics. This propagates the wrong assumption that women neurotologists are somehow the medical/educational branch of our field.

What are the downsides of excluding women from the podium? The ramifications are extensive. First, for the woman, it is disheartening to say the least when she works hard, produces science, and develops her expertise but is consistently overlooked for men who often have not achieved as much. Failure to recognize women (and people of color) in this manner prevents them from being considered key opinion leaders. This

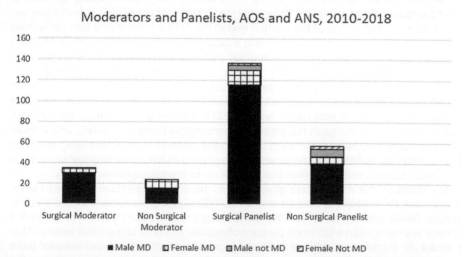

Fig. 2. Moderators and panelists, by sex and by degree, AOS and ANS, 2010 to 2018. "Surgical" means moderating or serving on a surgical panel; "nonsurgical" means moderating or serving on a nonsurgical panel. "Not MD" panelists held a variety of PhD degrees.

translates directly to less research[4,5] or consultant[6] funding, and a stunning drop in likelihood of them being considered for departmental chair or other leadership positions. This problem of underrepresentation of women at scientific meetings is, of course, not limited to our field.[7] Exclusion of women and people of color sends a clear message to those in practice and to trainees: "You are not welcome here as a teacher or full colleague. You may pay the entrance fee and sit there to learn from the worthy ones."

An argument I hear often, even in 2018, is that women are focused on children and family life. Luckily for society, many of us are raising wonderful families AND running busy surgical practices AND doing game-changing research AND writing papers. We are also disproportionately handed the uncompensated burden (pleasant though it may be, it is a burden of time, energy, and money) of educating the residents and medical students.[8] There are data to show that academic productivity of many women lags for a short while during the most intense periods of childbirth and early child rearing but catches up and surpasses that of men later.[9] Discounting a woman's potential early on is a huge cause of the leak, nay, water main break, from the academic pipeline. Societal data[10] show that low-income women lose 4% of their income per child and high-income women lose 10% of their income per child, whereas men gain at least 6% per child. So not only are we discounted professionally, we are penalized financially. Many women in surgical fields therefore chose not to have families. Those of us who made the choice to have children did so knowing the barriers we would face.

So, let's get back to that Fall 2017 microphone. Earlier in the day, in my role as immediate past president, I had raised the subject of manels at the American Academy of Otolaryngology-Head and Neck Surgery (AAO-HNS) Board of Directors meeting, and the board of directors decided to add language regarding sex and URM status on the program applications for the annual meeting from 2018 and going forward. One of my male colleagues, now newly attuned to manels, texted me to get into the ANS to see what he saw, cognizant now for the first time. The women in the ANS room had each other's email addresses in a single email thread, because we had had a networking event the evening before. If that meeting was in a movie or TV show, the rest of the attendees would have seen email bubbles rising up from all over the room. "What is this?!?" "Why only men?!?" "What the heck?!?" (and other unprintable expletives). One of the women texted the ANS Administrator that something was wrong with the panel. I typed in, with a picture of the manel, "If you're at ANS and this bothers you, make sure you note it on your evaluation form. #NoMoreManels." This oft-trending hashtag on Twitter was supported by others. The more I sat there, the more the panel went on, the more I realized that it has been more than 2 decades of me providing this same feedback (an observation echoed by at least one other woman on the thread) and here I was, in 2017, watching EIGHT men on a manel, seeing the 1 woman surgeon relegated to a nonsurgical topic, and seeing only 2 Asian American UIM and NO people from URM on the podium at all. Channeling my inner Linda Brodsky, buffeted by the power of my sisters in the room and my seniority in our field, I summoned the power that got me up to the microphone that day.

My words at that microphone gave voice to the unfairness I have witnessed since 1988. Back then, all of the women attending ANS and AOS could have fit into a Volkswagen Beetle and driven off into the sunset together. We didn't. Our numbers have grown. We have been welcomed by our colleagues, but only to a certain extent. After I spoke up, 2 otherwise rational male colleagues approached me and asked if there were any qualified women members of the ANS who could have been invited on the panel, and if we actually do skull base surgery. Yes, and yes. The membership process is the same for all of us.

I am proud to say that the leadership of our societies, both ANS and AOS, have answered the clarion call. Both societies' councils worked on the diversity resolution that is now an integral part of the mission statement of each society. We all owe a debt of gratitude to Dr Roberto Cueva, president of AOS, for drafting the statement, to Dr Moises Arriaga, president of the ANS, and to the councils of each society for fine-tuning and approving the statement, ensuring that it conveys the importance of inclusion and diversity on every single program to our membership and to our future.

Both unconscious and overt biases are difficult to identify and even more difficult to eliminate.[11] I commend the leadership of our societies, both AOS and ANS, for hearing my words, no matter how unpleasant my words made them feel, and for acting in a deliberate manner to eliminate bias from our programs and enable all of our members to have the same opportunities to shine. After the actions of the AAO-HNS, the AOS, and the ANS, similar actions have been taken by many of our sister societies in otolaryngology. As we turn the page to a more egalitarian tomorrow, I am proud to be part of these groups that are leading the way.

DISCLOSURE

The author has nothing to disclose.

REFERENCES

1. Sherwood J. On the radar: manel. Oxford Dictionary Blog. Available at: https://blog.oxforddictionaries.com/2017/07/05/on-the-radar-manel/. Accessed October 1, 2018.
2. AAMC Executive Council. The status of the new AAMC definition of "underrepresented in medicine" following the Supreme Court's decision in Grutter. Available at: https://www.aamc.org/download/54278/data/urm.pdf-. Accessed October 1, 2018.
3. Toh E, Angeli S, Cosetti M, et al. ANS inclusion and diversity initiative. St. Petersburg (FL): American Neurotology Society; 2018.
4. Eloy JA, Svider PF, Kovalerchik O, et al. Gender differences in successful NIH grant funding in otolaryngology. Otolaryngol Head Neck Surg 2013;149:77–83.
5. Lennon CJ, Hunter JB, Mistry AM, et al. NIH funding within otolaryngology: 2005-2014. Otolaryngol Head Neck Surg 2017;157:774–80.
6. Eloy JA, Bobian M, Svider PF, et al. Association of gender with financial relationships between industry and academic otolaryngologists. JAMA Otolaryngol Head Neck Surg 2017;143:796–802.
7. Kalejta RF, Palmenberg AC. Gender parity trends for invited speakers at four prominent virology conference series. J Virol 2017;91: e00739–17.
8. Willett LL, Halvorsen AJ, McDonald FS, et al. Gender differences in salary of internal medicine residency directors: a national survey. Am J Med 2015;128: 659–65.
9. Eloy JA, Svider P, Chandrasekhar SS, et al. Gender disparities in scholarly productivity within academic otolaryngology departments. Otolaryngol Head Neck Surg 2013;148:215–22.
10. England P, Bearak J, Budig MJ, et al. Do highly paid, highly skilled women experience the largest motherhood penalty? Am Sociol Rev 2016;81:1161–89.
11. Koch AJ, D'Mello SD, Sackett PR. A meta-analysis of gender stereotypes and bias in experimental simulations of employment decision making. J Appl Psychol 2015;100:128–61.

Printed and bound by CPI Group (UK) Ltd, Croydon, CR0 4YY

03/10/2024

01040406-0011